PRACTICAL
ELECTROMYOGRAPHY

This volume is one of the series,
Rehabilitation Medicine Library,
Edited by John V. Basmajian.

---

*New books and new editions published, in press or in preparation for this
series:*

* Originally published as part of the Physical Medicine Library, edited by
Sidney Licht.

Practical Electromyography

Edited by

ERNEST W. JOHNSON

M.D.

Professor and Chairman
Department of Physical Medicine
The Ohio State University
Columbus, Ohio

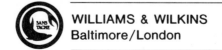

WILLIAMS & WILKINS
Baltimore/London

Made in the United States of America

Library of Congress Cataloging in Publication Data

Main entry under title:

Practical electromyography.

  (Rehabilitation medicine library)
  Includes index.
  1. Electromyography. 2. Neuromuscular diseases—Diagnosis. I. Johnson, Ernest W., 1924-
II. Licht, Sidney Herman, 1907- Electrodiagnosis and electromyography. III. Series. [DNLM:
1. Electrodiagnosis. 2. Electromyography. WE500.3 S693]
RC77.5.L52 1979   616.7′4′0754   79-4421
ISBN 0-683-04464-8

Composed and printed at the
Waverly Press, Inc.
Mt. Royal and Guilford Aves.
Baltimore, Md. 21202, U.S.A.

DEDICATION

This volume is dedicated to all the physiatrists who trained at Ohio State University, Department of Physical Medicine.

Foreword by Series Editor

Clinical or diagnostic electromyography has gone through enormous growth since Sidney Licht produced his book *Electromyography and Electrodiagnosis* in his series of volumes. Later, to help in the production of that outstanding book, he recruited Ernest Johnson. When the time came for me to choose an editor to update the book in the new *Rehabilitation Medicine Library* there was an excellent reason in addition to that obvious one for choosing Dr. Johnson—he had become one of the world's leading exponents of diagnostic EMG.

As the work of revision proceeded, it became obvious that a new book was emerging with little or no genetic connection with the old book. This fact led in turn to the new title, *Practical Electromyography*, which is a clear description of its intent and content. Dr. Johnson chose wisely from among his many former students in electromyography and rehabilitation medicine and his present and past associates to assemble an outstanding group of authoritative writers. This is the *state-of-the-art* in electromyography for both specialists and others who need a broad view of the subject. Details there are in abundance for those who need them. Yet, these many data are used to illuminate rather than to obscure the main message. As an old-time electromyographer, I am impressed.

Practical Electromyography is a unique book written by deeply involved and intelligent specialists who are both scientists and practitioners combined. The book should remain a practical manual and text-book for years to come.

JOHN V. BASMAJIAN

Preface

Sidney Licht was pretty proud when he edited the first book solely for physiatrists on electromyography in 1950. Since then, two revised and enlarged editions have been published and now, with the change of publisher from Elizabeth Licht to The Williams & Wilkins Company and the series editor from Sidney Licht to John V. Basmajian, it is meet and right to alter the format and substance as a new edition.

I have chosen to change the title to *Practical Electromyography*. This is for two principal reasons. The first is that clearly the title should reflect the content. Further it is a given that the content must be the responsibility of the editor. For the past 17 years, I have given a continuing education course in electromyography each year (occasionally two). All have been oversubscribed, so I have gradually increased the enrollment from 25 to now 50 students, and the next course will have over 100. I have attempted to restrict the applicants to experienced electromyographers—that is, physicians, usually physiatrists or neurologists, who are doing electromyography everyday in their practice. Each course begins and ends with an examination. This is a mechanism to assess the limitations of the students attending the course and, also, to give some indication of what they have learned during the 3-day intensive course. The experiences gained from these examinations have been a revelation about the common assumptions of those who teach electromyography.

The most serious deficiency is not theoretical knowledge but rather the identified voids, including surface anatomy and certain practical aspects of electrode placement as well as the techniques of needle electromyography. Similarly, understanding and interpretation of subtle abnormalities were invariably lacking in a majority of the physicians enrolled in the courses.

My restriction of enrollees to physicians has been challenged occasionally, but it must remain absolute. The electromyographic examination is an essential extension of the history and physical examination relevant to neuromuscular diseases. It must be planned only after a careful history and physical and it is dynamic—that is, the electromyographic examination must be modified during its actual performance as abnormalities are revealed. Only a practicing physician with both theoretical and clinical knowledge of neuromuscular diseases, including their differential diagnosis, is an appropriate electromyographer. While an assistant may be helpful in certain instances, I am convinced that the recording of dynamic electromyographic data for later interpretation by the physician-specialist can, and often does, lead to erroneous conclusions.

There are those who would criticize my use of the term "electromyography" as incorrectly describing the contents of the book and would recommend "clinical neurophysiology or electroneuromyography." I accept their semantic implications but reject their suggestion. Historically, traditionally, and practically (if not semantically), the term electromyography has currency when describing the determinations of motor and sensory conduction studies, reflexology and other frequently done data gathering about the electrical phenomenon occurring in the afferent and efferent nervous system.

After all, the phrase motor nerve conduction velocity is technically incorrect—a more appropriate term would be motor nerve impulse propagation rate—but historic and common usage prevails!

Obviously the book editor must be responsible for everything in the book. While the chapter authors properly deserve credit, the concepts presented in this volume are thoroughly and inescapably mine, whether by adoption or conception, and I will stand by them (at least until the next edition)!

The only chapter with which I did not tinker is the one on history by Dr. Sidney Licht, who, I may confess now, provided me some 20 years ago with the initial acceleration for this task of editing. He pointed out that editing is both hard work and low-paying. I can now confirm both of these statements.

To whom it is directed is a universal requisite of all book introductions. Mine, i.e., *Practical Electromyography*, must be considered a book for physicians-specialists who wish to solidify their base of clinical electromyography. The book is specifically directed to raising the level of everyday diagnostic electromyography. Our collective desire is to establish an acceptable level of electrodiagnosis by those physicians who are "into it" and can't seem to find time to polish their techniques with continuing education courses.

Some concepts presented may be authoritarian rather than authoritative, but they represent the distillate of over 20 years of electromyography in a clinical setting where decisions of management were guided by the results!

This is where the scalpel meets the skin or, more appropriately, where the electrode enters the muscle! While theoretical considerations are always necessary as background, one must ascend to practical notions when discussing electromyography with the surgeon who contemplates the potential (no pun intended) of nerve exploration, when and where to take a biopsy, what mode of management is optional, etc. The "practical" assumes primacy when immediate management decisions are beckoning.

My naivete, admittedly profound, does not permit me the musing that only physician-specialists will read the book; not so—hope is that others, perhaps less qualfied as electromyographers, will assiduously study the volume and decide that this specialized field of medicine may be more complex than was previously realized.

In any event, the interpretation of electromyography must rest with the performing electromyographer for both effectiveness and correctness. Lacking these two characteristics, the electromyogram is a procedure recorded in the medical chart without substance or value for the patient, and this is the person who is most important in the transaction.

ERNEST W. JOHNSON, M.D.
Book Editor

Acknowledgments

In addition to all the chapter editors, my appreciation extends to Fred Shephard, medical illustrator extraordinaire who put up with my idiosyncrasies, the three editors with The William & Wilkins Company ending with James L. Sangston, and John V. Basmajian, the series editor who cautioned me about the gap between good intentions and slow delivery with multiple-authored texts.

My wife, Joann who was patient with the papers spread out on the family room floor and the distractions during the "Hardy Boys" and "Hawaii Five-O."

Kay Adelsberger and Susan Heffelfinger, who did much of the typing and put up with my irascible and ubiquitous soft point pen.

John Basmajian deserves more than a bouquet for his confidence (well placed, I hope) in me.

My deep appreciation goes to Sidney Licht—more than a mentor—for his enthusiastic encouragement in my literary efforts.

All deserve my thanks and recognition for pushing me on to a completed text.

ERNEST W. JOHNSON, M.D.

Contributors

Michael A. Alexander, M.D.,
Assistant Professor, Department of Pediatrics and Physical Medicine, Ohio State University Hospitals

Randall L. Braddom, M.D.,
Associate Professor and Director, Department of Physical Medicine and Rehabilitation, University of Cincinnati

Ernest W. Johnson, M.D.,
Professor and Chairman, Department of Physical Medicine, Ohio State University

George H. Kraft, M.S., M.D.,
Professor, Department of Rehabilitation Medicine, University of Washington

Sidney Licht, M.D.,
Curator, Physical Medicine Collections, Yale University Medical Library, New Haven, Connecticut; Clinical Professor, University of Miami School of Medicine, Miami, Florida

Ian C. MacLean, M.D.,
Associate Professor of Clinical Rehabilitation Medicine and Director of Medical Education, Department of Rehabilitation Medicine, Northwestern University Medical School

John L. Melvin, M.D.,
Professor and Chairman, Department of Physical Medicine and Rehabilitation, The Medical College of Wisconsin, Milwaukee, Wisconsin

Lynn M. Mikolich, M.D.,
Decatur, Georgia

Watson D. Parker, M.D.,
Assistant Professor, Department of Physical Medicine, Iowa State University

John Petty, Jr., M.D.,
Wilmington, Ohio

David Piero, M.D.,
Clinical Assistant Professor, Department of Physical Medicine and Rehabilitation, Ohio State University Hospitals

Stuart Reiner, M.E.E.,
President of Teca Corporation, Pleasantville, New York

Joseph B. Rogoff, M.D.,
Professor, Rehabilitation Medicine, New York Medical College

John Schuchmann, M.D.,
Assistant Professor, Department of Physical Medicine and Rehabilitation, University of Cincinnati Medical Center, Cincinnati, Ohio

Margaret Turk, M.D.,
Assistant Professor, Department of Physical Medicine, Ohio State University Hospitals

John R. Warmolts, M.D.,
Associate Professor of Neurology, Department of Medicine, The Ohio State University College of Medicine

Robert J. Weber, M.D.,
Assistant Professor, Department of Physical Medicine, Ohio State University; Director of Physical Medicine Services, University Hospitals, Columbus, Ohio

Harold P. Weingarden, M.D.,
Director of Research and Education, Chief of Electro Diagnostic Services, Memorial Rehabilitation Foundation, Santa Barbara, California

David O. Wiechers, M.D.,
Assistant Professor, Department of Physical Medicine and Rehabilitation, Ohio State University Hospitals

Contents

1

Electromyography Examination

ERNEST W. JOHNSON, M.D.
WATSON D. PARKER, M.D.

Patients with a variety of complaints are referred for electrodiagnostic evaluations (1). These complaints include pain, weakness, limp, sensory disturbances, atrophy, and fatigue. Every electrodiagnostic examination begins with the patient giving a major complaint. The electromyographer then must develop the history of the complaint and evaluate the pertinent system.

The physical examination is necessary to identify the areas of dysfunction and other neurological deficits. These findings then provide the basis for planning the electromyogram. EMG evaluation of areas of probable weakness is initiated. As the EMG findings are revealed, the exploration is modified to provide the necessary data in combination with the history and physical to provide a probable clinical diagnosis.

For optimal relaxation of the patient, it is necessary to explain the procedure but not to go into specific details or to show the needle electrode. Many patients equate the length of the needle with the degree of pain. Suggesting that the patient will see the action of his muscles on television may relax the tension. In all instances, to get relaxation of a desired muscle, use a maneuver (or ask the patient) to contract the antagonist. To get relaxation in the paraspinals, a poke in the abdomen will cause contraction of the antagonist (Fig. 1.1). Side-lying positioning may be helpful also. Prone positioning is very helpful for many EMG examinations. The muscles with the greatest probability of abnormality should be explored first. For example, the paraspinals or the posterior neck muscles in radiculopathy may be the most productive to examine initially. The weakest muscle should be checked first, followed by the areas which appear normal. This will identify the distribution of the abnormality. The proper planning of the electrodiagnostic examination will maximize the information with the fewest electrode explorations.

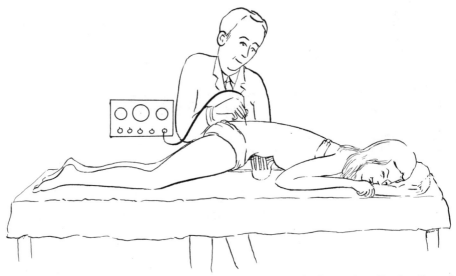

Fig. 1.1. Maneuver to obtain relaxation of the paraspinal muscles. Contraction of abdominals to resist the poking fingers causes relaxation of the antagonistic group-back extensors.

Begin with the muscle at rest. *All records will be oriented so that downward deflection indicates positivity.*

Step 1. Muscle at Rest

The calibration should be set at 50 μV/cm and the sweep speed at 5–10 msec/cm. The needle electrode should be thrust through the skin briskly. If the needle is of a very narrow caliber, it may be necessary to support the middle of the electrode with the index finger and thumb of the other hand in order that it not bend as it goes through the skin. Next, ask the patient for minimal movement to verify the location of the tip of the needle. Knowledge of surface anatomy and kinesiology is essential for the electromyographer.

Normal muscle is quiet and at rest (Fig. 1.2).

Occasionally fasciculation potentials will be seen in the normal individual. These are identified by their rate and rhythm of firing (Fig. 1.3). They generally activate at fewer than 5/sec and are quite irregular in their rhythm. This slow rate of firing and irregular rhythm distinguishes them from a motor unit potential under volitional control (Fig. 1.4).

It is conventional to classify fasciculation potentials by their shape. That is, they are either simple or complex. Simple fasciculations are di- or triphasic; complex fasciculations are polyphasic. These polyphasic fasciculations may be further divided into the usual polyphasic potentials and the so-called iterative or repetitive discharge polyphasic potentials. The latter is a motor unit potential which fires two, three, or four times in a row at a single activation, making a complex though symmetrical polyphasic potential.

Repetitive discharge or iterative fasciculation potentials are associated with myokymia, alkalotic states, and incipient tetany (2). Oftentimes a hyperventilating patient will demonstrate repetitive discharge fasciculations. Early in alkalosis, the volitional potentials are iterative and then, as the process progresses, these iterative discharges appear without voluntary control as fasciculation potentials. However, it should be noted that the first sign of the alkalotic state or incipient tetany will be a repetitive discharge potential under volitional control.

A motor unit potential which is ragged and has many spikes not crossing the isoelectric line is referred to as a disintegrative potential. These are seen in chronic motor unit diseases of a variety of types (3). It has been suggested that fasciculation potentials which are benign fire more slowly and are more commonly simple in shape. The so-called malignant fasciculations associated with amyotrophic lateral sclerosis may vary from moment to moment in amplitude and shape, as the neuromuscular transmission fails in some of the muscle fibers comprising that particular motor unit. Furthermore, it is extremely common for the fasciculation potential in amyotrophic lateral sclerosis to be highly polyphasic and large. Also, characteristic of this particularly malignant disease is an extremely low amplitude and short duration fasciculation potential, almost appearing as a fibrillation potential. The irregular rate of firing distinguishes these motor unit discharges as fasciculations. Benign fasciculations, that is, fasciculation potentials unassociated with other EMG abnormalities, are extremely frequent in the general population, particularly in the gastrocnemius, and must not be considered a characteristic of any disease.

Fibrillation potentials are identified by their initial positive deflection,

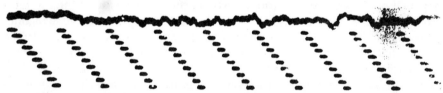

Fig. 1.2. Electrical silence with muscle at rest. Calibration: width of time signal, 50 µV; each dot, 1 msec.

- Fire Irregularly
- < 2 · 3/sec. Usually
- May Be Any Shape, Size
- Pathologic
  With Other EMG Abnormality

Fig. 1.3. Characteristics of a fasciculation potential.

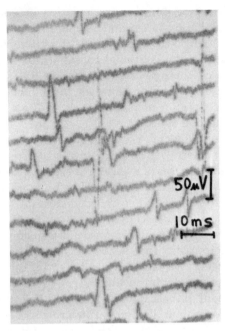

Fig. 1.4. Raster mode recording of fasciculation potentials in a patient with amyotrophic lateral sclerosis.

short duration, low amplitude, and regular rhythm (Fig. 1.5). They are usually di- or triphasic, less than 1.5 msec in duration and with an amplitude up to 600–800 μV, although they are usually under 200 μV (4). The amplitude depends on the instrumentation, particularly the exposed tip of the electrode. The rate of firing of fibrillation potentials is 2 to 20/sec and is regular. These single muscle fiber discharges are presumably the result of altered excitability of the muscle cell membrane so that the unstable membrane will activate when a variety of stimuli, including mechanical, chemical, or electrical, are present. Fibrillation potentials are seen in a variety of diseases but are not characteristic of any (Fig 1.6). It used to be thought that they were synonymous with denervation. We know now that this is not so, and they simply represent an altered state of the muscle cell membrane so that it depolarizes in a variety of circumstances. This could be the result of separation of the muscle fiber from its nerve supply; it is also present in altered electrolyte states, e.g., hypokalemia and hyperkalemia. Fibrillation potentials are present in inflammatory states of the muscle fiber, e.g., polymyositis, and are also seen in destructive processes of the muscle fiber, e.g., associated with intramuscular injections of a variety of substances (5).

In some individuals an intrinsic instability of the muscle cell membrane is present which formerly was called "EMG disease." This appears to be an autosomal dominant trait, which is probably a "forme fruste of myotonia congenita or paramyotonia congenita." These are spontaneously appearing positive sharp waves and fibrillation potentials when the electrode is inserted into the muscle.

Step 2. Insertional Activity

The calibration setting should be 50–100 μV/cm and a sweep speed of 5–10 msec/cm.

This is a highly controversial step in the performance of the EMG. Insertional activity is elicited by briskly moving the needle electrode through the muscle (Fig. 1.7) The injury potentials produced represent discharges of

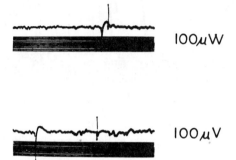

100μW

100μV

Fig. 1.5. Fibrillation potential and positive wave. Note initial positive deflection and short duration. Strip, 200 msec.

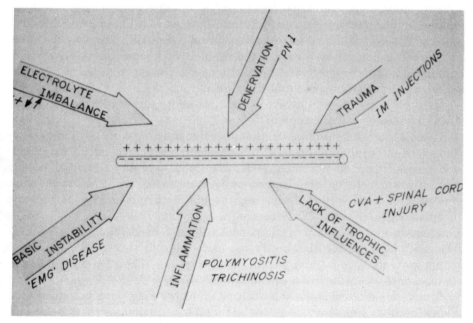

Fig. 1.6. Various conditions affecting muscle cell membrane stability, resulting in fibrillation potentials and positive waves.

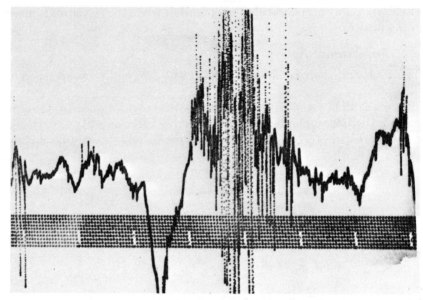

Fig. 1.7. Normal insertional activity in biceps brachii. Calibration: width of time signal, 100 μV; each dot, 1 msec.

the muscle cell membrane which are activated mechanically by movement of the needle. The character of the insertional activity is altered in a variety of neuromuscular conditions. For example, in early denervation it is prolonged and produces occasional positive sharp waves. These positive sharp waves are essentially the same as fibrillation potentials; however, they are an artifact produced by the tip of the needle (6), because the positive wave produced and recorded by the tip of the needle can be recorded simultaneously as a fibrillation potential by a second electrode at a short distance from the muscle fiber. Positive waves, therefore, are *early* indicators of unstable muscle cell membranes.

When reported as prolonged, this insertional activity, rather than being increased in duration, is "slurry" in its cessation when the needle electrode movement stops. In normal muscle, the burst of injury potentials stops abruptly when the needle electrode movements stop. If the electrode is in the area of muscle fiber endplates, the endplate spikes may present as positive sharp waves (7). Because the endplate spikes are single fiber discharges, and as the tip of the needle advances and is then situated into the area of the muscle fiber injury, the electrode will record the single fiber action potentials as positive sharp waves (Fig. 1.8). Their rhythm and rate of discharge will reflect that of endplate spikes (Fig 1.9).

Endplate electrical activity is of three types (8). First, endplate noise is a series of high frequency negative monophasic discharges of 8–10 μV in amplitude. It presents as a "sea shell" murmur or a widening of the noise level. As a result of the electrode tip disrupting a few packets of acetylcholine, it represents the subthreshold nonpropagated muscle cell membrane discharges.

Second, the tip of the needle may provoke enough acetylcholine to reach or exceed threshold of muscle cell membrane and thus result in a propagated single muscle fiber action potential. Since it arises at the endplate, its initial phase will be negative and its duration and amplitude will be the same as a fibrillation potential. Its rhythm will, however, be irregular since the discharges are dependent on the electrode (Fig. 1.10). As the needle electrode advances slightly and as the tip of the electrode records them from within the injured area of the muscle fiber, these single fiber endplate spikes will become positive sharp waves, the third type of endplate discharges.

Step 2 is the most abused by inexperienced electromyographers. It may

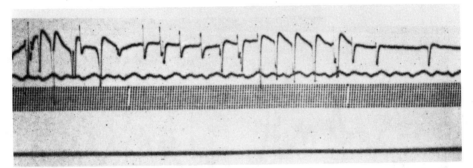

Fig. 1.8. Close up of endplate spikes changing to positive sharp waves. Needle is advanced slightly in vicinity of motor point. Width of time signal, 200µV; 10 lines, 10 msec.

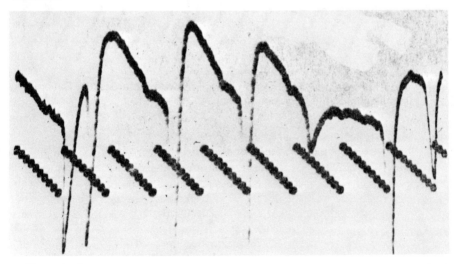

Fig. 1.9. Positive sharp waves recorded from motor point of abductor hallucis. Note the rhythm suggesting irregularity of endplate spike discharges. Calibration: width of time signal, 50 µV; each dot, 1 msec.

be overinterpreted as abnormal when the electrode is in small muscles of the hand and feet and likely in the vicinity of endplates or perhaps under-interpreted by less observant electromyographers when the disease process is minimal or the EMG is performed early in the course of a disease or injury.

At least 20 insertions at three different locations in the muscle should be completed before moving to other muscles. Since pathological muscle cell membrane irritability is on a continuum (Fig. 1.11) rather than a dichoto-mous process, abnormal insertional activity may be the earliest and the only EMG abnormality at certain important points in the disease or injury

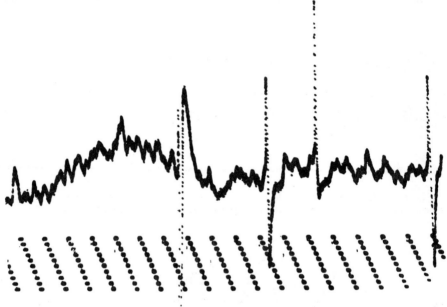

Fig. 1.10. Endplate spikes recorded in the first dorsal interosseus. Calibration: width of time signal, 50 µV; each dot, 1 msec.

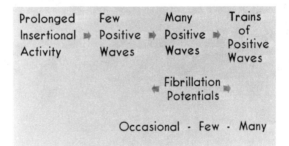

Fig. 1.11. Sequence of abnormal electrical activity resulting from a "sick" muscle cell and, thus, an unstable muscle cell membrane.

process (9). For example, 7–10 days after the onset of an acute radiculopathy, abnormal insertional activity consisting of a few positive waves may be the sole essential diagnostic EMG finding (Fig. 1.12). In mild disease states of the motor unit, abnormal insertional activity may be the most obvious EMG abnormality.

Whereas endplate spikes occur as a series of irregular single fiber discharges (Fig. 1.10), an irregular train of positive waves may not be of significance, since it could represent simply the tip of the electrode in the vicinity of endplates. On the other hand, two or three positive waves occurring after insertional activity stops may be highly significant in indicating early or minimal abnormal muscle fiber membrane instability.

Step 3. Minimal Contraction of the Muscle

With the location of the electrode tip in an identified muscle, the patient is asked just to think about contracting the muscle. Sweep speed should be set at 5–10 msec/cm and the voltage sensitivity at 100–200 μv/cm. Adjustments should be made to determine accurately the peak-to-peak amplitude of the motor unit potentials as well as the duration, shape, and number of motor action potentials.

Amplitude and duration of motor unit potentials vary in different muscles in normal individuals (Fig. 1.13). They are generally lower in amplitude and shorter in duration in the centrally placed muscles, and with longer duration

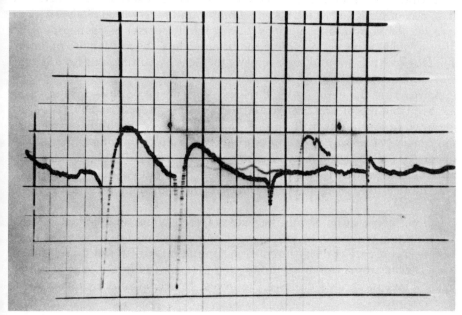

Fig. 1.12. A few positive waves seen as paraspinal muscles 9 days after acute onset of lumbar radiculopathy. Calibration: 50 μV per major vertical division; 30 msec per major horizontal division.

NORMAL AMPLITUDES OF MUP
──────── (μv) ────────

PECT. MAJ.	429 $\pm$ 12
BICEPS BR.	490 $\pm$ 11
GLUT. MAX.	533 $\pm$ 17
ABD. DIG. Q.	926 $\pm$ 63
GASTROC.	1133 $\pm$ 34
TRICEPS BR.	1157 $\pm$ 45
QUADS. FEM.	1217 $\pm$ 43

Fig. 1.13. Amplitudes of first recruited motor unit potentials in a normal individual (monopolar electrode). (Reprinted by permission from: R. McMorris, Thesis, University of Minnesota, 1952.)

and higher amplitude in the peripherally placed muscles (10). First recruited (i.e., low threshold) motor-unit potentials are the "tonic" motor units (type 1), generally of lower amplitude and shorter duration. Type 2 motor units are recruited later and are generally larger in amplitude and longer in duration. In normal conditions the motor units begin activation at a rate of 5/sec and increase the rate of firing as the effort is increased. Coincident with this increased rate of firing is the recruitment of additional motor units. A recruitment interval (11, 12) is that time between subsequent activation (i.e., rate of firing) at which a second motor unit is recruited. This varies in a variety of motor unit conditions. It is generally shorter in the neuropathic diseases and longer in myopathic conditions. Thus, the availability of motor units for recruitment and the necessity for early recruitment at lower firing rates occurs in "myopathy" (13).

However, in the neuropathic diseases the opposite occurs—that is, since the available motor units for recruitment are not present, each of the first recruited motor units will fire more rapidly (i.e., recruitment interval shortened) before the second motor unit is recruited. Varying amplitude of the motor unit potential may be observed at low rates of firing. This results from blocking at the myoneural junction of some muscle fibers comprising that motor unit. A signal delay line will help to demonstrate this (see Chapter 15).

Careful observation should be made of each motor unit potential (Fig. 1.14). Descriptions should include peak-to-peak amplitude, duration, number of phases, rate and rhythm of firing, variation in amplitude, and shape. Note that in step 3 the motor units examined are the first recruited motor units. Thus, in various diseases the lowest threshold motor units are the first recruited.

Step 4. Maximal Effort

In order that maximal effort be made, the electrode should be relatively superficial in the muscle, minimizing discomfort. Also, the muscle should be

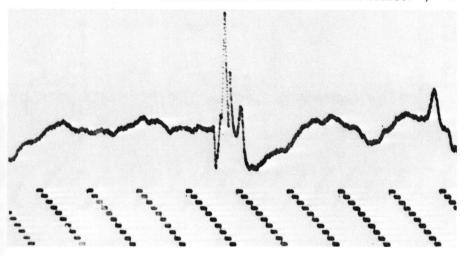

Fig. 1.14. A single motor unit potential (5 Hz) movement of electrode slightly changes shape to triphasic.

a one-joint muscle since maximal effort is difficult to elicit in a recumbent patient in a muscle which goes over several joints. For example, the vastus medialis is more appropriate than the rectus femoris muscle; also, the anterior tibial muscle is preferable to the semitendinosus muscle for obtaining maximal contraction effort by the patient.

Amplification should be 500–1000 μv/cm at sweep speed of 10 msec/cm. The audio signal will give an indication of the duration of the motor-unit potentials; myopathic—short; and neuropathic—long duration. Also, in neuropathic conditions with a reduced number of motor units available for recruitment, each unit will fire rapidly, and the sound of each can be detected as a rapid-firing machine gun (14, 15) (Fig. 1.15). In a ratchety response, as one sees in hysterical paralysis, step 4 will present as groups of motor units discharging, clustered together and firing rhythmically. This is the electromyographic correlate of the ratchety response, which is pathognomonic of hysterical paralysis.

It is estimated that there are six to eight motor units whose electrical activity will be detected by the tip of the needle electrode. Thus, if only two units (or portions thereof) are recorded at maximal rates of firing 30–40/sec, the probability is a condition reducing the number of motor units in that area by two-thirds to three-quarters (Fig. 1.15).

Peak-to-peak amplitude should be determined. Much notching at the tips of the motor unit potentials suggest an increase proportion of polyphasic motor-unit potentials; so step 3 should be revisited to determine the actual proportion of polyphasic motor-unit potentials in various samples.

Step 5. Distribution of the EMG Abnormality

When an abnormality has been uncovered, its anatomic pattern must be determined. This presupposes that the electromyographer has a thorough

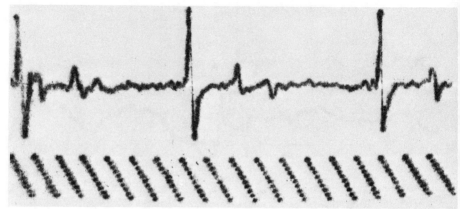

Fig. 1.15. Only one motor unit potential firing 15 Hz in ulnar nerve injury. First dorsal interosseous muscle calibration: width of time signal, 500 μV; each dot, 1 msec.

knowledge of surface and functional anatomy. Also, it is necessary that he have a detailed knowledge of the differential diagnostic conditions affecting the motor unit. The cord levels, plexus, and peripheral nerve distribution should be completely familiar to the electromyographer, and it is essential that a reliable anatomy text should be near the EMG instrument.

Conventional wisdom dictates examining contralateral muscles when EMG abnormalities are found. In generalized diseases all four extremities should be explored. Experience will suggest how many muscles should be explored for a negative examination.

Stereotyping the EMG examination is the usual error of the neophyte. Under no circumstances should the same group of muscles be explored in every patient. This is a common error in those electromyographers who use a printed list of muscles on their EMG report form. The sequence of the EMG must be dictated by the history and physical examination as well as the subsequently revealed EMG abnormalities.

In steps 1 to 4, each muscle should be explored in a proximal, middle, and distal area. At each area, circular individual movements of the electrode should be done at least 12 and probably 20 times. This is standard procedure for EMG exploration of a given muscle (Fig. 1.16).

Nerve stimulation studies probably should precede the needle exploration in certain instances, e.g., possible myasthenia gravis and certain entrapment syndromes, such as carpal tunnel syndrome and peripheral neuropathies. With proper experience and judgment, the electromyographer may vary the examination sequence for convenience of the patient or himself. Shortcuts in the five steps must await sufficient experience—in my judgment, after 2,000 EMG examinations have been completed.

Special Considerations of Anatomy

Accessible muscles for needle exploration include most of the 434 skeletal muscles in the body. A knowledge of functional anatomy, kinesiology, and

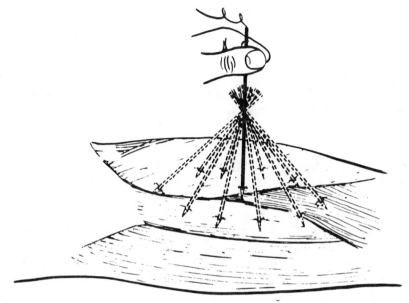

Fig. 1.16. Method of electromyographically exploring the muscle. This should be done in the proximal, central and distal position of each muscle studied.

surface anatomy is essential, as is the presence of an illustrated anatomic text near the electromyograph.

The *trapezius* and *facial muscles* are exceedingly thin so that an exploring electrode is likely to penetrate through the muscle unless meticulous care is taken. The *serratus anterior muscle* can be explored by placing two fingers in the intercostal spaces, thus straddling a rib, on the lateral chest and inserting the electrode down to the rib. This method will avoid an occasional complication of needle electromyography—penetrating the pleural cavity and resulting in a tension pneumothorax.

Similar care should be observed when exploring the *rectus abdominis* and the *external and internal oblique* portions of the abdominal muscles. The *diaphragm* may be reached in the posterior aspect just below the 12th rib, or in the midaxillary line just above the 11th rib. Relatively inaccessible muscles include the *posterior tibial,* the *supinator,* and the *short hip muscles.*

ANAL EMG

Cord levels of S3 and S4 innervate this muscle. It is explored at 12, 3, 6 and 9 o'clock with observations for positive sharp waves and fibrillation potentials, and also for the proportion of polyphasics and the number of motor-unit potentials at maximal contraction. The interference pattern is graded at 1–4 plus, with less than 3 plus as pathological, suggesting neurogenic disease. Calibration for maximal contraction is 200 µv/cm and 10 msec/cm.

EXTRINSIC EYE MUSCLES

It is necessary to anesthetize the conjunctiva for sampling these muscles, with one exception. The location and attachments of the inferior oblique muscle makes it accessible as the needle electrode is inserted through the skin at the inferior and nasal aspect of the orbit. These motor units are composed of only a few muscle fibers so that the amplitude and duration approach that of a single muscle fiber (16). Firing rates are exceedingly rapid up to 100 Hz.

FACIAL NERVE

Electromyographic study of the various affectations of the facial nerve generally involves exploration of at least four different muscles, e.g., frontalis, orbicularis oculi, mentalis, and posterior auricular. The latter muscle is supplied by the facial nerve just after it leaves the stylomastoid foramen. At this point the nerve is usually stimulated (we use needle stimulation). Best muscles for surface recording are the frontalis, orbicularis oculi, or one of the elongated muscles along the lateral aspect of the nose. Surface recording over the orbicularis oris will be confusing, since the masseter muscle response as it is volume-conducted will be recorded.

The *blink reflex* is elicited by stimulation over the supraorbital notch (V cranial N—afferent arm) and recording over the orbicularis oculi (efferent component). The early response will occur after a 9–11 msec latency and a

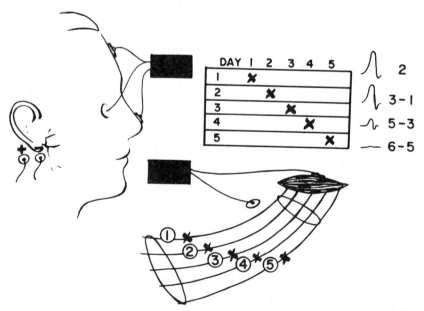

Fig. 1.17. Change in the surface-evoked potential as the facial nerve undergoes changes in Bell palsy. Since the distal segment remains excitable for 72–95 hr after Wallerian degeneration, as days elapse the number of excitable axons decreases. The pathological process involving the facial nerve is a longitudinal process; thus, different axons decreases are excitable for different days.

late response after a 28–32 msec latency. By recording bilaterally and stimulating each supraorbital muscle of V cranial nerve, the electromyographer may identify a block of either afferent or efferent arm of the blink reflex, e.g., angle tumor, etc. (17).

Bell palsy—idiopathic facial nerve compromise—can be diagnosed with appropriate electromyographic and nerve stimulation studies. Since the pathological process may extend over several days, it is essential that two or three serial studies be done to determine precisely the state of the nerve. Recall that the distal segment of a motor nerve which has been severed will remain excitable from 72 to 96 hr. The amplitude and duration of the evoked muscle response may be analyzed to give objective data to the referring physician. Clinically the facial paralysis may be complete, but the reversible (neurapraxic) portion will be demonstrated by electrically stimulating and noting the size of the response. Serial studies are necessary since the axon retains excitability even after beginning Wallerian degeneration (Fig. 1.17).

REFERENCES

1. JOHNSON, E., et al.: Use of electrodiagnostic examination in a University Hospital. *Arch. Phys. Med. Rehabil., 46:* 573, 1965.
2. KUGELBERG, E., AND COBB, W.: Repetitive discharges in human motor fibers during post schaemic state. *J. Neurol. Neurosurg. Psychiat., 14:* 88, 1954.
3. SCHWARTZ, M., et al.: The reinnervated motor unit in man. *J. Neurolog. Sci., 27:* 303, 1976.
4. JOHNSON, E., et al.: EMG abnormalities after intramuscular injections. *Arch. Phys. Med. Rehabil., 52:* 250, 1971.
5. LAMBERT, E., et al.: Studies on the origin of the positive wave in electromyography. *Newsletter Amer. Assoc. EMG EDX, 3:* 3, 1957.
6. STOHR, M.: Benign fibrillation potentials in normal muscle and their correlation with end-plate and denervation potentials. *J. Neurol. Neurosurg. Psychiat. 40:* 765, 1977.
7. WIEDERHOLT, W.: "End-plate noise" in electromyography. *Neurology, 20:* 214, 1970.
8. WIECHERS, D.: Mechanically provoked insertional activity before and after nerve section in rats. *Arch. Phys. Med. Rehabil., 58:* 402, 1977.
9. LAMBERT, E., AND McMORRIS, R.: Size of motor unit potentials in neuromuscular disorders. *Fed. Proc., 13:* 263, 1953.
10. PETAJAN, J., AND PHILIP, B.: Frequency control of motor unit action potentials. *Electroencephalogr. Clin. Neurophysiol., 27:* 66, 1969.
11. PETAJAN, J.: Clinical electromyographic studies of diseases of the motor unit. *Electroencephalogr. Clin. Neurophysiol., 36:* 395, 1974.
12. KUGELBERG, E.: Electromyograms in muscular disorders. *J. Neurol. Neurosurg. Psychiat., 10:* 122, 1947.
13. DENNY-BROWN, D.: Interpretation of the electromyogram. *Arch. Neurol. Psychiat., 61:* 99, 1949.
14. BUCHTAL, F., et al.: Motor unit territory in different human muscles. *Acta. Physiol. Scand. 45:* 72, 1959.
15. BAILEY, J., et al.: A clinical evaluation of electromyography of the anal sphincter. *Arch. Phys. Med. Rehabil., 51:* 403, 1970.
16. JENSAN, S. F.: Spontaneous electrical activity in denervated extraocular muscles. *Acta. Ophthalmol., 50:* 827, 1972.
17. KIMURA, J., et al.: Reflex response of orbicularis oculi muscle to supraorbital nerve stimulation. *Arch. Neurol., 21:* 193, 1969.
18. McMORRIS, R.: Amplitudes and durations of 1st recruited motor unit potentials. Thesis, Mayo Foundation, Graduate Education, University of Minnesota, 1952.

2

Motor Conduction

RANDALL L. BRADDOM, M.D.
JOHN SCHUCHMANN, M.D.

Brief History of Nerve Conduction Studies

The clinical use of nerve conduction studies is a relatively recent phenomenon, but the basic developments leading to the present state of knowledge have occurred over several centuries. In 1658, Jan Swammerdam observed twitches in an isolated frog muscle when its nerve was pinched or cut. In the late 1780s, Galvani discovered the relationship between electrical stimulation of a nerve and contraction of its muscle. A significant advance was made by Duchenne de Boulogne in 1833, when he found that muscles could be electrically stimulated percutaneously. In 1852, a German physiologist, Herman von Helmholtz, performed the first nerve conduction studies on humans when he crudely measured median nerve conduction velocity. In 1924, Erlanger et al. (1) reported their classical motor and sensory nerve conduction studies in the bullfrog and dog. They noted the changes in the configuration of the mixed nerve action potential as different lengths of nerve were stimulated. They found that the action potential appeared to be a mixture of several individual spikes, which they attributed to variation in the conduction velocity of the individual nerve fibers. In 1939 Hursh (2) and Gasser and Grundfest (3) reported studies of the relationship between nerve conduction velocity and nerve fiber diameter. They concluded that the conduction velocity was approximately proportional to the axon diameter. The clinical applicability of nerve conduction studies was greatly advanced in 1948, when Hodes et al. (4) published their studies of a series of normal subjects and patients with peripheral nerve injuries and hysterical paralysis. Their techniques for performing the nerve conduction studies were described, and normal values were presented for the ulnar, median, and radial nerves in the upper extremity and the tibial and peroneal nerves in the lower extremity. Their normal motor nerve conduction velocity values ranged from 46 to 67 m/sec. They also recognized the importance of the residual latency value in motor nerve conduction studies and attributed it to two factors: 1) a slower conduction velocity in the smaller terminal portions of the nerve, and 2) a delay in conduction at the neuromuscular junction.

Another milestone in the development of human nerve conduction studies was the report in 1949 by Dawson and Scott (5) of their studies involving the first measurement of percutaneous sensory nerve action potentials in humans. The ulnar and median nerves were studied, and they noted that the amplitude of the sensory evoked response varied in normal subjects from 10 to 60 μV. The clinical usefulness of nerve conduction studies was given further impetus in 1956, when Simpson (6) and Lambert (7) independently described the use of nerve conduction studies in diagnosing carpal tunnel syndrome.

Nerve conduction studies are now performed routinely in clinical practice, and more recent developments have included refinement of the instrumentation, standardization of techniques, and the evaluation of nerve conduction studies in both normal and pathological situations.

Basic Neurophysiology of Nerve Conduction

A complete discussion of the neurophysiology of nerve conduction is beyond the scope of this chapter. The reader is referred to Chapter 16 of this book and to textbooks of neurophysiology for a more complete discussion.

When a sufficient stimulus is applied to a nerve to cause the nerve transmembrane potential to change from its resting level of −90 mV to the threshold level, the membrane's conductance to ions increases dramatically. This change in conductivity causes a rapid reversal of the steady-state concentrations of sodium and potassium on both sides of the membrane, which results in depolarization of the membrane. In the steady-state, the Na+ concentration is high in the extracellular fluid and low in the intracellular fluid. The reverse is true for K+ ion concentrations. Changing the ionic concentrations causes a marked change in the potential (transmembrane potential) across the membrane. (The relationship of each ionic concentration to the transmembrane potential can be determined by the Nernst equation). The local depolarization of the membrane is propagated along the nerve by local circuit flow. The speed of conduction in an unmyelinated fiber increases as the cross-sectional area of the nerve increases, because the electrical resistance of the axoplasm decreases with increasing cross-sectional areas. Counteracting this effect is the fact that fiber membrane capacity per unit length is directly proportional to the diameter of the fiber, and increasing the capacity decreases speed of conduction. The net result of the decreasing resistance but increasing capacity is that the speed of conduction in unmyelinated fibers is approximately proportional to the square root of the diameter.

Vertebrate existence requires relatively small diameter nerves that have fast conduction velocities. Nature accomplished this by myelinating nerves.

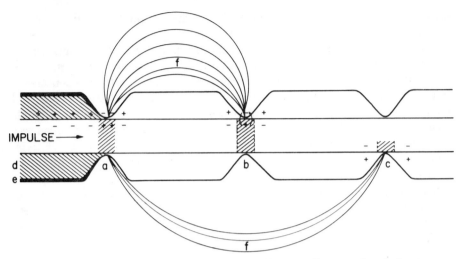

Fig. 2.1. Saltatory conduction in a myelinated nerve fiber. *a*, depolarized membrane at node of Ranvier; *b*, partially depolarized membrane at node of Ranvier (near threshold); *c*, beginning depolarization of membrane at node of Ranvier; *d*, myelin sheath; *e*, Schwann cell; *f*, electrical field. (Reprinted by permission from: J. A. Downey and R. C. Darling: *Physiological Basis of Rehabilitation Medicine*, W.B. Saunders Co., 1971.)

A myelinated nerve is covered by many Schwann cells. Each Schwann cell surrounds approximately a 2-mm section of the nerve axon (depending on the diameter of the nerve fiber) and wraps itself around the fiber approximately 100 times. The wrapping is so tight that there is less than 1 μ between the adjacent Schwann cell wrappings. Between the adjacent Schwann cell wrappings is a 1-μ gap where the axon membrane is in free communication with the interstitial fluid (Fig. 2.1). This gap in the myelin sheath is called the node of Ranvier. The sheathed portion of the nerve axon between the nodes of Ranvier is an internode. For reasons beyond the scope of this discussion, resting and action potentials are generated only at the nodes of Ranvier in myelinated fibers. Generation of a transmembrane potential requires energy; consequently, limiting this activity to the nodes of Ranvier conserves energy. As shown in Figure 2.1, depolarization of the axon membrane at one node of Ranvier causes local current flow to the next node of Ranvier. Impulse propagation in myelinated nerve fibers is basically a hopping of excitation from one node to the next (internodal regions are well insulated and relatively unexcitable). This is called saltatory conduction after the Latin word "saltare," meaning to dance. Saltatory conduction in myelinated fibers greatly increases conduction speed. Nerve conduction velocity of myelinated fibers is proportional to fiber diameter, with conduction velocity in meters per second being approximately six times the nerve fiber diameter in microns.

The nerve membrane repolarizes by an increase in potassium conductance and a decrease in sodium conductance. If depolarizing current is applied to a nerve at the end of an action potential before the reactivation of sodium conductance, the nerve will not depolarize again. At this time the nerve fiber is refractory to a stimulating current regardless of its strength (absolute refractory period). Slightly later in the course of repolarization the nerve can be stimulated, but the stimulating current must be greater than normal and the action potential generated will be smaller than normal (relative refractory period). A few milliseconds after depolarization, both the absolute and relative refractory periods cease and the nerve returns to a normal excitability state.

Nerve trunks are usually mixtures of myelinated and unmyelinated nerve fibers of various sizes. Unfortunately, there is confusion in the literature as to the best way to classify and name the various types of nerve fibers. Table 2.1 shows a useful classification of nerve fibers into four main categories. The A fibers are myelinated somatic afferent and efferent fibers. The B fibers are smaller myelinated efferent preganglionic axons found in autonomic nerves and are similar to A fibers, except that they do not have a negative after-potential. s.C. fibers are unmyelinated efferent postganglionic sympathetic axons. The s.C. group of unmyelinated fibers have pronounced negative and positive after-potentials. The d.r.C group are unmyelinated afferent axons found in peripheral nerves and dorsal roots. Nerve fibers in the d.r.C group have no negative after-potential but do have a large positive after-potential which converts with repetitive stimulation to a negative after-potential.

A Roman numeral system of designating nerves based on fiber diameter only was developed by Lloyd (10). In this classification, the A and B fibers are divided into three groups: group I includes fibers from 12 to 21 μ in diameter, group II from 6 to 12 μ, and group III from 1 to 6 μ. The C fibers are referred to in this system as group IV.

The Greek letters alpha, beta, gamma, delta, and epsilon are often used

TABLE 2.1. *Classification of Mammalian Nerve Fibers*[a]

Fiber diameter, μ	1–22	3	0.3–1.3	0.4–1.2
Conduction speed, m/sec	5–120	3–15	0.7–2.3	0.6–2.0
Spike duration, msec	0.4–0.5	1.2	2.0	2.0
Absolute refractory period, msec	0.4–1.0	1.2	2.0	2.0
Negative afterpotential amplitude,				
Percent of spike	3–5	None	3–5	None
Duration, msec	12–20		50–80	
Positive afterpotential amplitude,				
Percent of spike	0.2	1.5–4.0	1.5	—[b]
Duration, msec	40–60	100–300	300–1000	—[b]
Order of susceptibility to asphyxia	2	1	3	3
Velocity/diameter ratio	6	?	?	1.73 average

[a] From: T. C. Ruch, H. A. Patton, J. W. Woodlbury, and A. L. Towe (9).

[b] A post-spike positivity 10–30% of strike amplitude and decaying to half size in 50 msec is recorded from d.r.C. fibers. This after-positivity differs from the positive after-potential of other fibers.

to designate successive elevations of the compound action potential of the *A* fibers in a nerve trunk. These various portions of the compound action potential result from the fact that the various fibers conduct at different velocities proportional to their fiber diameter.

In clinical nerve conduction studies, stimulation of large nerve trunks evokes nerve action potentials that are recordable mainly from the large fibers (group A, type I). Generation of a complete compound action potential including the s.C and d.r.C fibers is a technique which is best done in vitro and is not generally feasible in clinical percutaneous nerve conduction studies. Clinical nerve conduction studies generally report the "fastest fiber" conduction velocity rather than the average conduction velocity of all the fibers in a mixed nerve.

The evoked response in motor conduction studies and the nerve action potential in sensory conduction studies become longer in duration as the segment of nerve over which the impulse passes is increased in length. This is referred to as "temporal dispersion" of the evoked response and is a normal phenomenon due to the mixture of fibers with different conduction velocities in the nerve trunk. Nerve conduction studies involve looking at an evoked response in relationship to a stimulus applied to the nerve at various stimulation distances. If the distance is changed, the evoked response will have a different shape.

In motor nerve conduction studies there is a difference in the distal latency that is observed and which would be predicted on the basis of the proximal nerve conduction velocity. If the nerve conduction velocity of the median nerve is 57 m/sec, the distal latency over an 8-cm distance should be 1.4 msec. The latency actually observed is 3.7 msec. This difference between the predicted distal latency and that which is observed is called the "residual latency." Buchthal and Rosenfalck (11) have pointed out that there is a residual latency in sensory nerve studies as well. If the median sensory fibers are stimulated at 14 cm, a mean latency of 3.2 msec is observed. This is longer than the calculated distal latency. With a nerve conduction velocity of 57 m/sec, a distal latency of 2.4 msec would be expected. The best explanation for the motor and sensory residual latencies is that the nerve fibers taper distally in terminal portions of extremities, reducing the nerve conduction velocity. In motor studies, the time required to cross the myoneural junction (0.5–1.0 msec) is also a factor.

Basic Technical Considerations

Clinical nerve conduction studies are usually done with commercial EMG apparatus that incorporates built-in nerve conduction equipment (see Chapter 15). Nerve conduction studies require the addition of a nerve stimulator to standard EMG apparatus. The stimulator must be synchronized with the cathode ray display so that the sweep is triggered slightly before the stimulus is delivered to the patient. This allows visualization of the stimulus "blip" and the response on one cathode ray sweep. The nerve stimulator should deliver square wave stimuli of various durations from a minimum of 0.1 msec to at least 1 msec. The stimulator should have a variable frequency of stimulation from 0.5 to 50 Hz. A manual switch or footplate switch that allows the clinician to deliver single stimuli is also useful. It is also convenient in clinical studies to have a moveable time marker so that latencies can be visually measured to within 1/10 of a millisecond.

A major design problem in nerve conduction equipment is preventing the stimulus voltage (up to 300 V) from interfering with the evoked response (often 30 μV or less in amplitude). Electronic considerations dictate that this be done by isolating the nerve stimulator from ground, which is accomplished in commercial equipment with an "isolation transformer." The secondary coil of the transformer supplying the stimulus output is not connected to ground intentionally (and is carefully isolated from it).

The EMG apparatus used in nerve conduction studies must have variable gain settings, since sensory responses as low as a few microvolts and motor responses as great as 20 mV are often obtained. The gain setting for a sensory nerve might be 20 μV per vertical division on the cathode ray tube screen. If the screen is divided into five vertical divisions, complete visualization of a 100-μV potential would be possible. The gain setting for a motor study is usually 1000 μV (1 mV) per vertical division. (As will be discussed later, the gain setting can affect the reading of the latency of the response).

The EMG apparatus must also have variable sweep speed settings, since the normal latencies seen in clinical practice range from a few milliseconds in nerve distal latency studies to 30 msec in H reflex studies. These latency values require sweep speeds, giving an elapsed time for one complete sweep across the screen of from 10 msec to 200 msec. The sweep speed should be adjusted to allow the expected potential to be seen in its entirety approximately in the center of the screen. After initial analysis of the response, the sweep speed can be adjusted to "spread out" or "compress" the response for further analysis.

The EMG apparatus used in nerve conduction studies must have the capacity to reject "common mode" signals. Common mode signals are those which occur at both the active recording and reference electrodes (see Chapter 15). Clinical EMG equipment must have a common mode rejection ratio of at least 100,000/1 and have a high input impedance (in the megohm range).

EMG apparatus requires a very high frequency response (10,000 Hz) to accurately portray potentials such as fibrillations. Nerve conduction studies do not require such a high frequency response, since the evoked responses are low frequency potentials of 2000 Hz or less. Some EMG equipment allows the clinician to manually set the frequency filter to reduce the frequency response to the level appropriate for nerve conduction studies. Some of the newer apparatus has preset filtration settings which change depending on whether the instrument is put in EMG or nerve conduction mode.

There are many types of stimulators available for use in conduction studies. Commercially available EMG equipment generally comes with a surface stimulator having a cathode and anode separated by a fixed inter-electrode distance of 1–3 cm (*K* of Fig. 2.2). The surface bipolar stimulator has the obvious clinical advantage of not requiring puncture of the skin. The surface stimulator is adequate for most clinical activities, but occasionally it is necessary to use needle stimulation. Needle stimulation involves the use of a monopolar needle electrode (most commonly Teflon-coated except at the tip; *B* of Fig. 2.2) as the cathode and a large surface electrode used as the anode (usually placed between the cathode and the active recording electrode; *A* of Fig. 2.2). This technique is useful when a nerve is too deep to be easily stimulated percutaneously or when a small stimulus intensity is desirable (it takes a greater stimulus voltage to stimulate a deep

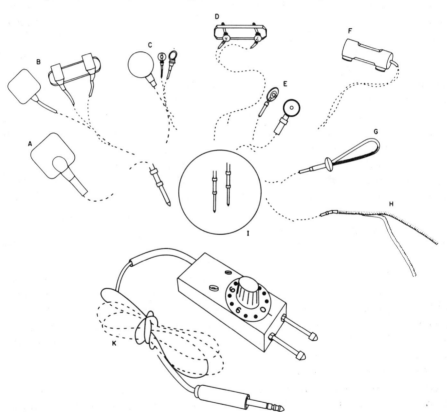

Fig. 2.2. Nerve conduction electrodes. (*A*) Lead or tin ground or reference place; (*B*) lead strips mounted on plastic bar with ground electrode; (*C*) Beckman electrodes with ground electrode; (*D*) Beckman electrodes on a plastic bar; (*E*) flat 1-cm electrodes (Teca Corp.); (*F*) flat electrodes on a plastic bar (Teca Corp.); (*G*) wire ring electrode (Teca Corp.); (*H*) pipe cleaner electrode; (*I*) 1 mm miniature tip plug; (*J*) 2-mm phone tip plug (unmarked plug to left of I); (*K*) bipolar surface stimulator (Teca Corp.).

nerve from the skin surface than from directly adjacent to it). Another means of stimulation is to place two monopolar needle electrodes adjacent to a nerve about 1–3 cm apart. This stimulation is analogous to the bipolar surface stimulator, except for applying the stimulus immediately adjacent to the nerve.

Regardless of the type of stimulator used, it is important for measurement reasons to know exactly where the stimulus is being applied to the nerve. There is some disagreement among electrodiagnosticians regarding the actual site of nerve stimulation. Some point out that it can advance from the cathode toward the active recording electrode in high voltage stimulation or even move in a retrograde direction to lie between the anode and cathode. For general clinical purposes, most agree that at usual stimulus intensities the point of initial stimulation is that portion of the nerve closest to the center of the cathode. In view of this, it is appropriate to orient the bipolar stimulator so that the cathode is closest to the active recording electrode. Placing the anode closest to the active recording electrode introduces a small measurement error in nerve conduction velocity determination. It may also produce "anodal block," in which the portion of the nerve under the anode becomes hyperpolarized and subsequently requires a higher than normal threshold stimulus for depolarization.

Some investigators routinely place a meter across the stimulation output electrodes to monitor the exact voltage or wattage delivered by the stimulator. This may be useful in research applications, but it does not appear to be helpful in routine clinical studies, because the only requirement of the square wave stimulus is that it must be supramaximal.

Recording electrodes are most commonly of the surface type in nerve conduction studies (B–H of Fig. 2.2). Surface electrodes are generally used for routine motor conduction studies, as they give a good overall picture of the evoked response and its maximal amplitude. Surface electrodes are also painless for the patient. The surface electrodes can be standard Beckman electrodes (C of Fig. 2.2) or round flat metal discs (E of Fig. 2.2). Other types of surface electrodes, such as silver strips, saline soaked cloth, saline soaked pipecleaners (H of Fig. 2.2), and metal spring electrodes (G of Fig. 2.2), can be used in specific applications (especially in sensory nerve conduction studies).

Needle electrodes can be placed directly in the muscle for recording the evoked potentials in small muscles where surface electrodes might give a response contaminated by volume conduction from adjacent muscles. The needle can be monopolar (B of Fig. 2.3) or coaxial (A of Fig. 2.3) and can be placed either directly in muscle or subcutaneously. If a monopolar needle is used as the active recording electrode, the reference electrode is usually a standard surface disc. Horning and associates (12) have pointed out that the type of recording electrode used can change the latency, shape, and amplitude of the evoked response. They preferred using surface recording electrodes as much as possible to obtain the shortest latency and the maximum amplitude. Both coaxial and monopolar intramuscular electrodes give initial defections of low amplitude that can be easily missed or misread. Moving the intramuscular needle electrode slightly can change the shape of the evoked response. Changing the needle from a superficial to deep location in the muscle can change the shape and also shorten the latency of the evoked response. Horning and associates pointed out that if needle electrodes must be used for any reason, the preferred technique is to use a coaxial needle placed deep in the muscle. Some sensory studies are best recorded by placing monopolar needle electrodes 1-4 cm apart adjacent to the nerve.

There is a host of optional nerve conduction study equipment available that can be helpful in some clinical studies and in many research activities. An electronic averager is capable of isolating potentials so low in amplitude that they are hidden in the equipment "noise." There is a minimum electronic internal noise level that is usually in the range of from 1 to 5 μV in most commercially available EMG equipment (see Chapter 15). One can view potentials as low as 0.1 μV in amplitude by using electronic averaging with large numbers of stimulations. An electronic averager works by aver-

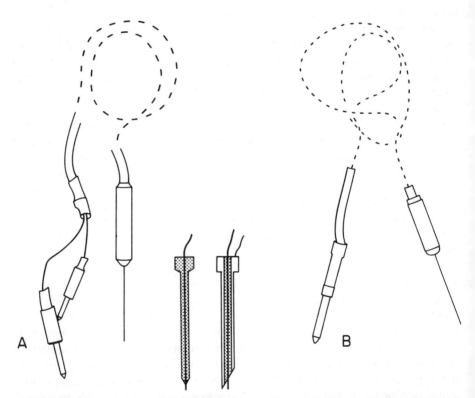

Fig. 2.3. Needle electrodes. (*A*) Coaxial or concentric electrode (see inset with two wires); (*B*) monopolar Teflon-coated electrode (see inset with one wire).

aging out all potentials which occur randomly over multiple sweeps. Since the internal noise of the machine and other extraneous potentials are random in nature, they average out over multiple sweeps and are reduced or eliminated. A very low amplitude but consistent potential such as the evoked response, will be "pulled out of the noise" by the averager.

A paired stimuli apparatus allows the delivery of two stimuli to a nerve separated by a time interval of from 1 to 100 msec. Paired stimuli are not generally clinically useful but are helpful in research applications, such as the H reflex paired stimuli recovery curve.

Another optional equipment item for nerve conduction studies is a storage scope. This will hold one or more sweeps of the cathode ray tube and allow indefinite visualization without photography. A single supramaximal stimulus with the evoked response held on a storage scope often prevents having to do multiple stimulations in determining latency and amplitude in an uncooperative patient. This equipment is particularly useful in pediatric clinical studies, since children often object to and resist multiple nerve stimuli.

Still another optional item in nerve conduction studies is a device that electronically or photographically makes a permanent record of the response. A fiberoptic recording device, such as that on the Teca TE-4 EMG machine (Teca Corp., White Plains, N.Y.), will print out the evoked responses on light sensitive paper that can be viewed and stored indefinitely. A Polaroid camera for direct photography of the evoked responses can also be used. A recent innovation is a device that electronically stores the cathode ray tube (CRT) sweep and replays it at a greatly reduced sweep speed to allow a mechanical pen writer to print it on inexpensive paper, such as ordinary EKG paper. Experienced clinicians generally do not find photographing of the evoked responses necessary, but it is useful in difficult diagnostic problems and in research activities.

The safety of the patient during nerve conduction studies must be assured (see Chapter 15). It would seem prudent both for the safety of the patient and for the medicolegal protection of the practitioner that all electrodiagnostic equipment is checked for excessive "leakage current." Most hospitals now have electrical safety teams who routinely inspect all hospital-owned electrical equipment for leakage currents. Hospitals across the nation have set different standards for maximum allowable leakage current but most commercial EMG manufacturers build their equipment to have a leakage of 100 μA or less. This can be tested with a "leakage meter," a device that hospital engineering departments should have.

For the safety of the patient and to facilitate interference-free studies, it is important to make certain that the EMG and nerve conduction apparatuses are plugged into a receptacle having a functioning ground. Electrical outlets can be tested to see if they do have a functioning ground with an inexpensive voltmeter. In ordinary grounded 60 Hz a.c. wall receptacles, one of the plug connectors should show 110 V between itself and ground, while the other connector should have zero volts between itself and ground. There should be 110 V between the two connectors. If this is not the case, the ground wire is not connected to earth ground and this should be corrected before doing clinical studies. The patient should not touch conductive objects in the room during the examination unless care has been taken to make certain that these conductive objects are at the same electrical potential as ground. This is made easier if the number of metallic objects in the room is held to a minimum by using wooden plinths and plastic or wooden furnishings. Some examining rooms have conductive materials that are grounded to a water pipe that may not be at zero volts (true earth ground). If patients grounded to the EMG machine touch such an object, they may be exposed to the potential difference between the two grounds.

We were unable to document any cases in the literature of patients being injured by the zero to 300 V stimuli used in nerve conduction studies. Certainly prudence is advised in doing nerve conduction studies on patients with cardiac pacemakers, especially since EMG equipment manufacturers do not recommend it and for medicolegal reasons are opposed to it. It is unlikely that ventricular fibrillation would result from nerve conduction studies, especially since the output of the stimulator in amperes or total watts is limited and is inversely proportional to the skin and tissue resistance ($I = E/R$).

As an aside, it should be remembered that the EMG machine can be used in cardiac emergencies as a makeshift EKG monitor. This is most readily done by attaching the reference electrode to any extremity, placing the active recording electrode on the chest, and slowing down the sweep speed so that one sweep takes 5 sec. The sensitivity setting should be 50–100 μV per centimeter or vertical division.

Sources of Error and Pitfalls

Although most of the techniques for performing nerve conduction studies are relatively simple, the clinician must be aware of potential sources of error that can lead to erroneous results and misdiagnoses. Potential errors in nerve conduction studies can arise from four general areas: anatomical factors, physiological factors, instrumentation errors, and technical errors.

ANATOMICAL FACTORS THAT MAY PRODUCE ERRORS

The clinician must be aware that variations from the "normal" anatomy can and frequently do occur. An anastomosis between the median and ulnar nerves in the forearm is frequent, reportely occurring in 15–25% of normal subjects. This anastomosis sends median fibers to the ulnar nerve, rather than from ulnar to median. This median to ulnar crossover is referred to as the Martin-Gruber anastomosis (13, 14). Its presence can be determined during routine median and ulnar nerve conduction studies. In the presence of the Martin-Gruber anastomosis, the amplitude of the evoked motor response is greater when the ulnar nerve is stimulated at the wrist than when it is stimulated at the elbow. This is because some ulnar fibers have crossed over to the ulnar nerve from the median nerve in the forearm.

The first dorsal interosseus muscle is usually innervated by the deep branch of the ulnar nerve, but in 3–10% of cases it is innervated partially or completely by the median nerve.

An anomalous nerve occasionally innervates the extensor digitorum brevis and is called the accessory deep peroneal nerve. It actually originates from the superficial branch of the peroneal nerve, not the deep branch as its name might suggest. The accessory deep peroneal nerve runs inferiorly along the posterior border of the peroneus brevis and passes posterior to the lateral malleolus. It then sends a branch to the extensor digitorum brevis muscle. In 1969, Lambert (15) reported that this anomaly should be suspected if the amplitude of the evoked motor response, when stimulating the peroneal nerve at the ankle, is less than when it is stimulated at the knee.

Other nerve anomalies occasionally occur. Gassel (16) suggested that, if confusion exists because of the possible presence of anomalous innervation, nerve conduction studies before and after local procaine nerve blocks can localize an anomalous pathway. He also pointed out that procaine diffuses quickly, so small carefully placed quantities should be used to avoid anesthetizing more than the desired nerve.

PHYSIOLOGICAL FACTORS THAT MAY PRODUCE ERRORS

Temperature

Nerve conduction velocity is related to the intraneural temperature, as nerve conduction velocity decreases approximately 2.4 m/sec for every centigrade degree of temperature decrease. This is based on the work of Henriksen (17), who varied the limb temperature while repeating nerve conduction studies. The temperatures were measured by a needle thermistor inserted to a depth of 2 cm into the proximal one-third of the forearm near the ulnar nerve. Nerve conduction velocity continues to decline with decreasing temperature until approximately 8°C, when nerve function ceases. Cooling also increases the duration of the relative and absolute refractory periods (18). Henriksen also reported studies in several patients with poliomyelitis who had apparent slowing of nerve conduction in the affected extremities. The nerve conduction velocities were normal when the limb was warmed, indicating that the slow conduction was due to the subnormal limb temperature rather than to nerve pathology. To alleviate this potential error, skin temperature should be routinely measured and the extremity warmed to normal when diminished temperatures occur.

Age

Motor nerve conduction velocity values at birth are approximately one-half of normal adult values. Nerve conduction velocity increases with age so that by 3 years of age it is in the low adult range and by 4 years of age it has reached normal adult values. The nerve conduction velocity then remains relatively stable until 60 years of age, when it begins to decrease at a rate of approximately 1.5% per decade (19). Sensory nerve conduction velocity and sensory evoked potential amplitude decrease more rapidly with age than the corresponding motor nerve responses (20, 21).

INSTRUMENTATION ERRORS

Modern electrodiagnostic equipment should be properly maintained and calibrated to minimize nerve conduction error due to equipment dysfunction. The most common error is having the time scale miscalibrated. Time scale calibration should be routinely evaluated, and a high index of suspicion should exist if the conduction values contradict what appears to be present clinically. Another potential error exists if the onset of the sweep is not synchronized so that it consistently occurs at the same point before the electrical stimulus.

Older electrodiagnostic equipment may have a variation in the sweep speed as the trace crosses the screen. Usually this gives a sweep that is accurate in the center of the screen but not at the edges. Some older equipment had the grid or graticule markings on a separate clear sheet in front of the CRT screen. If the graticule markings were used to measure the latency, a parallax error was likely unless the clinician sighted the latency from directly in front of the screen.

TECHNICAL ERRORS

The great majority of errors in nerve conduction studies are the result of various technical difficulties. These errors can be subdivided into two categories: errors in the performance of nerve conduction studies, and errors in interpretation of the results.

Errors in the Performance of Nerve Conduction Studies

Standardization of technique. In the electrodiagnostic evaluation of a patient, it is of extreme importance to be able to compare current nerve conduction values with those obtained at a previous examination and with values obtained from a normal population. For these comparisons to have any validity, it is imperative that nerve conduction studies be performed consistently with a standardized technique. Great care should be taken to consistently place the recording and stimulating electrodes at standardized sites. Where possible, a standardized distance between the active recording electrode and the stimulator should be used.

Errors in stimulation. Reversal of the stimulating cathode and anode can cause a latency reading error of 0.5 msec, giving an erroneously prolonged latency value. The stimulus should always be supramaximal. The stimulus intensity should be progressively increased until the maximum amplitude response is obtained. Then the stimulus should be further increased 25–50% to ensure a supramaximal stimulus. If a less than supramaximal stimulus is used, some of the fastest conducting fibers may not be stimulated. This would result in a falsely prolonged latency value. If too great a supramaximal stimulus is used, the nerve potentially can be stimulated distal to the actual position of the cathode, resulting in an erroneously short latency value. An extremely high supramaximal stimulus can also spread to adjacent nerves by volume conduction. This is especially likely between the median and ulnar nerves in the forearm and the tibial and peroneal nerves in the popliteal fossa. This spread of the stimulus can occur with either surface or needle stimulating electrodes but is more common with percutaneous stimulation.

Errors in recording. The type of recording electrode used can greatly alter the response that is obtained. Horning et al. (12) reported variations in distal latency values when studies were performed with intramuscular needle recording electrodes and surface recording electrodes. The shortest latency value over any given distance was generally recorded with a surface recording electrode. A needle electrode inserted deeply into the muscle recorded a slightly longer latency, while a superficially placed needle electrode recorded an even longer latency. Latencies recorded with monopolar needle electrodes were frequently quite difficult to measure because the initial deflection of the evoked response was often of extremely low amplitude. This could lead to an error of several milliseconds in the latency readings. They suggested that if a needle recording electrode must be used, it would be best to use a coaxial electrode placed deeply in the muscle.

Errors of amplification. An error can occur when the sensitivity of the amplifier is changed during the performance of a nerve conduction study. There is a tendency for a longer latency value to be recorded with low amplification rather than with high amplification. The amplification used should be consistent for all stimulating sites of a nerve and should also be consistent when prior results are compared with current studies. With very high amplification, it is possible to record a small negative deflection immediately prior to the onset of evoked motor response. This small potential is called the intramuscular nerve action potential (11, 22). The specific origin of the potential has not been absolutely clarified but it is thought to arise either from the motor or sensory axons.

Errors of measurement. Another important source of error is in the measurement of the exact distance over which the nerve is stimulated. Maynard and Stolov (23) found that when 20 experienced electromyographers carefully measured a distance on a hard surface, there was an average measurement error of 3.6 mm.

The technique of measurement and the position of the extremity are extremely important in reducing error, as was demonstrated in a study by Checkles et al. (24). They noted that the ulnar nerve has a tendency to fold upon itself at the elbow in full elbow extension. If measurement of the across-elbow segment is performed with the elbow fully extended, falsely low values for ulnar nerve conduction across the elbow are obtained. They discovered that the optimal position for measuring the across-elbow segment of the ulnar nerve was with the elbow in 70° of acute flexion.

Errors of latency reading. Despite the use of standardized techniques and a well calibrated instrument, potential error can still occur due to variation in reading the exact latency value. This was pointed out by Honet et al. (25), who determined the latency values from 25 Polaroid photographs of evoked responses and then calculated the conduction velocities. They noted a variation in the conduction velocities of 2.0–3.0 m/sec. This represents a coefficient of variation of approximately 4–5%, due just to the variability of reading the latency.

Errors in Interpretation of the Results

Volume conduction. A nerve stimulus can spread to nerves other than the one being tested. This causes the active recording electrode to detect action potentials which are generated near but not in the muscle being studied. Gassel (16) stimulated the tibial nerve at the ankle with recording electrodes placed over the extensor digitorum brevis muscle. In all of the 10 subjects he studied, a response was recorded from the extensor digitorum brevis with stimulation of the tibial nerve. To rule out anomalous innervation of the extensor digitorum brevis, a procaine block of the muscle was performed and the procedure repeated. A response was again recorded over the extensor digitorum brevis, which actually represented a volume conducted response from the adjacent foot muscles innervated by the tibial nerve. He also noted similar results in the abductor hallucis muscle when the deep peroneal nerve was stimulated due to volume conduction from the extensor digitorum brevis. Volume conduction causes confusion, especially in children, as their small extremities make it difficult to isolate the stimulus to one nerve. Volume conduction must be constantly considered as a potential source of error.

H reflex and F wave. With submaximal stimulation of the tibial nerve it is possible to record an H reflex from the calf muscles, and with supramaximal stimulation of the tibial and other nerves it is possible to record an F wave. These responses are greatly prolonged when compared with the direct motor response and can cause significant errors if they are interpreted as being direct motor responses.

The clinician performing nerve conduction studies should be aware of all of the above potential sources of error and should exercise extreme care in the performance of nerve conduction studies so that accurate, reliable, and reproducible results are obtained.

Median Nerve Motor Conduction

The median nerve arises from the medial and lateral cords of the brachial plexus. The nerve roots forming the lateral cord are primarily C5, C6 and C7, and the nerve roots forming the medial cord are primarily C8 and T1. In the arm, the median nerve runs in close proximity to the brachial artery.

In the proximal arm, it lies lateral to the brachial artery and then passes anterior to the artery to lie medial to it in the distal arm. In the cubital fossa, the median nerve lies behind the bicipital aponeurosis and in front of the brachialis muscle. The nerve enters the forearm between the two heads of the pronator teres, passes deep to the flexor digitorum superficialis, and then descends through the forearm deep to the flexor digitorum superficialis and superficial to the flexor digitorum profundus. The anterior interosseus branch arises from the posterior surface of the median nerve as it passes between the two heads of the pronator teres. This branch innervates the lateral portion of the flexor digitorum profundus, the flexor pollicis longus, and the pronator quadratus. The main trunk of the median nerve descends to the wrist, where it lies between the tendons of the flexor digitorum superficialis and the flexor carpi radialis. It passes deep to the flexor retinaculum (transverse carpal ligament) to enter the palm through the carpal canal (carpal tunnel). It then sends a motor branch to the superficial head of the flexor pollicis brevis, the abductor pollicis brevis, and the opponens pollicis. Palmar digital branches provide cutaneous sensation to the thumb, index, and middle fingers, as well as the lateral half of the ring finger. The palmar digital branches also give off motor fibers to the first and second lumbrical muscles.

Median nerve motor conduction studies are performed with the active recording electrode placed one-half the distance between the metacarpophalangeal joint of the thumb and the midpoint of the distal wrist crease. The reference electrode is placed distally on the thumb, and the ground electrode is placed over the palmar aspect of the ulnar border of the hand (Fig. 2.4). The patient should be in a supine position with the shoulder abducted approximately 10° and the elbow completely extended. The distal latency value is recorded with the cathode of the stimulator 8 cm proximal to the active electrode and located between the palmaris longus and flexor carpi radialis tendons. The median nerve can also be stimulated more proximally at various sites, such as 5 cm distal to the elbow, in the cubital fossa, 10 cm proximal to the elbow, and at Erb's point (26). The median nerve can be quickly located at the elbow just medial to the pulsation of the brachial artery. The location of the stimulator at Erb's point is at the angle formed by the clavicle and the posterolateral fibers of the sternocleidomastoid muscle. The lengths of the nerve segments can be accurately measured with a metal tape, except for the segment from Erb's point to above the elbow, which is best measured with obstetric calipers (26) (Fig. 2.5). Since the initial report of median nerve motor nerve conduction by Helmholtz in 1852, numerous authors have reported values for normal median nerve motor conduction. Many of these studies can be criticized because the nerve segments over which the stimulation was performed were nonstandardized. Many authors recommend using anatomical landmarks, such as the wrist crease, as sites of stimulation. Since hand size varies greatly in the general population, the use of anatomical landmarks as stimulation sites induces

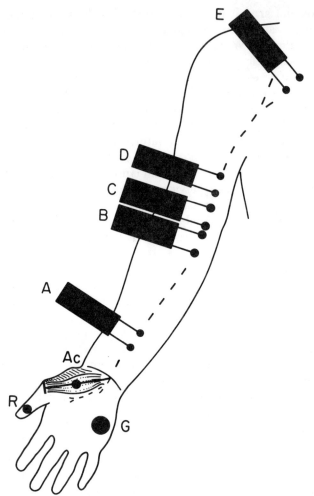

Fig. 2.4. Median motor nerve conduction study. *Ac*, active recording electrode; *R*, reference electrode; *G*, ground electrode; *A-E*, sites of median nerve stimulation.

significant variation into the latency determinations. The use of a standardized 8-cm stimulation distance for the distal latency circumvents this difficulty and allows data from individual patients to be accurately compared with values obtained from large series of normal persons (27). The values reported in Table 2.2 were obtained by using the above technique.

In the routine performance of median nerve conduction studies, one must be aware of the possible presence of the Martin-Gruber anastomosis. This is a neural communication between the median and ulnar nerves in the forearm present in approximately 15–25% of the general population (Fig. 2.6). The median nerve distal latency value would be abnormal with median nerve pathology at the wrist in a patient with a coexisting Martin-Gruber

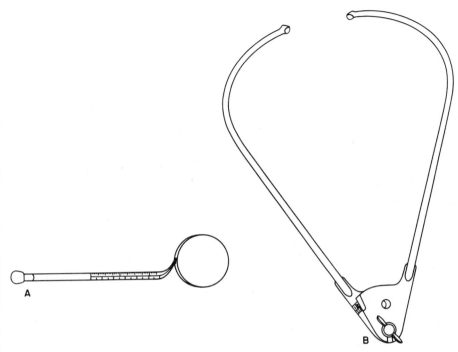

Fig. 2.5. Measurement equipment. (*A*) Steel tape; (*B*) obstetric calipers with points filed flat.

TABLE 2.2. *Median Nerve Motor Conduction (Normal Values)*

	Unit	Mean Value	Standard Deviation	Reference
Distal latency	msec	3.7	0.3	(27)
Conduction velocity	m/sec			
1. Below elbow to wrist		55.1	5.2	(26)
2. Elbow to wrist		58.6	3.8	
3. Erb's point to elbow		62.8	6.0	
4. Erb's point to above elbow		62.9	6.0	
Amplitude of evoked response (wrist stimulation)	mV	13.2	5.0	(27)
Duration of evoked response (wrist stimulation)	msec	7.5	1.5	(27)

anastomosis. When the median nerve is stimulated proximally at the elbow, a nearly normal proximal latency value can be obtained. This is because some of the fibers in the median nerve cross over into the ulnar nerve and give a response in the ulnar-innervated muscle that is volume conducted to the active recording electrode. A clue to the existence of a Martin-Gruber anastomosis is the presence of a larger amplitude and an initial positive deflection when stimulating the median nerve at the elbow rather than at

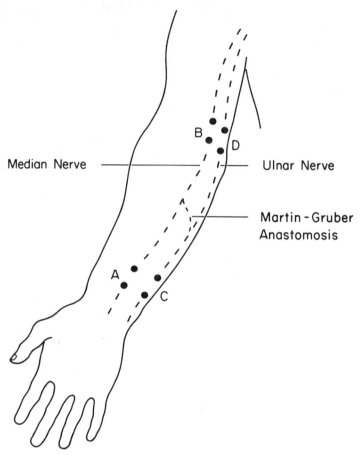

Fig. 2.6. Martin-Gruber anastomosis. *A*, Site of distal median stimulation; *B*, site of proximal median stimulation; *C*, site of distal ulnar stimulation; *D*, site of proximal ulnar stimulation.

the wrist. This is due to "ulnar" fibers contained in the proximal median nerve being stimulated, giving a volume conducted response from ulnar innervated muscles to the active recording electrode over the thenar eminence (13, 14).

Ulnar Nerve Motor Conduction

The ulnar nerve arises primarily from the C8 and T1 nerve roots and from the medial cord of the brachial plexus. It occasionally receives fibers from the seventh cervical nerve. It passes through the axilla on the medial side of the axillary artery. In the midarm, it pierces the medial intermuscular septum and descends anterior to the medial head of the triceps. At the elbow, it lies in a groove on the dorsum of the medial epicondyle. In the upper part of the forearm, it passes between the heads of the flexor carpi ulnaris and goes distally in the forearm in close association with this muscle. About 5 cm proximal to the wrist the nerve becomes superficial and gives off two cutaneous branches. The nerve then continues into the hand after passing through Guyon's canal. In the hand, the nerve divides into a superficial and deep branch. The superficial branch innervates the palmaris brevis, supplies sensory fibers to the skin on the medial side of the hand, and divides into the palmar digital nerves, which give sensory supply to the small finger and medial aspect of the ring finger. The deep branch gives fibers to the interossei and the third and fourth lumbricals before it ends by supplying the adductor pollicis, the first palmar interosseous, and the deep head of the flexor pollicis brevis muscles.

For the routine performance of ulnar nerve motor conduction studies, the active recording electrode is placed over the main bulk of the hypothenar musculature (Fig. 2.7). To accurately pinpoint this location, marks are placed along the medial border of the hand at the distal wrist crease and at the metacarpophalangeal joint. The distance between these two points is

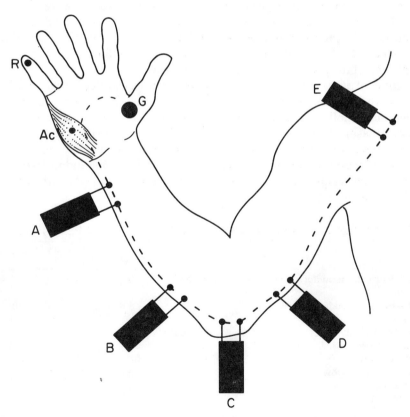

Fig. 2.7. Ulnar nerve motor conduction studies. *Ac*, active recording electrode; *R*, reference electrode; *G*, ground electrode; *A-E*, sites of stimulation.

measured and bisected for placement of the active recording electrode at the midpoint. The reference electrode is placed distally on the small finger and the ground electrode is located on the lateral aspect of the hand. The best position for testing the ulnar nerve is with the patient supine, with the shoulder in approximately 45° of abduction and the elbow acutely flexed to 70°. To avoid error, both the stimulation and measurement of the nerve segments should be done in this position. The distal latency response is evoked with the cathode of the stimulator exactly 8 cm proximal to the active recording electrode and just lateral to the tendon of the flexor carpi ulnaris. The ulnar nerve can also be stimulated more proximally at sites along its course, as reported by Jebsen (26). He stimulated the nerve at a point 5 cm distal to the elbow, at the elbow, 10 cm proximal to the elbow, and supraclavically. When measuring the nerve segment across the elbow, care must be taken to keep the elbow in 70° of acute flexion. The course of the nerve should be measured as closely as possible around the elbow. Checkles et al. (24) found that falsely low conduction values were obtained when ulnar conduction across the elbow was performed with the elbow extended. They noted that accurate and reproducible values were obtained when the elbow was maintained in 70° of acute flexion. Cadaver dissections demonstrated that the ulnar nerve was folded upon itself when the elbow was extended. With 70° of acute flexion of the elbow, the nerve was straightened but not overstretched along its course.

At times it is necessary to assess conduction in the deep branch of the ulnar nerve. For this procedure the active recording electrode is placed over the adductor pollicis muscle (best located over the lateral portion of the palmar crease). The nerve is stimulated as in the routine procedure described above. Many authors have reported values for normal ulnar nerve motor conduction, but many of these studies had a nonstandardized technique. Normal values based on the standardized technique described above are listed in Table 2.3.

TABLE 2.3. *Ulnar Nerve Motor Conduction (Normal Values)*

	Unit	Mean Value	Standard Deviation	Reference
Distal latency (to abductor digiti quinti)	msec	3.2	0.5	—[a]
Distal latency (to adductor pollicus)	msec	3.4	0.6	(28)
Conduction velocity	m/sec			
1. Below elbow to wrist		59.4	5.3	(26)
2. Elbow to wrist		57.9	4.3	(26)
3. Erb's point to elbow		58.4	4.1	(26)
4. Erb's point to above elbow		61.3	5.4	(26)
5. Across elbow		62.7	5.5	(24)

[a] Schuchmann, unpublished data.

Nerve Root Stimulation

The brachial plexus, as well as the subclavian artery and vein, leaves the thorax by arching over the first rib between the scalenus anticus and scalenus medius muscles. Compression of this neurovascular bundle between the scalenus anticus and medius is thought to be one etiology of the thoracic outlet syndrome (scalenus anticus syndrome) (29–31). Ulnar nerve conduction studies are generally performed to ascertain the presence of the thoracic outlet syndrome (32). Slowing of ulnar conduction in the segment from Erb's point to above the elbow is erroneously thought to represent a finding compatible with the thoracic outlet syndrome. Stimulation at Erb's point is actually distal to the site of the pathology, consequently this technique is imprecise. It has been recently appreciated that cervical nerve roots can be directly stimulated by a needle electrode inserted through the posterior neck into the area where the roots exit from the intervertebral foramina (Fig. 2.8). To stimulate the C8 nerve root, for example, the spinous process of the C7 vertebrae is palpated, and the needle stimulating electrode is inserted approximately 1 cm lateral and caudad to the superior portion of the spinous process. The stimulating electrode is inserted until it touches the inferior aspect of the transverse process, where it is in the immediate

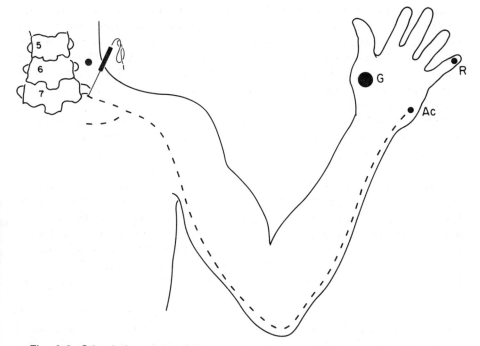

Fig. 2.8. Stimulation of the C8 nerve root with recording over ulnar innervated muscles. *Ac*, active recording electrode; *R*, reference electrode; *G*, ground electrode.

proximity of the C8 nerve root. Stimulation of the nerve root is performed using a standard supramaximal technique with the active recording electrode placed over the hypothenar muscles as for routine ulnar conduction studies. The study has not been adequately standardized to be able to report normal values, but this technique does appear to be of more value in determining the presence of the thoracic outlet syndrome than ordinary conduction studies of the ulnar nerve. *Editor's Note:* A side-to-side difference of more than 1 msec is suggestive of thoracic outlet syndrome.

Radial Motor Conduction

The radial nerve is somewhat more difficult to study than the median and ulnar nerves because there are no radially innervated muscles in the hand and because stimulation sites are less easily demarcated. In spite of the relative difficulty of radial motor studies, it is important that the clinician develop a reliable technique, because radial nerve dysfunction is frequently seen in clinical practice.

The radial nerve is the terminal branch of the posterior cord and begins at approximately the level of the glenohumeral joint. It runs posterior and medial to the proximal humerus but gradually spirals around the midportion of the humerus to occupy an anterolateral position between the brachioradialis muscle and the biceps tendon in the distal arm. After reaching the forearm, the radial nerve divides into the superficial radial nerve (sensory only) and the posterior interosseus nerve (motor only). The posterior interosseus nerve penetrates the supinator muscle and the interosseus membrane and terminates by innervating the extensor indicis proprius muscle in the distal forearm.

Different authors have selected various sites along the radial nerve for motor stimulation. They have also chosen different radial muscles from which to record the evoked response. Gassel and Diamantopolous (33) used concentric needle recording electrodes in the anconeus, extensor digitorum communis, brachioradialis, and triceps muscles. They used surface bipolar stimulation at Erb's point, in the midarm as the radial nerve passes into the spiral groove (approximately 4 cm posterior to the insertion of the deltoid), and distally approximately 5 cm above and slightly posterior to the lateral epicondyle of the humerus. They recorded nerve conduction velocity values of 74 m/sec (S.D., 6.7 m/sec) to the brachioradialis, 72 m/sec (S.D., 6.1 m/sec) to the extensor digitorum communis, and 66 m/sec (S.D., 9.2 m/sec) to the anconeus.

Trojaborg and Sindrup (34) stimulated the radial nerve at three sites with a pair of needle electrodes insulated except at their tips. They stimulated the nerve in the forearm 8 cm proximal to the styloid process of the ulna, where the nerve can often be palpated just lateral to the extensor carpi ulnaris muscle. They also stimulated at the elbow in the groove between the brachioradialis muscle and the biceps tendon 6 cm proximal to the lateral epicondyle of the humerus. They also stimulated in the axilla in the groove between the coracobrachialis and the medial edge of the triceps (18 cm proximal to the medial epicondyle of the humerus). They used concentric needle electrodes to record the responses in the triceps, brachioradialis, extensor digitorum communis, extensor pollicus longus, and extensor indicis. In a small number of normal subjects ($n = 10$) they found a conduction velocity between the axilla and the elbow of 69 m/sec, regardless of whether the conduction was measured to the brachioradialis, extensor digitorium communis, extensor pollicus longus, or extensor indicis muscles. They found that the conduction velocity of the radial motor fibers between the elbow and the forearm was consistently 10% lower than in the proximal segment of the nerve.

While many other methods of doing motor conduction studies of the radial nerve are reported in the literature, perhaps the most clinically practical is that suggested by Jebsen (35) (Fig. 2.9). In this method, surface stimulation of the radial nerve is done with the subject in a supine position, with the arm abducted approximately 10°, the elbow flexed 10–15°, and the forearm pronated. The evoked response is recorded by a coaxial electrode in the extensor indicis muscle. The radial nerve is stimulated 3–4 cm proximal to the site of the needle insertion in the extensor indicis muscle, next approximately 5–6 cm proximal to the lateral epicondyle, where the radial nerve lies in the groove between the brachialis and brachioradialis muscle, and then at Erb's point. Gassel and Diamantopolous (33) measured the distance from the stimulation point site at Erb's point to the stimulation site proximal to the elbow with obstetric calipers whose edges were filed flat (Fig. 2.5). This was found both by Gassel and Diamantopolous and by Jebsen in cadaveric studies to be a more accurate reflection of the true nerve length over this segment than would be surface tape measurements. Jebsen also noted that the relative degree of abduction and adduction of the arm affected the accuracy of the calipers measurement. Abducting the arm at 40° increased the calipers measurement of the distance by 1.4 cm over that obtained in 10° of abduction. The distal distance was measured as accurately by a metal tape as by calipers.

Jebsen (35) found in 98 radial nerves of 49 normal subjects that the mean proximal conduction velocity was 72 m/sec (S.D., 6.3 m/sec). The mean distal conduction velocity of the radial motor fibers was 61.6 m/sec (S.D., 5.9 m/sec). The proximal velocity was consistently faster than the distal velocity (only 7 of the 98 radial nerves tested had a distal velocity faster than the proximal).

Unfortunately none of the studies of radial nerve motor conduction velocity reports a standardized distal latency such as has been done for most other nerves. A standardized distal latency is especially useful information in the study of peripheral neuropathy, since most peripheral neuropathies

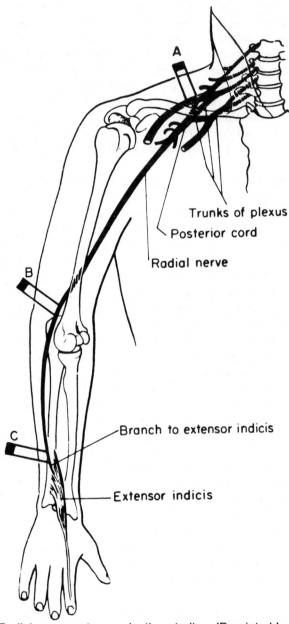

Trunks of plexus
Posterior cord
Radial nerve

Branch to extensor indicis

Extensor indicis

Fig. 2.9. Radial nerve motor conduction studies. (Reprinted by permission from: R. H. Jebsen: *Arch. Phys. Med. Rehabil., 47:* 597, 1966.)

produce prolongation of the distal latency before actual slowing of nerve conduction proximally. Pending the reporting of a well standardized distal latency, clinicians are advised to develop their own standardized distal latency data.

Motor Studies of the Musculocutaneous Nerve

The musculocutaneous nerve arises from the lateral cord of the brachial plexus. After sending a branch to innervate the coracobrachialis muscle, it pierces this muscle and continues down the arm to innervate the biceps brachii and the brachialis muscles. It terminates in the forearm as a sensory branch called the lateral cutaneous nerve of the forearm.

The musculocutaneous nerve is rarely studied in clinical practice because of the infrequency of isolated involvement of this nerve. Three cases of specific injury to the musculocutaneous nerve as it courses through the coracobrachialis muscle were recently reported by Braddom and Wolfe (36). The injury to the musculocutaneous nerve in these cases appeared to be due to heavy exercise causing trauma to the portion of the nerve that passes through the coracobrachialis muscle. The most frequent indication for study of the musculocutaneous nerve is in brachial plexus lesions in which it is only one of many nerves being tested.

Techniques for studying the musculocutaneous nerve have been reported by a number of investigators. One of the first studies of latencies to muscles of the shoulder girdle was by Redford (37). He reported latency values from stimulation of the musculocutaneous nerve in the axilla to recording electrodes over the biceps brachii. Similar reporting of latencies were done by Gassel (38), Vacek and Drugova (39), and Kraft (40), with the exception that the latency was determined by stimulation at Erb's point rather than by stimulation of individual nerves in the axilla. These elected to use latencies rather than to calculate nerve conduction velocities because of the difficulty of stimulating the musculocutaneous nerve at two locations. Gassel reported mean values for latency to the biceps brachii that varied with the length of the segment of nerve. At 20 cm the latency was 4.6 msec (S.D., 0.6 msec), at 24 cm it was 4.7 msec (S.D., 0.6 msec) and at 28 cm it was 5.0 msec (S.D., 0.5 msec). Kraft reported a mean latency to the biceps brachii of 4.5 msec (S.D., 0.6 msec) with a normal range of 3.3–5.7 msec. He placed all latency values together but noted that the distance from the site of stimulation to the active recording electrode varied from 23.5 to 29.0 cm in his subjects (calipers measurement). The studies of Gassel, Vacek and Drugova, and Kraft are useful also because they give techniques and standardized values for similar studies of the axillary and suprascapular nerves in addition to the musculocutaneous.

Trojaborg (41) reported a technique for determining both motor and sensory conduction velocities in the musculocutaneous nerve. The motor technique requires that the musculocutaneous nerve be stimulated with a needle electrode at Erb's point and in the axilla. The musculocutaneous nerve in the axilla is located between the axillary artery on its medial aspect and the coracobrachialis muscle on its lateral aspect (just above the level of the tendon of the latissimus dorsi). The action potentials are recorded with concentric needle electrodes placed in the biceps brachii in the area giving a maximal response. The motor nerve conduction values were studied in 51 normal subjects from 15 to 74 years of age. The nerve conduction velocity between the stimulation site at Erb's point and the stimulation site in the axilla ranged from 70 m/sec in the 15–24-year-old age group to 58 m/sec in the 65–74-year-old group. The mean value for all ages was 64 m/sec. The nerve conduction varied greatly with age and decreased 2 m/sec per decade of age. It is apparent that the choice of which of the above techniques the clinician uses to study the musculocutaneous nerve should relate to the type of clinical problem and the equipment that is available.

Peroneal Nerve Motor Conduction Studies

The common peroneal nerve is derived from the ventral rami of L4, L5, and S1 and from the lateral division of the sciatic nerve. In the lower thigh, the common peroneal nerve separates from the sciatic nerve and passes along the lateral border of the popliteal fossa. It wraps around the lateral neck of the fibula and then divides into its two terminal branches, the superficial and deep peroneal nerves. The deep peroneal nerve passes down the leg deep to the extensor digitorum longus muscle and in front of the interosseous membrane. It innervates the tibialis anterior, the extensor hallucis longus, the extensor digitorum longus, the peroneus tertius muscles, and the extensor digitorium brevis. The superficial peroneal nerve passes down the leg between the peronei and the extensor digitorum longus muscles and innervates the peroneus longus and peroneus brevis muscles.

For peroneal nerve conduction studies, the active recording electrode is placed over the main bulk of the extensor digitorum brevis muscle. This is located in the anterolateral aspect of the proximal midtarsal area. The reference electrode is placed distally over the small toe and the ground electrode is placed over the medial portion of the foot (Fig. 2.10). The stimulating cathode is placed 8 cm proximal to the active recording electrode to provide a standardized distal latency segment. The peroneal nerve is also stimulated proximally at the fibular head and in the popliteal fossa. As shown by Checkles et al. (42), there is no significant difference between measuring the peroneal nerve segment with a surface metal tape or with calipers. The normal values for peroneal nerve motor conduction are listed in Table 2.4.

Lambert (15) noted that, in peroneal nerve conduction studies, the amplitude of the evoked response when stimulating at the ankle was occasionally less than when stimulating at the fibular head. In these patients, stimulation posterior to the lateral malleolus produced an evoked response in the extensor digitorum brevis muscle. This phenomenon was found to be due to the presence of an anomalous nerve branch, the accessory deep

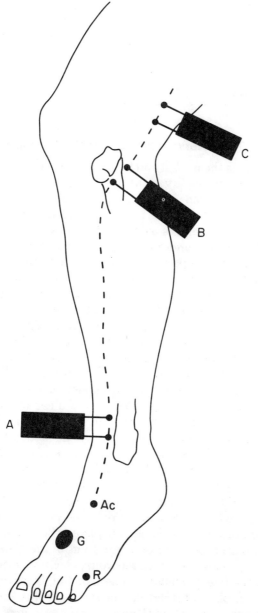

Fig. 2.10. Peroneal nerve motor conduction studies. *Ac*, active recording electrodes; *R*, reference electrode; *G*, ground electrode; *A-C*, sites of stimulation.

peroneal nerve. This nerve originates from the superficial peroneal nerve and is felt to be present in approximately 22% of normal limbs. This common anomaly should be constantly considered when performing routine peroneal nerve conduction studies.

TABLE 2.4. *Peroneal Nerve Motor Conduction (Normal Values)*

	Unit	Mean Value	Standard Deviation	Reference
Distal latency	msec	4.3	0.6	(43)
Conduction velocity	m/sec			
1. Below fibular head		52	4.0	(43)
2. Popliteal fossa to ankle		51.1	6.3	(42)

Tibial Nerve Motor Conduction Studies

The tibial nerve is the medial and larger of the two branches of the sciatic nerve which separate at a variable distance above the popliteal fossa underneath the long head of the biceps femoris muscle. After coursing through the center of the popliteal fossa, the tibial nerve gradually moves medially in relation to the tibia as it continues down the leg. It goes around the medial malleolus and under the flexor retinaculum through the "tarsal tunnel." Immediately after passing beneath the flexor retinaculum, the tibial nerve divides into three branches. The first is the calcaneal branch, which provides both deep and superficial sensation to the heel. The other two branches are the medial and lateral plantar nerves, which innervate all intrinsic muscles of the foot except the extensor digitorum brevis. These nerves also provide sensory fibers to the sole and the toes. The medial plantar nerve is analogous to the median nerve in the hand, in that it supplies cutaneous sensation to the 3½ medial digits and to the abductor hallucis, flexor digitorum brevis, flexor hallucis brevis, and one lumbrical. The lateral plantar nerve is analogous to the ulnar nerve in the hand, in that it supplies the cutaneous branches to the lateral 1½ digits and innervates the muscles of the sole not supplied by the medial plantar nerve.

One of the most reproducible techniques for studying the tibial nerve is that reported by Johnson and Ortiz (44). They found that the abductor hallucis was a convenient muscle from which to record an evoked response. The motor point of the abductor hallucis is located 1 cm behind and below the navicular tubercle, which is easily palpated on the medial aspect of the foot (Fig. 2.11). For studying the lateral plantar branch of the tibial nerve, they suggested recording over the motor point of the abductor digiti quinti pedis muscle by placing the active recording electrode directly beneath the anterior tip of the lateral malleolus one-half the distance to the sole. The tibial nerve is stimulated behind the medial malleolus and at the popliteal crease. In 100 normal subjects of all ages they found a tibial nerve conduction velocity of 50.9 m/sec (S.D., 7.16 m/sec). The distal latency of the medial and lateral plantar nerves was determined at numerous foot temperatures. At approximately 26.5°C, the distal latency of the medial plantar nerve was 5.32 msec with a standard deviation of 0.82 msec. The lateral plantar nerve had a latency of 5.8 msec with a standard deviation of 0.84 msec.

Braddom and Johnson (45) later refined this technique for the medial plantar branch in 100 normal subjects of all ages by standardizing an 8-cm distance from the point of cathodal stimulation behind the medial malleolus to the active recording electrode on the abductor hallucis. These studies were done without warming or cooling the foot in a laboratory with an ambient temperature of 21°C. The subjects had an average age of 39 years (S.D., 16 years). The tibial distal latency measured in the medial plantar nerve was 4.8 msec with a standard deviation of 0.8 msec. The tibial nerve conduction velocity was 49.8 m/sec with a standard deviation of 6.0 m/sec.

Sciatic Motor Conduction Studies

The sciatic nerve originates mainly from spinal segments L5 and S1 but also gets some fibers from L4 and S2. The sciatic nerve is the largest nerve trunk in the body. A close examination of the sciatic nerve shows that it is actually two nerves tightly sheathed together. These two nerves are the lateral and medial divisions of the sciatic nerve, which distally become the common peroneal and tibial nerves, respectively. The sciatic nerve leaves the pelvis by way of the greater sciatic foramen. The piriformis muscle largely fills the greater sciatic foramen and the sciatic nerve normally runs under it. In approximately 12% of normal subjects, the peroneal (lateral) division of the sciatic nerve passes through the piriformis muscle, and in approximately 0.5%, it passes above the piriformis muscle. The sciatic nerve is covered proximally by the gluteus maximus in its course midway between the ischial tuberosity and the greater trochanter. The nerve is most super-ficial just after it exits from under the gluteus maximus and before it goes

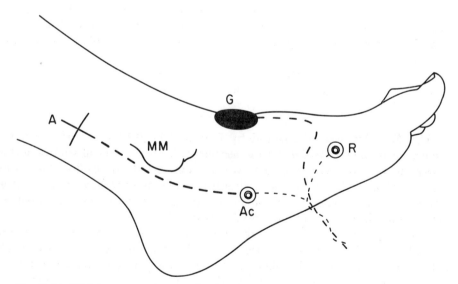

Fig. 2.11. Tibial nerve motor conduction studies. *Ac*, active recording electrode; *R*, reference electrode; *G*, ground electrode; *MM*, medial malleolus; *A*, stimulation site.

deep to the long head of the biceps femoris. The nerve then continues down the center of the posterior thigh until it divides into its tibial and peroneal nerve components above the popliteal fossa.

Nerve conduction studies of the sciatic nerve are infrequently performed, probably because the nerve is difficult to stimulate with a surface stimulator. The sciatic nerve can be studied using the active recording sites listed above for either the peroneal or tibial nerves. Perhaps the easiest technique is to place the recording electrodes for a tibial nerve conduction study with the active recording electrode over the abductor hallucis. After stimulating with a surface stimulator behind the medial malleolus and at the popliteal crease in the usual manner for a tibial nerve conduction study, a needle electrode is inserted into the proximal thigh adjacent to the sciatic nerve at the inferior margin of the gluteus maximus. Yap and Hirota (46) found this proximal site to be most easily stimulated with a needle electrode as surface stimulation required very large stimuli and painful pressure and even then was often unsuccessful. The evoked response in the abductor hallucis may have been higher in amplitude after stimulation of the sciatic nerve as compared to the stimulation of the tibial nerve in the popliteal space. This difference is probably related to volume conduction from nearby peroneal muscles since the proximal sciatic stimulation excites both the peroneal and tibial components of the sciatic nerve.

Yap and Hirota (46) reported values for the sciatic nerve in the segment from the inferior gluteal margin to the popliteal fossa of 53.8 m/sec (S.D., 3.3 m/sec) in 19 individuals. Some clinicians prefer to stimulate the sciatic nerve and record the evoked response over such large muscles as the hamstrings or the gastrocnemius. Except in unusual clinical and some research situations, the sciatic nerve is probably more easily studied by placing the active recording electrode over a peroneal or a tibially innervated intrinsic muscle of the foot as described above.

Some prefer to study the sciatic nerve indirectly by using the H reflex. The H reflex technique for this is described below.

H Reflex

The H reflex was discovered by Hoffman in 1918 (47) and given its eponymic name by Magladery and associates in their classical studies of the early 1950s (48–52). In the last two decades, the H reflex has been the subject of literally hundreds of literature reports that have suggested a myriad of clinical uses. Many of these clinical uses were recently classified and summarized by Braddom and Johnson (53).

The neurophysiology of the H reflex is still disputed but most investigators consider it to be a monosynaptic reflex. There is also disagreement as to where it can normally be elicited, but it is most easily and consistently elicitable in muscles innervated by the S1 roots and the tibial nerve. In infancy, the H reflex can be elicited in almost any skeletal muscle on stimulation of the appropriate peripheral nerve. The H reflex is gradually "suppressed" until approximately one year of age, when it is elicitable consistently only in muscles innervated by the S1 root and the tibial nerve. Some have described the H reflex as nothing more than an electronic Achilles tendon reflex in which the I-a fibers from the nuclear bag receptors of the muscle spindle system are directly electrically stimulated. When a muscle is stretched by a hammer striking its tendon, the annulospiral endings of the nuclear bag fibers transmit afferent stimuli along I-a fibers to alpha motor neurons innervating that muscle. These I-a fibers facilitate the alpha motor neurons and cause them to discharge, which shortens the muscle to restore its original length. Although the H reflex appears to use part of this muscle stretch reflex pathway, it is not exactly analogous to a muscle stretch reflex for a number of reasons. One reason is that the H reflex is normally consistently elicitable only in the tibial nerve and S1 root distribution, while muscle stretch reflexes are present everywhere. Another reason is that it is possible for the muscle stretch reflexes and the H reflex to dissociate in some situations. Although a person with brisk muscle stretch reflexes will generally have an easily elicitable H reflex of high amplitude, it is possible for patients to have reduced muscle stretch reflexes but a normal amplitude H reflex in acute spinal shock and after treatment with diazepam. This can occur after recovery from a xylocaine nerve block when the gamma efferent fibers are still blocked but the I-a and alpha motor neuron fibers are functional.

The H reflex is best elicited by submaximal stimuli. It is theorized that a supramaximal stimulus given to a mixed nerve, such as the tibial nerve, suppresses the H reflex by causing motor fiber antidromic impulses, which depolarize the anterior horn cells. The impulses in the I-a fibers reaching the anterior horn cells are then unable to discharge the anterior horn cells because they are in a refractory state. Consequently the H reflex should be elicited with a stimulus that is just strong enough to stimulate the I-a fibers without providing a strong antidromic motor stimulus.

The H reflex is also suppressed by high frequency stimuli; consequently, the stimulus frequency should not be more than 1/sec. This suppression phenomenon can be used in paired stimuli studies in which the patient is given two stimuli separated by variable lengths of time (milliseconds). The amplitude of the initial H reflex is compared with that of the second. This data can be plotted on what is called an H reflex recovery curve (Fig. 2.12). Although the physiology of the H reflex recovery curve is beyond the scope of this discussion, it should be pointed out that the recovery curve is abnormal in patients with any type of upper motor neuron dysfunction. The curve has even been used to predict the effect of L-dopa and thalamotomy in parkinsonism (54).

The H reflex latency can be easily measured in a standardized manner using the method of Braddom and Johnson (45). The distance between the tibial nerve at the popliteal crease and the tibial nerve at the uppermost portion of the medial malleolus is marked and then bisected (Fig. 2.13). This

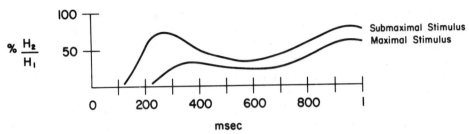

Fig. 2.12. H reflex pair stimuli recovery curve. The tibial nerve is given a pair of stimuli separated by various intervals in milliseconds. The amplitude of the second H reflex response is compared to the first one as a percentage.

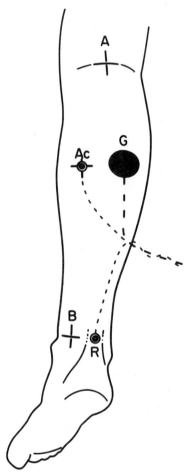

Fig. 2.13. H reflex study electrode placement. *Ac*, active recording electrode; *R*, reference electrode; *G*, ground; *B*, mark placed across the tibial nerve at the superior border of the medial malleolus; *A*, site of stimulation of tibial nerve at the popliteal crease.

gives a standard point for placement of the active recording electrode over the medial gastrocnemius. Submaximally stimulating the tibial nerve at the popliteal crease gives an evoked response which, in 100 normal subjects of all ages, had a mean latency of 29.8 msec (S.D., 2.74 msec). The H reflex latency was found to be highly correlated with leg length (r = 0.561) and age (r = 0.441). An analysis of the simultaneous regression of the H latency on age and leg length produced the formula: H latency (milliseconds) = 9.14 + 0.46 leg length (centimeters) + 0.1 age (years). This formula allows the clinician to predict expected H reflex latency.

Perhaps one of the most useful clinical applications of the H reflex is in unilateral S1 radiculopathy. In 25 normal subjects of all ages, Braddom and Johnson (45) noted that the H reflex latency could be measured in both legs of the subject with a mean difference of only 0.3 msec. The Pearson r correlation coefficient between the bilaterally elicited H reflex latencies was 0.993. The standard error of estimating the H latency of one leg from that of the other was only 0.40 msec.

Three standard errors (1.20 msec) encompass 99% of the statistical error inherent in estimating the H latency of one leg from the other in the same patient (this assumes careful clinical technique). A difference of more than 1.2 msec in a patient would indicate an abnormal situation. This could be due to a unilateral injury of the tibial nerve, sciatic nerve, or S1 nerve roots. Of course other factors, such as a marked difference in leg length, should be considered. Braddom and Johnson (45) subsequently found in 25 patients with unilateral S1 radiculopathy that all showed either a prolongation or absence of the H reflex latency on the affected side. Further clinical work in this regard has verified these findings. Recently, Schuchmann (43) repeated this H reflex technique in both legs of patients with unilateral L5 radiculopathy and found that there was no significant difference in the latencies. This shows that a prolongation or absence of the H reflex unilaterally in a patient with the clinical stigmata of lumbosacral radiculopathy is very suggestive of radiculopathy at the S1 level (Fig. 2.14).

The H reflex can be elicited in almost any muscle of a patient with a central nervous system lesion at or below the midbrain stem. A lesion at or below this level seemingly releases the inhibition of the H reflex that is normally present in adults. In a complete spinal cord quadriplegic, stimulation of almost any mixed nerve below the lesion gives an easily elicitable H reflex.

The H reflex can be used to study nerve conduction velocity over a long segment of nerve. The H reflex latency is a relatively poor indicator of peripheral neuropathy since most of the H reflex pathway is proximal. It becomes prolonged in peripheral neuropathy but usually only after the distal sensory and motor studies demonstrate significant abnormalities. The H reflex can be used to study proximal conduction and is helpful in conditions which are believed to begin as proximal nerve dysfunctions such as the Guillain-Barré syndrome.

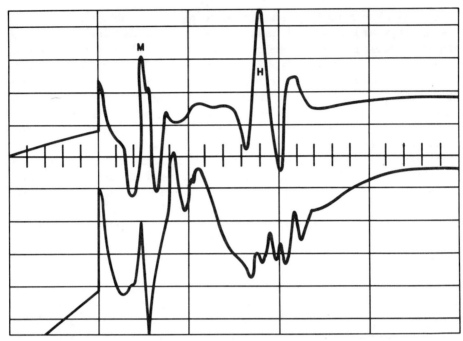

Fig. 2.14. H reflex elicited in both lower extremities in a patient with unilateral S1 radiculopathy. The top trace shows the H reflex on the unaffected side with a latency of 29.8 msec and an amplitude of 1000 μV. The lower trace shows the H reflex on the affected side with a latency of 32.1 msec and an amplitude of 200 μV. (200 μV per vertical division and 20 msec per major horizontal division.)

The F Wave

Magladery and associates first noted and named the F wave in the early 1950s (48–52). The F wave is called a wave rather than a reflex because most investigators feel it does not involve a synapse. It has been assumed that the F wave results when an antidromic motor fiber impulse physiologically rebounds off the anterior horn cells and orthodromically returns to cause muscle contraction. Only motor fibers are required to elicit an F wave, as interruption of the posterior roots does not abolish it. Many investigators have noted that the F wave has a variable latency as well as amplitude and shape. Whether this represents an unresolved problem in technique or whether it indicates that the F wave is actually a multisynaptic reflex is currently a matter of debate.

The F wave is most easily elicited by placing the recording electrode over an intrinsic muscle of the hand or foot and supramaximally stimulating the appropriate motor nerve. The frequency of stimulation does not alter the F wave as it does the H reflex, but a stimulation frequency of 1/sec is recommended. The F wave has a latency that is approximately the same as the H reflex over the same nerve segment.

In muscles where it is possible to obtain an H reflex, care must be taken to separate the H reflex and the F wave. It should be remembered that the H reflex is suppressed by supramaximal stimulation, while the F wave is seen only with supramaximal stimulation (Fig. 2.15). Consequently a late wave should not be considered to be an F wave until the stimulus intensity has been raised sufficiently to eliminate the possibility of an H reflex. The shape of the F wave and the H reflex may be similar, as both are being produced by the firing of a portion of the same group of alpha motor neurons. The H reflex is usually high in amplitude (often as high as 10 mV over the gastrocnemius), whereas the F wave is usually less than 200 μV.

The F wave is useful at times in determining whether brachial plexus

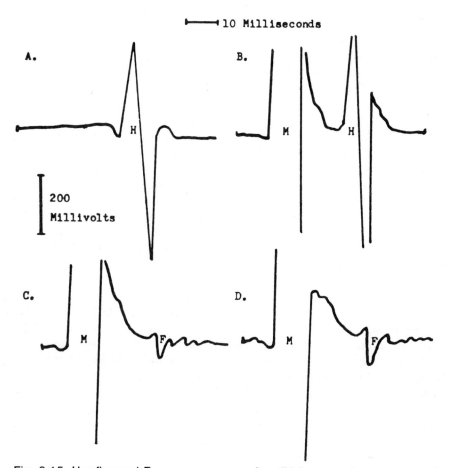

Fig. 2.15. H reflex and F wave responses after tibial nerve stimulation with the active recording electrode over the abductor hallucis muscle. (A) H reflex at low intensity stimulus strength; (B) M response and H reflex at stronger stimulus strength; (C) F wave appears after even stronger stimulus; (D) F wave is slightly larger after supramaximal stimulus. (Reprinted by permission from: R. L. Braddom and E. W. Johnson: Arch. Phys. Med. Rehabil., 55: 161, 1974.)

injuries involve motor root avulsions, particularly at the C8 and T1 levels (which innervate hand intrinsic muscles). The F wave appears to also be of value in detecting thoracic outlet syndrome (lower trunk of brachial plexus) and may be useful in lumbosacral root compromise.

Femoral Nerve

The femoral nerve is the largest branch of the lumbar plexus and arises from the dorsal division of the ventral primary rami of the second, third, and fourth lumbar nerves. It penetrates the psoas major muscle and emerges at its distal lateral border and passes inferiorly between it and the iliacus. After passing behind the inguinal ligament to enter the thigh, it splits into several divisions: 1) medial cutaneous nerve, 2) intermediate cutaneous nerve, 3) saphenous nerve, and 4) muscular branches. The major muscular branches innervate the quadriceps femoris muscle. Johnson et al. (55) noted from anatomic dissections that the vastus medialis was the most accessible superficial muscle innervated by the femoral nerve. The motor branch to the vastus medialis travels in a nearly direct course, such that surface measurements correlate well with actual nerve length. They recommended that the active recording electrode be placed over the center of the vastus medialis muscle. The reference electrode should be placed over the quadriceps tendon just proximal to the patella, and the ground electrode should be placed between the stimulating and recording electrodes (Fig. 2.16). The sites of stimulation used by them were superior to the inguinal ligament, inferior to the inguinal ligament, and in Hunter's canal along the medial aspect of the thigh. Stimulation of the femoral nerve in Hunter's canal was quite difficult, with the results being unsatisfactory. Results obtained from stimulation of the nerve above and below the inguinal ligament were reproducible and were found to be useful techniques in assessing the presence of femoral neuropathy. The values obtained by Johnson et al. are listed in Table 2.5.

The mean delay noted across the inguinal ligament was 1.1 msec. The mean overall length of the nerve segment studied was 35.4 ± 1.9 cm, with the mean distance across the inguinal ligament being 5.5 ± 1.6 cm.

The technique described above is difficult in obese patients and can be made more reliable by using needle stimulating and recording electrodes. In 1963, Gassel (56) reported a study in which he stimulated the femoral nerve with a needle electrode just distal to the inguinal ligament. A needle recording electrode was located in the anterior thigh. A mean motor latency over a 14-cm distance was reported to be 3.7 ± 0.1 msec. The mean latency value over 30 cm was 6.0 ± 0.15 msec, and the mean conduction velocity between these two points was 70 ± 7.8 m/sec.

Facial Nerve

The facial nerve emerges from the medulla oblongata close to the inferior cerebellar peduncle. It courses anteriorly and enters the internal auditory meatus. It runs anterolaterally until it reaches the geniculate ganglion, at

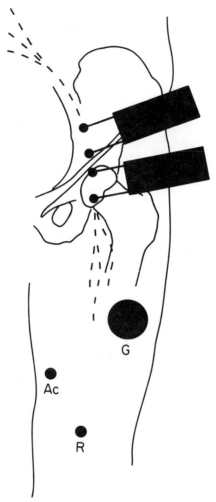

Fig. 2.16. Femoral nerve motor conduction studies. *Ac*, active recording electrode; *R*, reference electrode; *G*, ground electrode. Note stimulators placed above and below the inguinal ligament.

which time it curves posteriorly and inferiorly into the facial canal. The nerve emerges from the stylomastoid foramen and, after giving off a branch to the posterior belly of the digastric and the stylohyoid muscle, enters the center of the parotid gland. It then divides into five terminal branches (temporal, zygomatic, buccal, mandibular, and cervical) which are distributed to the muscles of facial expression.

The extracranial portion of the facial nerve is quite accessible for routine performance of nerve conduction studies. The facial nerve is best stimulated just below the ear and anterior to the mastoid process. The nerve can be stimulated either percutaneously or with a needle electrode. The active recording electrode can be either a surface electrode placed over one of the facial muscles or a coaxial needle electrode inserted into a facial muscle. Muscles commonly used as recording sites include the frontalis, orbicularis oculi, nasalis, and orbicularis oris (Fig. 2.17). When surface recording elec-

TABLE 2.5. *Femoral Nerve Motor Conduction (Normal Values)*

	Unit	Mean Value	Standard Deviation	Reference
Latency	msec			(55)
1. Above inguinal ligament		7.1	0.7	
2. Below inguinal ligament		6.0	0.7	
Conduction velocity	m/sec	69.4	9.2	(55)

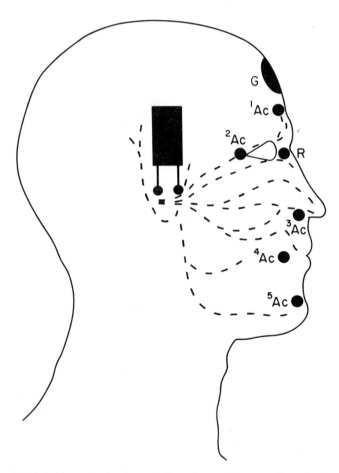

Fig. 2.17. Facial nerve conduction studies. *Ac*, active recording electrode site; *R*, reference electrode; *G*, ground electrode; *1*, frontalis muscle; *2*, orbicularis oculi muscle; *3*, nasalis muscle; *4*, orbicularis oris muscle; *5*, mentalis muscle.

trodes are used, the reference electrode is generally placed over the base of the nose with the ground electrode on the forehead (57, 58). Taverner (59) studied the facial nerve in 110 normal subjects and reported a mean latency value of 2.7 msec with a standard deviation of 0.36 msec. There was no significant difference between the right and left latency values. He concluded that a distal latency value greater than 4 msec was abnormal. Halar et al. (60) reported a facial nerve mean latency value in normals of 3.33 msec with a standard deviation of 0.38 msec. They also noted no significant right-left latency difference.

Nerve conduction velocity values for the facial nerve are generally not calculated because of the branching nature of the facial nerve and its relatively short length. Distal latency values more accurately reflect facial nerve function than nerve conduction values.

The Blink Reflex
(Orbicularis Oculi Reflex)

The blink reflex was first described in 1896 by Overend. It is a multifaceted reflex that involves neural components of the fifth and seventh cranial nerves, as well as other neurological centers. In 1952, Kugelberg (61) studied the response of the orbicularis oculi muscle to a tap over the brow. He noted two different responses: an early ipsilateral response with a latency of 12 msec and a late bilateral response with a latency ranging between 21 and 40 msec. The early response is thought to be transmitted through a simple reflex arc with the afferent limb involving the main sensory nucleus of the trigeminal nerve and the efferent component involving the facial nerve. The late bilateral reflex is thought to be transmitted through a multisynaptic arc with the exact neural route of transmission unclear at this time, but it is probably transmitted through the spinal tract of the trigeminal nerve with secondary trigeminal pathways ascending to connect with both the ipsilateral and contralateral facial nuclei in the pons.

To perform the blink reflex study, active recording electrodes are placed over both the right and left orbicularis oculi muscles. The reference electrodes are placed on each side of the nose and the ground electrodes on the inferior aspect of the chin (Fig. 2.18). The technique as described by Kimura et al. (62) involves the use of a two-channel amplifier for simultaneous recording of bilateral responses. They stimulated the supraorbital nerve percutaneously with the cathode over the supraorbital foramen. An initial stimulus intensity of approximately 50 V with a duration of 0.1 msec should be used and then increased slowly to the intensity giving the maximal evoked response. For the early reflex response, the mean latency between stimulation and recording of the response from the ipsilateral orbicularis oculi muscle was found to be 10.6 msec with a standard deviation of 0.82 msec. The mean right-left difference was 0.31 msec for the early reflex response, and any difference in right-left latency greater than 1.2 msec was considered to be abnormal. The late reflex response can be recorded bilat-

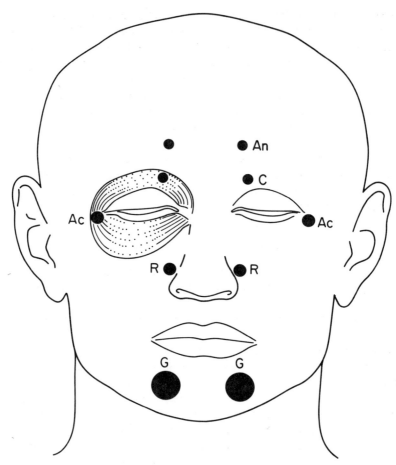

Fig. 2.18. The blink reflex study electrode sites. *Ac*, active recording electrode; *R*, reference electrode; *G*, ground electrode; *An*, anode of stimulator; *C*, cathode of stimulator.

erally following unilateral nerve stimulation. The ipsilateral mean latency was 31.3 msec with a standard deviation of 3.3 msec, and the contralateral mean latency was 31.6 msec with a standard deviation of 3.78 msec (determined by averaging results from 10 individual records). Normally the ipsilateral-contralateral difference in the late reflex response was less than 5 msec. These results are similar to those of Bender et al. (63). Bender noted that the best results were obtained when he used a stimulus duration of 0.7 msec and an intensity of approximately 40–80 V. The blink reflex has not been widely used clinically. It is of potential value in documenting trigeminal and facial nerve involvement in patients with acoustic neuromas (64). It also is useful in assessing proximal function of the trigeminal and facial nerves in pathological states, including Bell's palsy.

The Interpretation and Use of Motor Conduction Studies

It is important to remember that nerve conduction velocity studies, like all electrodiagnostic studies, are merely an extension of the physical examination. They are not substitutes for clinical skill or knowledge. There is little value in doing nerve conduction studies unless they are preceded by a history and physical that guide their selection. There are many nerves in the body and the clinician cannot reasonably study all of them in any one patient. The successful use of nerve conduction studies requires the combination of many factors, including a skilled clinician, accurately calibrated equipment, carefully standardized techniques, and a constant remembrance of the common sources of error.

A knowledge of basic neurophysiology and neuropathology is imperative in understanding the results of nerve conduction studies. A demyelinating neuropathy, such as diabetic peripheral neuropathy, gives early slowing of fiber conduction, but an axonal neuropathy, such as alcoholic peripheral neuropathy, gives an early reduction of the amplitude of the evoked response. A neuropathy of acute onset, such as that of the Guillain-Barré syndrome, may not show slowing the peripheral nerve conduction for 2 or 3 weeks, even when the patient is obviously weak. The first nerve conduction parameter to be abnormal in Guillain-Barré syndrome may be a temporal dispersion of the evoked response, rather than slowing of the conduction velocity. Common anatomic variations such as the Martin-Gruber anastomosis between the median and ulnar nerves and the accessory deep peroneal nerve must be recognized by the clinician to avoid diagnostic confusion. It must be kept in mind that neurapraxic lesions may not show abnormalities unless conduction is studied through the segment of neurapraxia. A nerve undergoing complete Wallerian degeneration can be stimulated for up to 72 hr, an important fact to be kept in mind when interpreting nerve conduction results early in the course of a nerve injury. The clinician must also understand the statistical nature of nerve conduction studies and the limitations of statistical techniques. The effect on nerve conduction of age and temperature must be constantly remembered in interpreting nerve conduction studies.

Nerve conduction studies are an important part of the electrodiagnostic examination. When appropriately used they can greatly increase the clinical diagnostic armamentarium of the electromyographer.

REFERENCES

1. ERLANGER, J., GASSER, H. S., AND BISHOP, G. H.: The compound nature of the action current of nerve as disclosed by the cathode ray oscillograph. *Amer. J. Physiol.*, *70:* 624, 1924.
2. HURSH, J. B.: Conduction velocity and diameter of nerve fibers. *Amer. J. Physiol.*, *127:* 131, 1939.
3. GASSER H. S., AND GRUNDFEST, H.: Axon diameters in relation to the spike dimensions and the conduction velocity in mammalian A fibers. *Amer. J. Physiol.*, *127:* 393, 1939.
4. HODES, R., LARRABEE, M. G., AND GERMAN, W.: The human electromyogram in response

to nerve stimulation and the conduction velocity of motor axons. *Arch. Neurol. Psychiat.,* *60:* 340, 1948.

5. DAWSON, G. D., AND SCOTT, J. W.: The recording of nerve action potentials through skin in man. *J. Neurol. Neurosurg. Psychiat., 12:* 259, 1949.

6. SIMPSON, J. A.: Electrical signs in the diagnosis of carpal tunnel and related syndromes. *J. Neurol. Neurosurg. Psychiat., 19:* 275, 1956.

7. LAMBERT, E. H.: Electromyography and electric stimulation of peripheral nerves and muscle. In *Clinical Examination in Neurology.* Philadelphia: W. B. Saunders Co., 1956.

8. DOWNEY, J. A., AND DARLING, R. C.: *Physiological Basis of Rehabilitation Medicine.* Philadelphia: W. B. Saunders Co., 1971.

9. RUCH, T. C., PATTON, H. D., WOODBURY, J. W., AND TOWE, A. L.: *Neurophysiology.* Philadelphia: W. B. Saunders Co., 1965.

10. LLOYD, D. P. C.: Neuron patterns controlling transmission of ipsilateral hind limb reflexes in cat. *J. Neurophysiol., 6:* 292, 1943.

11. BUCHTAL, F., AND ROSENFALCK, A.: Evoked action potentials and conduction velocity in human sensory nerves. *Brain Res. 3:* 1, 1966.

12. HORNING, M. R., KRAFT, G. H., AND GUY, A.: Latencies recorded by intramuscular needle electrodes in different portions of a muscle: Variation and comparison with surface electrodes. *Arch. Phys. Med. Rehabil., 53:* 206, 1972.

13. IYER, V., AND FENICHEL, G. M.: Normal median nerve proximal latency in carpal tunnel syndrome: A clue to coexisting Martin-Gruber anastomosis. *J. Neurol. Neurosurg. Psychiat., 39:* 449, 1976.

14. KIMURA, J., MURPHY, J. M., AND VARDA, D. J.: Electrophysiological study of anomalous innervation of intrinsic hand muscles. *Arch. Neurol., 33:* 842, 1976.

15. LAMBERT, E. H.: The accessory deep peroneal nerve. *Neurology, 19:* 1169, 1969.

16. GASSEL, M. M.: Sources of error in motor nerve conduction studies. *Neurology, 14:* 825, 1964.

17. HENRIKSEN, J. D.: Conduction velocity of motor nerves in normal subjects and patients with neuromuscular disorders. M. S. Thesis, University of Minnesota, Minneapolis, 1956.

18. CHATFIELD, P. O.: Effects of cooling on nerve conduction in a hibernator (golden hamster) and non-hibernator (albino rat). *Amer. J. Physiol., 155:* 179, 1948.

19. NORRIS, A. H., SHOCK, N. W., AND WAGMAN, I. H.: Age changes in the maximum conduction velocity of motor fibers of human ulnar nerves. *J. Appl. Physiol., 5:* 589, 1953.

20. LAFRATTA, C. W., AND CANESTRARI, R. E.: A comparison of sensory and motor nerve conduction velocities as related to age. *Arch. Phys. Med. Rehabil., 47:* 286, 1966.

21. LAFRATTA, C. W.: Relation of age to amplitude of evoked antidromic sensory nerve potentials. *Arch. Phys. Med. Rehabil., 53:* 388, 1972.

22. GUTMANN, L.: The intramuscular nerve action potential. *J. Neurol. Neurosurg. Psychiat., 32:* 193, 1969.

23. MAYNARD, F. M., AND STOLOV, W. C.: Experimental error in determination of nerve conduction velocity. *Arch. Phys. Med Rehabil., 53:* 362, 1972.

24. CHECKLES, N. S., RUSSAKOV, A. D., AND PIERO, D. L.: Ulnar nerve conduction velocity—Effect of elbow position on measurement. *Arch. Phys. Med. Rehabil., 52:* 362, 1971.

25. HONET, J. C., JEBSEN, R. H., AND PERRIN, E. B.: Variability of nerve conduction velocity determinations in normal persons. *Arch. Phys. Med Rehabil., 49:* 650, 1968.

26. JEBSEN, R. H.: Motor conduction velocities in the median and ulnar nerves. *Arch. Phys. Med. Rehabil., 48:* 185, 1967.

27. MELVIN, J. L., SCHUCHMANN, J. A., AND LANESE, R. R.: Diagnostic specificity of motor and sensory nerve conduction variables in the carpal tunnel syndrome. *Arch. Phys. Med Rehabil., 54:* 69, 1973.

28. JOHNSON, E. W., AND MELVIN, J. L.: Sensory conduction studies of median and ulnar nerves. *Arch. Phys. Med. Rehabil., 48:* 25, 1967.

29. NICHOLS, H. M.: Anatomic structures of the thoracic outlet. *Clin. Orthop. Related Res., 51:* 17, 1967.

30. LORD, J. W., AND ROSATI, L. M.: Thoracic-outlet syndromes. *Clin. Symposia, 23:* 2, 1971.
31. URSCHEL, H. C., AND RAZZUK, M. A.: Management of the thoracic-outlet syndrome. *N. Engl. J. Med., 286:* 1140, 1972.
32. CALDWELL, J. W., CRANE, C. R., AND KRUSEN, E. M.: Nerve conduction studies: An aid in the diagnosis of the thoracic outlet syndrome. *S. Med. J. 64:* 210, 1971.
33. GASSEL, M. M., AND DIAMANTOPOULOS, E.: Pattern of conduction times in the distribution of the radial nerve—A clinical and electrophysiological study. *Neurology, 14:* 222, 1964.
34. TROJABORG, W., SINDRUP, E. H.: Motor and sensory conduction in different segments of the radial nerve in normal subjects. *J. Neurol. Neurosurg. Psychiat., 32:* 354, 1969.
35. JEBSEN, R. H.: Motor conduction velocity in proximal and distal segments of the radial nerve. *Arch. Phys. Med. Rehabil., 47:* 597, 1966.
36. BRADDOM, R., AND WOLFE, C.: Musculocutaneous nerve injury after heavy exercise. *Arch. Phys. Med. Rehabil., 59:* 290, 1978.
37. REDFORD, J. W. B.: Conduction time in motor fibres of nerves which innervate proximal muscles of extremities in normal persons and in patients with neuromuscular diseases. Thesis, University of Minnesota, Minneapolis, 1958.
38. GASSEL, M. M.: A test of nerve conduction to muscles of the shoulder girdle as an aid in the diagnosis of proximal neurogenic and muscular disease. *J. Neurol. Neurosurg. Psychiat., 27:* 200, 1964.
39. VACEK, J., AND DRUGOVA, B.: Proximalni amyotrofie-elektromyograficka stimulace erbove badu. *Cesk. Neurol. 30:* 183, 1967.
40. KRAFT, G. H.: Axillary, musculocutaneous and suprascapular nerve latency studies. *Arch. Phys. Med. Rehabil., 53:* 383, 1953.
41. TROJABORG, W.: Motor and sensory conduction in the musculocutaneous nerve. *J. Neurol. Neurosurg. Psychiat., 39:* 890, 1976.
42. CHECKLES, N. S., BAILEY, J. A., AND JOHNSON, E. W.: Tape and caliper surface measurement in determination of peroneal nerve conduction velocity. *Arch. Phys. Med. Rehabil., 50:* 214, 1969.
43. SCHUCHMANN, J. A.: H reflex latency in radiculopathy. *Arch. Phys. Med. Rehabil., 59:* 185, 1978.
44. JOHNSON, E. W., AND ORTIZ, P. R.: Electrodiagnosis of tarsal tunnel syndrome. *Arch. Phys. Med. Rehabil., 47:* 776, 1966.
45. BRADDOM, R. L., AND JOHNSON, E. W.: Standardization of H reflex and diagnostic use in S1 radiculopathy. *Arch. Phys. Med. Rehabil., 55:* 161, 1974.
46. YAP, C. B., AND HIROTA, T.: Sciatic nerve motor conduction velocity study. *J. Neurol. Neurosurg. Psychiat., 30:* 233, 1967.
47. HOFFMANN, P.: Uber die Beziehungen der Sehnenreflexe zur willkurlichen bewegung and zum tonus. *Z. Biol., 68:* 351, 1918.
48. MAGLADERY, J. W., AND McDOUGAL, D. B., JR.: Electrophysiological studies of nerve and reflex activity in normal man: I. Identification of certain reflexes in electromyogram and conduction velocity of peripheral nerve fibres. *Bull. Johns Hopkins Hosp., 86:* 265, 1950.
49. MAGLADERY, J. W., PORTER, W. E., PARK, A. M., et al.: Electrophysiological studies of nerve and reflex activity in normal man: IV. Two neurone reflex and identification of certain action potentials from spinal roots and cord. *Bull. Johns Hopkins Hosp., 88:* 499, 1951.
50. MAGLADERY, R. D., TEASDALL, A. M., PARK, A. M., et al.: Electrophysiological studies of reflex activity in patients with lesions of the nervous system: I. Comparison of spinal motoneurone excitability following afferent nerve volleys in normal persons and patients with upper motor neurone lesions. *Bull. Johns Hopkins Hosp., 91:* 219, 1952.
51. LANGUTH, H. W., TEASDALL, R. D., AND MAGLADERY, J. W.: Electrophysiological studies of reflex activity in patients with lesions of the nervous system: III. Motoneurone excitability following afferent nerve volleys in patients with rostrally adjacent spinal cord damage. *Bull. Johns Hopkins Hosp., 91:* 257, 1952.
52. TEASDALL, R. D., LANGUTH, H. W., AND MAGLADERY, J. W.: Electrophysiological studies

of reflex activity in patients with lesions of nervous system: IV. A note on the tendon jerk. *Bull. Johns Hopkins Hosp., 91:* 267, 1952.

53. BRADDOM, R. L., AND JOHNSON, E. W.: H reflex: Review and classification with suggested clinical uses. *Arch. Phys. Med. Rehabil., 55:* 412, 1974.

54. FUJITA, S., AND COOPER, I. S.: Effects of l-dopa on the H-reflex in parkinsonism. *J. Amer. Geriat. Soc., 19:* 289, 1971.

55. JOHNSON, E. W., WOOD, P. K., AND POWERS, J. J.: Femoral nerve conduction studies. *Arch. Phys. Med. Rehabil., 49:* 528, 1968.

56. GASSEL, M. M.: A study of femoral nerve conduction time. *Arch. Neurol., 9:* 607, 1963.

57. JOHNSON, E. W., AND WAYLONIS, G. W.: Facial nerve conduction delay in patients with diabetes mellitus. *Arch. Phys. Med. Rehabil., 45:* 131, 1964.

58. WAYLONIS, G. W., AND JOHNSON, E. W.: Facial nerve conduction delay. *Arch. Phys. Med. Rehabil., 45:* 539, 1964.

59. TAVERNER, D.: Electrodiagnosis in facial palsy. *Arch. Otolaryngol., 81:* 470, 1965.

60. HALAR, E., TAYLOR, N., AND KAO, T.: Facial nerve conduction latency in hemiplegic and hypertensive patients. *Arch. Phys. Med. Rehabil., 53:* 509, 1972.

61. KUGELBERG, E.: Facial reflexes. *Brain, 75:* 385, 1952.

62. KIMURA, J., POWERS, J. M., AND VAN ALLEN, M. W.: Reflex response of obicularis occuli muscle to supraorbital nerve stimulation. *Arch. Neurol., 21:* 193, 1969.

63. BENDER, L. F., MAYNARD, F. M., AND HASTINGS, S. V.: The blink reflex as a diagnostic procedure. *Arch. Phys. Med. Rehabil., 50:* 27, 1969.

64. LYON, L. W., AND VAN ALLEN, M. W.: Alterations of the orbicularis occuli reflex by acoustic neuroma. *Arch. Otolaryngol., 95:* 100, 1972.

ADDITIONAL REFERENCES

BAER, R. D., AND JOHNSON, E. W.: Motor nerve conduction velocities in normal children. *Arch. Phys. Med. Rehabil., 46:* 698, 1965.

DIBENEDETTO, M.: Sensory nerve conduction in lower extremities. *Arch. Phys. Med. Rehabil., 51:* 253, 1970.

GRANT, J. C. B., AND BASMAJIAN, J. V.: *Grant's Method of Anatomy.* Baltimore: The Williams & Wilkins Co., 1965.

JOHNSON, E. W., AND MELVIN J. L.: Nerve conduction studies (unpublished report).

KAPLAN, P. E.: Sensory and motor residual latency measurements in healthy patients and patients with neuropathy—Part 1. *J. Neurol. Neurosurg. Psychiat., 39:* 338, 1976.

MAYER, R. F., AND FELDMAN, R. G.: Observations on the nature of the F wave in man. *Neurology, 17:* 147, 1967.

SCHUCHMANN, J. A.: Sural nerve conduction: A standardized technique. *Arch. Phys. Med. Rehabil., 58:* 166, 1977.

SHIOZAWA, R., AND MAUER, H.: In vivo human sural nerve action potentials. *J. Appl. Physiol., 26:* 623, 1969.

SMORTO, M. P., AND BASMAJIAN, J. V.: *Clinical Electroneurography.* Baltimore: The Williams & Wilkins Co., 1972.

TEASDALL, R. D., PARK, A. M., LANGUTH, H. W., et al.: Electrophysiological studies of reflex activity in patients with lesions of nervous system: II. Disclosure of normally suppressed monosynaptic reflex discharge of spinal motoneurones by lesions of lower brain-stem and spinal cord. *Bull. Johns Hopkins Hosp., 91:* 245, 1952.

3

Sensory Conduction

JOHN SCHUCHMANN, M.D.
RANDALL L. BRADDOM, M.D.

The reader is referred to Chapter 2 for an overview of the history, neurophysiology, basic technical considerations, and common sources of error in nerve conduction studies.

Many disorders of the peripheral nerve begin, or are most noticeable, as sensory abnormalities. Methods of performing reliable and reproducible sensory nerve conduction studies have been a high priority in the development of electrophysiologic studies of neural conduction. In 1949, Dawson and Scott (1) made a significant breakthrough when they recorded sensory nerve action potentials in humans. A delay in the development of sensory nerve conduction techniques resulted from the fact that the amplitude of the evoked sensory nerve response is often 20 μV or less. These small amplitude evoked responses occasionally can be obscured by the intrinsic noise of the amplifer. With the use of carefully standardized techniques and the availability of signal averaging devices, more and more sensory nerves are now being adequately studied. Sensory nerve conduction studies, as currently performed, measure conduction along the myelinated group I-a nerve fibers. Impulses are propagated along these fibers by saltatory conduction. Sensory nerve conduction studies differ from motor nerve conduction studies in that no neuromuscular junction or muscle is involved. The nerve is stimulated at one point along its course, and the sensory nerve action potential is recorded at a different site along the same nerve. When a sensory nerve is stimulated, the impulse is propagated both proximally in an orthodromic direction and distally in an antidromic direction. The studies of Johnson and Melvin (2) demonstrated that there is no significant difference in the rate of orthodromic and antidromic conduction. Because of this, similar values are obtained when sensory nerve conduction studies are performed antidromically or othodromically.

The basic technique of sensory nerve conduction studies involves placing the active recording electrode over a sensory branch of the nerve to be studied. The reference electrode is placed at least 4 cm distal to the active recording electrode. The ground electrode is usually placed between the stimulating and recording electrodes. Since the sensory evoked response is often low in amplitude with a slow initial deflection from the baseline, the latency values are usually measured from the onset of the stimulus artifact to the peak of the negative deflection of the sensory action potential. Measuring to the peak of the negative deflection gives more reliable and reproducible results than those obtained by measuring to the initial negative deflection. It should be remembered that when the latency is measured to the peak of the sensory action potential, an average conduction of the group I-a fibers is obtained, rather than the conduction velocity of the fastest fibers.

Of the various conduction parameters obtained from sensory nerve studies, most authors feel that the latency and conduction values are the most clinically useful. Some authors stress that the amplitude of the evoked response is the most significant parameter. The amplitude of the response, however, appears to have more variability than the latency and conduction values. The amplitude varies greatly with the technique used, while the latency and conduction values demonstrate less variability.

As in motor nerve conduction studies, it is imperative that standardized techniques be used for sensory nerve conduction studies. The distance between the active recording electrode and the stimulating cathode should be standardized. Many of the errors common to sensory nerve conduction studies are identical to those obtained with motor nerve conduction studies. Please see the previous chapter on motor nerve conduction studies for a discussion of these potential errors. Although sensory nerves are numerous, they are often quite small and difficult to study with current electrophysiologic techniques. Reproducible techniques have been developed for the median, ulnar, and radial nerves in the upper extremity and the lateral femoral cutaneous and sural nerves in the lower extremity. With the advent of averaging techniques, other sensory nerves and their branches have been studied, but a description of all these techniques is beyond the scope of this text.

Median Nerve Sensory Conduction

Median nerve sensory conduction studies are widely performed in clinical practice because they are relatively easy to perform, are reproducible, and provide very useful information in such common problems as carpal tunnel syndrome and peripheral neuropathy.

The pertinent anatomy of the median nerve is reviewed in the chapter on motor nerve conduction studies (Chapter 2). Median nerve sensory conduction studies across the carpal canal can be performed adequately with either an orthodromic or antidromic technique. In orthodromic median nerve sensory conduction techniques, the active recording electrodes should be mounted 4 cm apart on a plastic block (D and F of Fig. 2.2). These electrodes are then placed over the median nerve at the wrist with the plastic bar oriented such that the active recording electrode is the most distal. The distance between the active recording electrode and stimulating cathode should be exactly 14 cm. The stimulating electrodes can be used to excite the digital sensory branches of the median nerve in the index and middle fingers simultaneously or in either of these fingers separately.

For the antidromic technique the active recording and reference electrodes (*G* and *H* of Fig. 2.2) are placed 4 cm apart over the digital nerve branches of the index and middle fingers with the stimulating cathode placed exactly 14 cm proximal to the active recording electrode (Fig. 3.1). The ground electrode is placed over the palmar aspect of the ulnar border in the hand in both the orthodromic and antidromic techniques. The median nerve can also be stimulated at the elbow at the same sites used for motor nerve conduction studies (See Chapter 2 on median motor conduction studies.)

Accurate comparison and interpretation of results requires that standard-

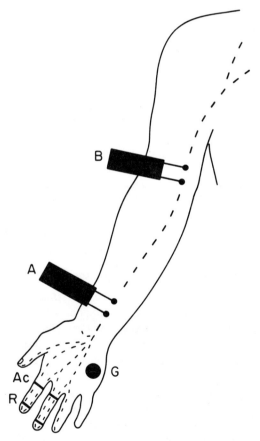

Fig. 3.1. Median nerve antidromic sensory conduction studies. *Ac*, active recording digital electrode, *R*, reference digital electrode; *G*, ground; *A-B*, sites of median nerve stimulation.

ized techniques such as those just described be routinely used for all median nerve sensory conduction studies. Normal values obtained from using the above technique are presented in Table 3.1.

Ulnar Nerve Sensory Conduction

The anatomy of the ulnar nerve is presented in Chapter 2 on motor nerve conduction studies. The ulnar nerve innervates most of the hand intrinsic muscles. If an antidromic technique is used to study ulnar sensory conduction, both the motor and sensory fibers of the ulnar nerve are stimulated and a high amplitude motor response may obscure the much smaller sensory response. Because of this, studies of ulnar nerve sensory conduction are best performed with an orthodromic technique. In the ulnar orthodromic sensory conduction technique, the stimulating cathode is located on the digital branches of the small and/or ring fingers (Fig. 3.2). (Two types of stimulating electrodes are illustrated in *G* and *H* of Fig. 2.2). The anode is placed 4 cm distal to the cathode. The active recording and reference electrodes are mounted 4 cm apart on a plastic block (*D* and *F* of Fig. 2.2). The active recording electrode is placed exactly 14 cm proximal to the cathode and over the ulnar nerve at the wrist. Mounting the active recording and reference electrodes in a plastic block helps one tape the electrodes down tightly over the ulnar nerve to obtain a more satisfactory recording of the evoked response. The recording electrodes can also be moved proximally around the elbow to obtain forearm ulnar nerve sensory conduction velocity values.

At times it is possible to obtain a satisfactory antidromic ulnar nerve sensory response. In the antidromic technique, the active recording and reference electrodes should be placed 4 cm apart and as far distally on the small and ring fingers as possible. The ulnar nerve is then stimulated at a point 14 cm proximal to the active recording electrode. The nerve can also be stimulated at the elbow to determine the forearm conduction velocity. Normal values for ulnar nerve sensory conduction are listed in Table 3.2.

Radial Nerve Sensory Conduction

The sensory fibers of the radial nerve are not studied as often in clinical practice as are those of the median and ulnar nerves because of the greater difficulty in technique. A major problem is that the radial nerve has four separate sensory branches. The posterior cutaneous nerve of the arm exits from the radial nerve in the upper arm, the lateral cutaneous nerve of the arm comes from the radial nerve in the midarm and the posterior cutaneous nerve of the forearm leaves the radial nerve slightly above the elbow. The final sensory branch begins just below the elbow when the radial nerve splits to form a motor branch called the posterior interosseus nerve and a sensory branch called the superficial radial nerve. Most of the techniques described in the literature for studying the sensory fibers of the radial nerve actually study only the superficial radial nerve.

The first clinically practical method for studying the sensory fibers of the radial nerve was introduced by Downie and Scott in 1964 (5) and then improved in 1967 (6). In their technique described in 1967, the active recording electrode was placed on the largest terminal branch of the superficial radial nerve as it crosses the tendon of the extensor pollicus longus. If this point is difficult to locate, they suggested simply placing the active

TABLE 3.1. *Median Nerve Sensory Conduction Studies (Normal Values)*

	Unit	Mean Value	Standard Deviation	Reference
Distal latency	msec	3.2	0.2	(3)
Conduction velocity, forearm	m/sec	56.9	4.0	(3)
Amplitude of evoked response (wrist stimulation)	μV	41.6	25.0	(3)
Duration of evoked response (wrist stimulation)	msec	1.8	0.4	(3)

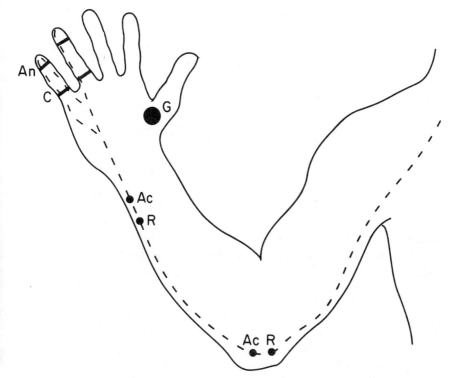

Fig. 3.2. Ulnar nerve sensory conduction studies. *An*, anodal digital stimulating electrode; *C*, cathodal digital stimulating electrode; *G*, ground electrode; *Ac*, active recording electrode; *R*, reference electrode.

TABLE 3.2. *Ulnar Nerve Sensory Conduction (Normal Values)*

	Unit	Mean Value	Standard Deviation	Range	Reference
Distal latency	msec	3.2	0.25		(4)
Conduction velocity, forearm	m/sec	57.0	5.0		(4)
Amplitude of evoked response	μV			15–50	(2)

recording electrode 1 cm distal to the extensor retinaculum. Their electrodes were silver discs 1 cm in diameter mounted 2.5 cm apart on a plastic bar (similar to *F* of Fig. 2.2).

A bipolar stimulator should be placed over the superficial radial nerve in the midforearm. Reversing this procedure gives an orthodromic technique. They reported radial sensory conduction values of 47–64 m/sec with a mean of 53.8 m/sec in 50 normal subjects of all ages. The latency was read to the peak of the evoked response, and the stimulation distance was read as that from the center of the stimulating rods to the center of the recording electrodes.

In 1969, Trojaborg and Sindrup (7) reported another technique of sensory studies of the radial nerve. They placed surface stimulating electrodes on the proximal phalanx of the thumb, with the cathode and anode separated by a 2 cm distance. A needle electrode (cathode) is placed near the superficial radial nerve at the wrist with an adjacent surface anode. They also placed needle electrodes adjacent to the radial nerve at the elbow and in the axilla. The latency was measured to the onset of the response rather than to its peak. In 23 normal subjects the conduction velocity of the radial sensory fibers from the thumb to the wrist was 58 m/sec (S.D., 6 m/sec). The sensory conduction velocity in the wrist to elbow segment was 66 m/sec (S.D., 3.5 m/sec). The elbow to axilla segment had a conduction velocity of 67 m/sec (S.D., 6.5 m/sec). The amplitudes of these sensory potentials are quite small (especially proximally), and averaging techniques are usually required, since some are 20 μV or less in amplitude. It should be noted that stimulation of the radial sensory fibers by surface electrodes over the proximal phalanx of the thumb also stimulates some sensory fibers of the median nerve. It would be possible in a complete radial nerve injury to stimulate at the thumb and record a sensory potential at the axilla from median sensory fibers rather than from the radial. For this reason Trojaborg and Sindrup preferred to stimulate the radial sensory fibers at the wrist when recording was to be done at the elbow and axilla.

In our clinical experience, determining the distal latency of the radial sensory fibers is a relatively easy technique which does not require averaging equipment. This technique is that of placing metal ring or pipe cleaner recording electrodes (*G* and *H* of Fig. 2.2) on the proximal phalanx of the thumb with a 4-cm separation. The superficial branch of the radial nerve is then percutaneously stimulated over the dorsal aspect of the wrist, with the cathode exactly 14 cm proximal to the active recording electrode. The latency is read to the peak of the response. Unpublished data of Johnson and Melvin indicates that the mean latency is 3.3 msec (S.D., 0.4 msec) (4).

Due to the difficulty of studying the sensory fibers of the radial nerve proximal to the wrist, we do not normally attempt it in our laboratory except with the use of averaging techniques. Needle electrodes are placed at the elbow and axilla as in the technique of Trojaborg and Sindrup (7). A surface stimulator is then placed over the superficial radial nerve on the dorsum of the wrist with the stimulator oriented such that the cathode is closest to the active recording electrode. At times the radial sensory nerve potentials can be found and measured by superimposing a number of cathode ray sweeps. Most of the time, however, electronic averaging of from 50–500 sweeps is necessary to delineate the sensory nerve action potentials. The normal values accepted in our laboratory are those reported above by Trojaborg and Sindrup. Generally we find that many clinical problems whose dianosis would be aided by proximal radial sensory studies are unilateral, making it feasible to compare the results obtained in the affected limb with those in the opposite limb.

Lateral Femoral Cutaneous Nerve Conduction

The lateral femoral cutaneous nerve has been of interest to electrodiagnosticians for many years because of the common clinical syndrome of meralgia paresthetica.

The lateral femoral cutaneous nerve of the thigh is a sensory nerve derived from the posterior roots of the spinal segments L2 and L3. It emerges from the lateral surface of the psoas muscle to cross the iliacus muscle beneath the iliac fascia. It then passes 1 cm medial to the anterior superior iliac spine, as it courses beneath the inguinal ligament. At this point, it is occasionally possible to elicit a Tinel's Sign in patients with meralgia paresthetica. Approximately 12 cm inferior to the anterior superior iliac spine, the nerve becomes superficial and divides into a large anterior branch and a somewhat smaller posterior or lateral branch.

Butler et al. (8) reported a clinically useful technique for studying the lateral femoral cutaneous nerve both orthodromically and antidromically (Fig. 3.3). The nerve is stimulated antidromically above the inguinal ligament with a monopolar Teflon-coated needle electrode (cathode). The nerve action potential is recorded 12 cm below the stimulating point over the anterior branch of the lateral femoral cutaneous nerve. The active recording electrodes consisted of two strips of lead fastened 4 cm apart on plastic bars (B of Fig. 2.2). Each lead strip was 1.2 cm wide and 1.9 cm long. They reversed the procedure by stimulating the anterior branch of the lateral femoral cutaneous nerve with the lead strip electrodes and using a Teflon-coated monopolar needle as the active recording electrode adjacent to the lateral femoral cutaneous nerve above the inguinal ligament. In 24 normal

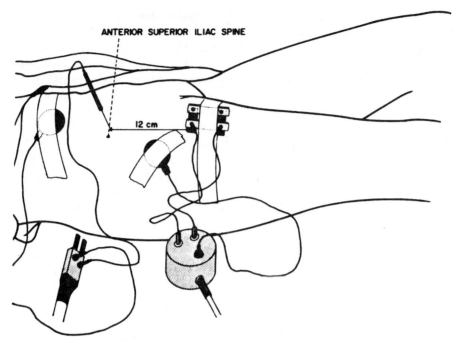

Fig. 3.3. Lateral femoral cutaneous nerve conduction studies. Note position of needle electrode and the lead strip electrodes. (Reprinted by permission from: E. T. Butler, E. W. Johnson, and Z. A. Kaye: *Arch. Phys. Med. Rehabil., 55:* 31, 1974.)

subjects of all ages, they found a mean latency over this 12-cm segment of 2.6 msec (S.D., 0.2 msec) (Fig. 3.4). The amplitude of the nerve action potential was from 10–25 μV. The mean conduction velocity was 47.9 m/sec (S.D., 3.7 m/sec). In a case report of a patient with unilateral meralgia paresthetica, Butler et al. noted an absence of the lateral femoral cutaneous nerve potential on the affected side with a normal potential on the opposite side.

The lateral femoral cutaneous nerve technique requires considerable practice on the part of the electrodiagnostician. The exact anatomy of the nerve is sufficiently variable that it is often necessary to try both the orthodromic and antidromic technique and even use averaging equipment to obtain the response. The response is usually absent in patients with meralgia paresthetica, so sufficient proficiency is needed to be certain that the absence is due to pathology rather than to deficient technique.

Sural Nerve Conduction

The sural nerve is formed by a union of the medial sural cutaneous nerve and the communicating branch of the common peroneal nerve. It arises at a variable level in the popliteal fossa and passes distally between the two heads of the gastrocnemius. It runs beneath the deep fascia until it reaches the proximal tendo achillis, where it perforates the fascia and passes behind the lateral malleolus. It supplies the skin along the distal dorsolateral aspect of the leg and the lateral aspect of the foot.

The active recording electrode and reference electrode are mounted 4 cm apart on a plastic block (*D* and *F* of Fig. 2.2) and are placed over the sural nerve as it passes around the lateral malleolus (Fig. 3.5). Antidromic evoked responses can be recorded with surface stimulation 10, 14, 17, and 20 cm proximal to the active recording electrode. The most reproducible results are obtained when stimulating over the 14- and 17-cm distances. At the 10-cm point, technical difficulty can be experienced, with the shock artifact obscuring the evoked response (9). In subjects of short stature and in some with long and broad distal gastrocnemius muscles, it may be difficult to obtain an evoked response at the 20-cm distance, probably due to the fact that the sural nerve lies deep beneath the two heads of the gastrocnemius muscle.

Nerve conduction velocity values can be calculated from the data obtained but offer no clinical advantage over the latency values. This is done by dividing the distance by the latency minus .1 msec (latency of activation). Normal values for sural nerve conduction studies are listed in Table 3.3.

Interpretation and Use of Sensory Conduction Studies

The reader is referred to the section on the Interpretation and Use of Motor Conduction Studies in Chapter 2, since most of those statements apply to sensory as well as motor conduction studies. Several factors

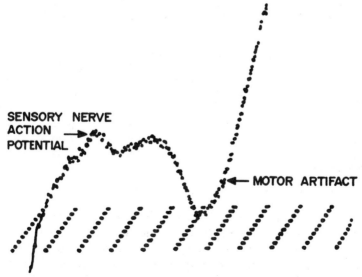

SENSORY NERVE ACTION POTENTIAL

MOTOR ARTIFACT

Fig. 3.4. Lateral femoral cutaneous nerve conduction study evoked response. Slanted dotted lines represent 1 msec. (Reprinted by permission from: E. T. Butler, E. W. Johnson, and Z. A. Kaye: *Arch. Phys. Med. Rehabil., 55:* 31, 1974.)

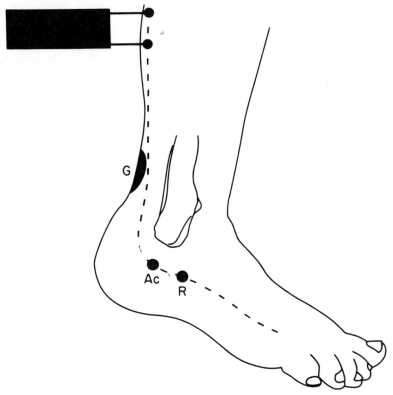

Fig. 3.5. Sural conduction study. *Ac*, active recording electrode; *R*, reference electrode; *G*, ground. Note position of recording electrodes under the lateral malleolus.

TABLE 3.3. *Sural Nerve Conduction (Normal Values)*

	Unit	Mean Value	Standard Deviation	Reference
Distal latency	msec			
1. Over 10 cm.		2.84	0.27	(10)
2. Over 14 cm.		3.50	0.25	
3. Over 17 cm.		4.02	0.30	
4. Over 20 cm.		4.58	0.36	
Amplitude of evoked response	μV	23.7	3.8	(11)

complicate the routine use and clinical interpretation of sensory nerve conduction studies. These include the facts that sensory nerves are more affected by the age of the patient than are motor nerves, sensory nerve conduction techniques are generally more difficult to perform than are motor nerve conduction techniques, sensory evoked responses are quite small in relation to motor evoked responses, and averaging techniques are more likely to be necessary in sensory studies than in motor studies (Fig.

3.6). The clinician must be proficient in performing sensory nerve conduction studies to ensure that an absent or abnormal response is due to pathology rather than to deficient technique. The clinician must also constantly consider the possibility of volume conduction of the stimulus from the nerve under study to an adjacent nerve or volume conduction of an evoked muscle response to the active recording electrode. This can occasionally happen in sensory nerve conduction studies if the clinician greatly increases the stimulus intensity in an attempt to obtain an elusive sensory nerve action potential.

After the techniques for sensory nerve conduction studies are practiced

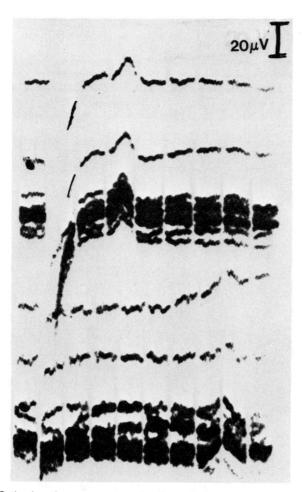

Fig. 3.6. Orthodromic sensory conduction of ulnar nerve. Top three sweeps recording at wrist; third is repeated sweeps (10) to average out the noise. Bottom three sweeps recording at elbow; sixth is average of 10 sweeps superimposed to identify the nerve action potential. Calibration: sweep is interrupted at 1 msec intervals; 20 μv calibrated in upper right. Shock applied after 1-msec delay.

sufficiently to be clinically reliable and reproducible, the clinician will find them to be of great help in electrodiagnostic practice.

REFERENCES

1. DAWSON, G. D., AND SCOTT, J. W.: The recording of nerve action potentials through skin in man. *J. Neurol. Neurosurg. Psychiat., 12:* 259, 1949.
2. JOHNSON, E. W., AND MELVIN, J. L.: Sensory conduction studies of median and ulnar nerves. *Arch. Phys. Med. Rehabil., 48:* 25, 1967.
3. MELVIN, J. L., SCHUCHMANN, J. A., AND LANESE, R. R.: Diagnostic specificity of motor and sensory nerve conduction variables in the carpal tunnel syndrome. *Arch. Phys. Med. Rehabil., 54:* 69, 1973.
4. JOHNSON, E. W., AND MELVIN, J. L.: Nerve conduction studies (unpublished data).
5. DOWNIE, A. W., AND SCOTT, T. R.: Radial nerve conduction studies. *Neurology, 14:* 839, 1964.
6. DOWNIE, A. W., AND SCOTT, T. R.: An improved technique for radial nerve conduction studies. *J. Neurol. Neurosurg. Psychiat., 30:* 332, 1967.
7. TROJABORG, W., AND SINDRUP, E. H.: Motor and sensory conduction in different segments of the radial nerve in normal subjects. *J. Neurol. Neurosurg. Psychiat., 32:* 354, 1969.
8. BUTLER, E. T., JOHNSON, E. W., AND KAY, Z. A.: Normal conduction velocity in the lateral femoral cutaneous nerve. *Arch. Phys. Med. Rehabil., 55:* 31, 1974.
9. SHIOZAWA, R., AND MAUER, H.: In vivo human sural nerve action potentials. *J. Appl. Physiol. 26:* 623, 1969.
10. SCHUCHMANN, J. A.: Sural nerve conduction: A standardized technique. *Arch. Phys. Med. Rehabil., 58:* 166, 1977.
11. DIBENEDETTO, M: Sensory nerve conduction in lower extremities. *Arch. Phys. Med. Rehabil., 51:* 253, 1970.

4

Neuromuscular Junction

IAN C. MACLEAN, M.D.

The neuromuscular synapse is the first example of chemical synaptic transmission to be confirmed. It is entirely due to a chemical mediator called acetylcholine (ACh) as originally proposed by Dale and his colleagues in the early 1930s. Dale and Loewi were conjointly awarded the Nobel prize in 1936 (Loewi for his studies of chemical transmission during vagal inhibition of the heart).

For many years, electrodiagnostic techniques have been used to detect myasthenia gravis. Then, in 1956, Lambert and colleagues (1) described a new disorder of neuromuscular transmission that is associated with carcinoma of the lung. The two syndromes have very different pathophysiological characteristics. It was thought that it would be a simple matter to distinguish them electrodiagnostically, but it was found that abnormalities suggesting myasthenia gravis can be seen in certain muscles and those suggesting myasthenic syndrome in other muscles of the same patient. Transitional stages between the two disorders have also been described. To add to the confusion, it is now known that a variety of diseases can result in defective neuromuscular transmission.

Since several types of defects of neuromuscular transmission are possible, our goal is to identify them by elucidating their specific electrophysiologic characteristics; however, present EMG differences are usually only quantitative. Single fiber EMG has added another dimension and microelectrode evaluation of miniature endplate potentials offers great promise, but it is not practical to use either of these techniques on a routine basis. It is evident that as we strive toward more precision in our analysis of neuromuscular transmission defects, more specific tests will need to be developed.

Morphology of the Neuromuscular Junction

The motor unit (Fig. 4.1) is composed of a motoneuron and all the muscle fibers that neuron innervates. The function of the neuromuscular junction is to transfer impulses from the very small motor nerve endings to the much larger muscle fibers, thus initiating muscle fiber contraction.

The structure of the junctional apparatus (Fig. 4.2) includes a nerve

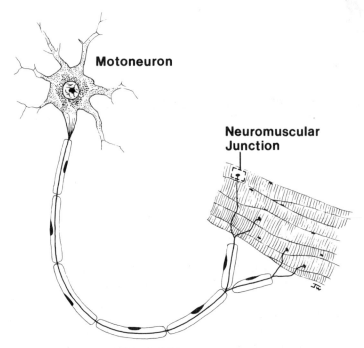

Fig. 4.1. The motor unit.

terminal, a motor endplate, and a synaptic cleft of about 400 Å that separates the two. The nerve terminal is an unmyelinated extension of the axon, and the axoplasm contains numerous spherical structures about 500 Å in diameter known as synaptic vesicles, which contain prepackaged ACh. Mitochondria are also abundant in the nerve terminal.

The motor endplate is a structural enlargement of the muscle fiber that forms a trough or groove into which fits the terminal nerve ending. The endplate consists of the postsynaptic membrane which has many infoldings and is continuous with the muscle fiber membrane. The sarcoplasm underlying it contains large numbers of mitochondria, as well as muscle nuclei. Because of extensive infoldings of the postsynaptic membrane, the motor endplate has a much larger surface area than the nerve terminal it envelops.

Physiological Mechanisms

When a nerve impulse is initiated, it travels down to its nonmyelinated terminals and starts up an impulse in the muscle fibers. The electrical activity of the nerve impulse arriving at the terminals is insufficient in itself to depolarize the muscle fiber directly by its action current; instead, a chemical mediator, ACh, is transferred across the synaptic cleft, probably by diffusion. There the ACh reacts with receptor molecules in the postsynaptic membrane and alters the properties of the membrane so that it becomes highly permeable to small cations. The result is a local depolari-

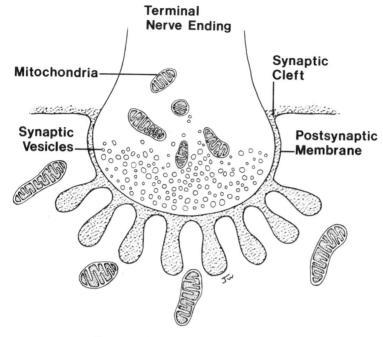

Fig. 4.2. The neuromuscular junction.

zation of the postsynaptic membrane known as the endplate potential. It reaches a threshold of excitation of the muscle fiber and triggers a propagated impulse which travels at a constant speed away from the junction and is associated with muscle fiber contraction. This series of events is summarized in Figure 4.3. That brief description of the process of neuromuscular transmission requires elaboration before proceeding to a discussion of defects in the system and electrodiagnostic methods of detecting them.

ACH STORAGE

Motor nerve fibers and their endings are known to contain ACh, as well as choline acetyltransferase, which is needed for its synthesis. Once synthesized, the ACh is stored in the synaptic vesicles of the motor nerve terminal, each vesicle containing about 10,000 molecules.

QUANTAL LIBERATION OF ACH

Liberation of the contents of a vesicle into the synaptic cleft is referred to as a quantal emission. A single depolarization of a presynaptic terminal results in the release of a large number of quanta. Since it is an all-or-none phenomenon, nerve terminal depolarization does not vary significantly, but the liberation of quanta of ACh is totally dependent on an influx of calcium ions into the nerve terminal. How calcium triggers the release of the transmitter is not well understood, but a reduction in external calcium diminishes ACh liberation. The synaptic vesicle, once it has liberated its

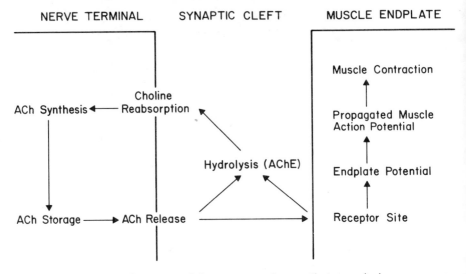

Fig. 4.3. Summary of the process of synaptic transmission.

contents, remains in the nerve terminal, is refilled with ACh, and becomes available for reuse.

DEPOLARIZATION OF THE POSTSYNAPTIC MEMBRANE

As ACh is released, it diffuses across the synaptic cleft. Some is hydrolyzed in the process, but the remainder reacts with receptor sites on the postjunctional membrane. This causes, at that site, a sudden permeability of the membrane to sodium, potassium, and other cations which are affected simultaneously and to about the same extent. Little or no change in permeability of the endplate to anions is produced. The intensity of the effect increases with the local concentration of ACh and the available receptor molecules.

MINIATURE ENDPLATE POTENTIALS

The resting potential across the muscle membrane is about 90 mV, inside negative, which, during the brief periods of increased permeability to small cations, shifts toward zero. In the resting state, quantal emissions occur in a random fashion, resulting in low amplitude excitations at the endplate on the order of about 0.5 mV. These are nonpropagated responses known as miniature endplate potentials (MEPP). When this sequence of irregularly recurring small potentials was first observed in the early 1950s by Fatt and Katz, they referred to the phenomenon as biological noise. It is now known that these potentials result from the spontaneous release of quanta of ACh.

THE ENDPLATE POTENTIAL

With the arrival of an impulse at a nerve terminal, 100–200 quanta are normally released, causing a local depolarization of the postsynaptic membrane; this is known as an endplate potential (EPP). In the early 1940s, Kuttler first elucidated the nature of the EPP in his classic study of a single nerve-muscle preparation. It is nonpropagated, spreads simply by the cable properties of the muscle fiber, and so is decremented progressively in space and time, becoming nearly depleted at 3–4 mm from the endplate. It has no refractory period. An excitation that occurs before total decay from a previous excitation will result in summation along the whole length of the electronic extension of the EPP. Each quantum produces the equivalent of an MEPP, but because of the enormous emission associated with the nerve impulse, the quantal composition is not normally revealed.

THE MUSCLE ACTION POTENTIAL

In the process of depolarization, the EPP reaches a critical threshold. A propagated action spike develops along the length of the muscle fiber, resulting in a shift of the internal potential from negativity to positivity. This is the muscle action potential that spreads in both directions along the muscle fiber away from the endplate and triggers mechanical contraction. Until sufficient internal negativity is restored, the muscle fiber remains refractory to a subsequent impulse.

As seen in Figure 4.4, the recording at the endplate reveals the EPP with the muscle action potential superimposed. At 1 and 2 mm from the endplate, the effect of the EPP becomes less evident since it is nonpropagated. However, the muscle spike is larger, presumably because the transmitter action on the endplate prevents the impulse from attaining as high a reversal point as elsewhere along the muscle membrane.

The time sequence of neuromuscular transmission is of interest. Following the arrival of the nerve impulse, no electrical change is seen in the muscle fiber for about 0.5–0.8 msec. Another 0.5 msec is required for the EPP to reach the threshold of excitation of the muscle fiber. These findings are totally consistent with the chemical nature of transmission at the neuromuscular synapse.

HYDROLYSIS AND RESYNTHESIS OF ACH

Acetylcholine esterase, a powerful enzyme that hydrolyzes ACh, is highly concentrated at the neuromuscular junction, especially on its postsynaptic surface. As ACh is released into the synaptic cleft, part is rapidly hydrolyzed into choline and acetic acid and part attaches to the receptor sites on the postsynaptic membrane, staying there 1–2 msec before breaking free to be destroyed by acetylcholine esterase. The choline is then recycled. It enters the nerve terminal where the enzyme choline acetyltransferase combines it with acetic acid to reform ACh for replenishing the synaptic vesicles. Thus, postsynaptic hydrolysis of ACh serves both to terminate the local action of the transmitter and to provide free choline which can be reabsorbed and resynthesized in the presynaptic terminal.

It appears that for continuous replenishment of ACh, nerve terminals

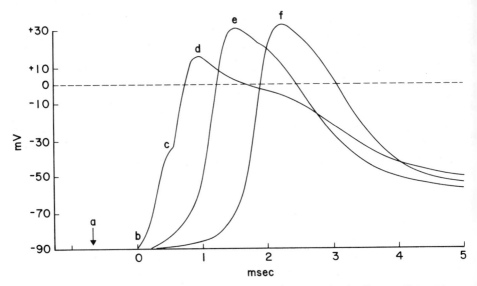

Fig. 4.4. The microelectrode recordings of a single muscle fiber action potential. *a*, arrival of nerve impulse at nerve terminal; *b*, onset of endplate potential; *c*, threshold for propagated muscle action potential; *d–f*, action potential recorded intracellularly at 0, 1, and 2 mm from the motor endplate. (Adapted from: J. C. Eccles: *The Understanding of the Brain*, p. 40, McGraw-Hill, New York, 1973.)

depend largely upon a process that enables them to absorb choline from the extracellular space. It is possible that this may be brought about by a specific transport mechanism built into the presynaptic membrane.

SAFETY FACTOR FOR NEUROMUSCULAR TRANSMISSION

Many components of the mechanism for neuromuscular transmission exist. If one or more components is altered by a disease process, the efficiency of the entire mechanism can be diminished.

There are three basic components that operate presynaptically. First, the number of quanta released with each impulse could be reduced or the size of the quanta could be altered. Normally these are quite uniform. Second, the quantity of available stores of ACh could be reduced or the system for resynthesis and replenishment of stores could be impaired. Under ordinary circumstances, there is a mechanism for rapid replenishment; otherwise the reserve supply would last only a few minutes. A single impulse, however, results in a decrease of available stores that persists for a number of seconds. Third, the release of ACh is intimately associated with the influx of calcium into the nerve terminal. With each impulse some calcium remains for up to 200 msec. If a subsequent impulse arrives at the nerve terminal during this period, the additional calcium boosts the liberation of transmitter. The probability of release of ACh during repetitive depolarization of the nerve terminal depends mainly on two opposing factors: the long-acting effect on available stores and the short-acting effect of calcium binding in the terminal.

On the postsynaptic side, an alteration of the number of receptor sites or their sensitivity to ACh could seriously impair neuromuscular transmission because of the effect on EPP amplitude. The amplitude has a significant normal variation, but because it is well above threshold for initiation of the propagated muscle action potential, no neuromuscular block occurs. Normally the threshold of the muscle action potential is quite stable, but if a disease process were to produce an elevation in threshold, a transmission defect would result.

In the absence of disease, the impulse propagation from nerve to muscle has an effective safety factor, so that under a wide range of normal biological conditions the nerve cell can fire impulses and all the muscle fibers it innervates will contract.

Explanation of the physiological basis of neuromuscular transmission is covered in greater depth elsewhere (2, 3), and the experiments leading to the concepts discussed above are analyzed in detail.

Electrodiagnostic Techniques

It is known that several diseases may cause abnormalities of neuromuscular transmission. Sometimes, as in severe generalized myasthenia gravis which responds to edrophonium, the diagnosis is clear without the support of electrical studies. However, when muscle weakness is minimal, fluctuating or localized, electrodiagnostic procedures can frequently be helpful. Even in syndromes that appear to be easily recognized, electrical studies add weight to the diagnosis, provide objective documentation, and offer a monitoring method for following the course of the disease.

Several methods have been described as useful in detecting defects of neuromuscular transmission, some simple, others quite complicated. The last few years have shown many advances in the clinical application of techniques for studying neurophysiological phenomena. This, combined with a better understanding of pathophysiological mechanisms, has allowed an expansion of our ability to diagnose diseases that alter neuromuscular transmission.

NEEDLE ELECTRODE EXAMINATION

Perhaps the easiest and least uncomfortable test for detecting a neuromuscular transmission defect is evaluation of the motor unit action potential by insertion of a standard needle electrode into a muscle. The patient is then asked to produce a minimal voluntary contraction, and the firing series of a single motor unit is observed and recorded. If every muscle fiber of the motor unit depolarizes with each nerve impulse, and if the needle is absolutely stationary within the motor unit territory, then the amplitude, duration, and configuration of each successive action potential of the same motor unit will be identical. Actually a variation of up to 5% in amplitude can occur normally.

SINGLE SUPRAMAXIMAL STIMULATION

Several investigators have evaluated the muscle response to a single supramaximal nerve stimulation in relation to abnormality of neuromuscular transmission (4, 5). Although the amplitude is clearly below normal range in patients with myasthenic syndrome and a few with myasthenia gravis, the value of this test by itself is very limited. It virtually always requires supplemental studies to confirm a diagnosis, and therefore should be used only to raise the electromyographer's index of suspicion that an abnormality may exist. One's time and effort is more fruitfully spent on other parts of the examination.

REPETITIVE STIMULATION

Various methods of stimulating nerves repetitively and recording responses from muscle have been developed and are gradually being scrutinized and standardized for more accurate interpretation in the diagnosis of neuromuscular transmission defects (5, 6). Jolly (7), in 1895, described a technique of observation of muscle fatigue during repetitive electrical stimulation. Although based on sound principles, the method was crude by present standards, but the conclusions he was able to reach were remarkable for his time. The method continues to generate interest (8), although it is no longer widely used.

Today, as a result of the development of electronic equipment that can accurately record the parameters of the evoked compound muscle action potential, it is possible to demonstrate slight deviations from the normal muscle response. To accomplish this, the electromyographer must pay careful attention to the details of the procedure or confusing and erroneous results may be obtained.

Step 1. Selection of Area to be Studied

Repetitive stimulation can be performed on any combination of nerve and muscle that is anatomically available. For instance, it is technically very simple to stimulate the ulnar nerve at the wrist and record from the hypothenar muscles of the hand. There may be many times, however, when it would be more desirable to stimulate the third cranial nerve and record from the extraocular muscles, but this is technically impossible with present methods. Therefore, one must choose nerve-muscle combinations that are accessible. The location of the recording electrode must be near the motor point so as to permit recording of a large, well synchronized potential with an initial negative deflection. Stimuli should be square wave pulses of 50–500 μsec duration.

There are advantages and disadvantages to the use of each nerve-muscle unit that might be studied. The degree of technical difficulty must be considered, and this is often directly related to reliability of results. Since yield of abnormality can be greater in one area than another depending on the disease process, selection must also be based on the clinical picture. It would not be uncommon for a proximal muscle to be more abnormal than a distal one, yet more difficult to test and more uncomfortable for the patient. Thus, the decision as to which nerve-muscle combinations to examine must be based on clinical judgment.

Perhaps the most commonly examined combination is stimulation of the ulnar nerve at the wrist with the response recorded from the hypothenar muscles. This may be the simplest test to perform, and the response is highly reliable. However, the area is often less involved in the disease process; therefore, normal results do not necessarily mean the patient is normal. The median nerve-thenar test is similar but technically more difficult because there is more movement.

A useful combination is median nerve-flexor carpi radialis, which is technically easy although the yield of abnormality is variable. If a more proximal group is desired, the musculocutaneous (from axilla)-biceps combination is excellent both in terms of yield and technical ease. The deltoid and infraspinatus are possible sites from which to record and require brachial plexus stimulation in the supraclavicular fossa.

In the lower limb, a combination that is technically easy to use is peroneal-anterior tibial. If a more proximal group is desired, femoral-quadriceps is possible.

When bulbar symptoms predominate and electrophysiological abnormalities have not been detected in the limbs, the facial nerve can be used with surface electrodes over frontalis, orbicularis oculi or nasalis.

Step 2. Application of Electrodes

To avoid serious error, one must be certain that both the stimulating and recording electrodes are securely fastened to the patient in a manner that eliminates all movement between the electrodes and the nerve or muscle underlying them. If surface electrodes are used, the skin should be clean and dry; alcohol or other solvent is useful. Only the smallest dot of electrode paste should be used for each site so as to avoid extension of the paste beyond the diameter of the electrode. Each electrode should be secured to the skin with ample quantities of adhesive tape; Velcro straps or similar devices are not adequate for this purpose.

Some investigators feel that to avoid errors, short subcutaneous needle electrodes should be used to record from the muscle. If these are used, care must be taken to avoid piercing the fascia with the needle, since contraction of the muscle will then cause movement of the electrode. With the tip in place subcutaneously, the electrode should be securely anchored with adhesive tape.

For nerve stimulation, needle electrodes can also be used. With the tip of the cathode in close proximity to the nerve, only very small amounts of current are required; but if the needle is not correctly placed, local muscle contraction in the area of the electrode or gross body movements produced by nerve stimulation can easily cause the needle to shift. This can result in a change from supra- to submaximal stimulation of the nerve and lead to errors in interpretation. Whether needle or surface electrodes are used, they should not be held by hand.

In this step of the procedure, emphasis must be on immobilizing the limb being examined and anchoring the electrodes in relation to that limb so as to minimize movement between electrodes and the underlying nerves and muscles. This will avoid spurious alterations in recorded responses that might be misconstrued as a true decrement. Examination for base line movements can confirm this false decremental response.

Step 3. Supramaximal Stimulation

With each stimulus, adequate current must pass through the nerve to depolarize all the motor axons in the nerve trunk being stimulated. To determine the desired intensity, the current is increased gradually. When the first motor axon is depolarized, a threshold response is recorded, and as the intensity becomes greater, the compound muscle action potential increases. When the current intensity is just sufficient to depolarize all the motor nerve fibers, the evoked potential reaches its maximum. For the purposes of these studies, it is necessary always to have this maximal evoked response to ensure a constant standard input to all neuromuscular junctions. To be certain this response occurs with each stimulus, the current intensity is increased at least 25–50% above that required for a maximal response. Periodically throughout the course of the examination, the electromyographer must determine that the stimulus has remained supramaximal.

Step 4. Frequency and Duration of Stimulation

The range of frequency of repetitive stimulation generally considered for use in detecting defects in neuromuscular transmission by electrophysiologic determinations is 1–50/sec. (Higher frequencies may be more suitable for evaluating mechanical parameters of muscle contraction.) The recovery cycle following a single stimulus is such that at 1/sec stimulation many patients with mild to moderate myasthenia gravis will not show a defect, while at 10/sec a facilitation of quantal ejection can confuse or obscure a typical myasthenic decrement. Therefore, Desmedt (9) has advocated 3/sec stimulation and has shown that the decrement does not progress significantly beyond the fifth stimulus. He has based his studies on five stimuli at 3/sec. To avoid long term activity-dependent alterations in the level of neuromuscular block, these trains of stimuli are applied at intervals of not less than 30 sec.

Repetitive stimulation at rates of 10–50/sec is usually unnecessary and should be reserved for specific indications, especially since discomfort of the patient increases with the frequency. These rapid rates can demonstrate the abnormality in diseases that respond to facilitation, such as the myasthenic syndrome of Eaton-Lambert or botulinum intoxication. A more comfortable method of inducing facilitation is to stimulate at a rate of 2 or 3/sec, for 30 sec, exercise the muscle being tested, and then repeat the 2 or 3/sec stimulation immediately. An increase in the evoked response of a few percent can be seen normally, but a marked increase is indicative of the myasthenic syndrome. They are also helpful in detecting abnormality of the motor nerve terminal.

Step 5. Mode of Display

The muscle response to repetitive nerve stimulation can be displayed and recorded in various ways (Fig. 4.5). There are a few basic requisites that are essential. First, the display must separate each response sequentially so that amplitudes and configurations of the evoked potentials can be compared. Second, there must be a method of permanently recording the responses so that time can be devoted to accurate measurements of the potentials. It is not sufficient to estimate alterations that may appear transiently during a brief sweep across an oscilloscope.

Step 6. Evaluation of the Evoked Responses

With the safety factors that exist in the normal individual to preserve neuromuscular transmission at maximum, there should never be a decrement, at least theoretically, that would not be considered abnormal. However, for reasons that are still unknown, decrements as large as −8% (6) occur in normal subjects during slow repetitive stimulation (1–10/sec), so it

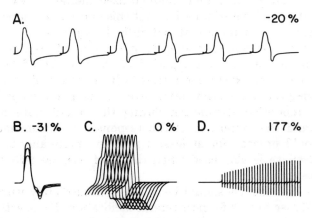

Fig. 4.5. Some modes of display of repetitively evoked compound muscle action potentials. (A) Each potential displayed individually forming a sequential series, (B) responses superimposed resulting in difficulty recognizing sequence and presenting some problems with analysis of configurations of individual potentials; (C) a method providing sequential representation and the ability to analyze each response; (D) a technique useful for checking alterations in amplitude but inadequate for noting duration and configuration.

is generally considered that a -10% decrement is required before abnormality can be established. With rapid repetitive stimulation (10–50/sec), incremental responses are usually noted in normal subjects and may be as great as 40% (5). However, this is due to synchronization, and the area under the evoked response does not change. To calculate percentage change, increment or decrement, a comparison is made between the amplitude of the first evoked compound muscle action potential (P_1) and the amplitude of a subsequent potential (P_S) in the same train of responses according to the following formula:

$$\% = \frac{100\ (P_S - P_1)}{P_1}$$

True increments and decrements occur smoothly in a geometrical progression from one evoked response to the next. If alterations in amplitude occur erratically, there is a technical error in performance of the procedure. The results must be discarded, the source of error eliminated, and the procedure repeated.

Step 7. Exercise Testing

The tests of repetitive stimulation described above are performed first on rested muscle. The muscle is then exercised with the duration being adjusted to the clinical picture and results of electrodiagnostic testing at that point. The exercise is always a maximal voluntary isometric contraction. Patients do not find this difficult to maintain for 15–20 sec, but when 1–2 min of exercise are required, they are best divided into 20-sec periods with intervals of not more than 5 sec. A more standardized method of exercise can be achieved with repetitive stimulation, but this is probably unnecessary and the discomfort to the patient makes it difficult to justify.

If myasthenic syndrome is suspected and the initial responses are of low amplitude, a vigorous 10–15-sec period of exercise should be utilized. A similar period of exercise is recommended whenever a significant decrement appears during the initial stimulation, even if the amplitude is large. However, when repetitive stimulation during the rested state produces no decrement and the amplitude of the responses is within normal range, exercise should proceed for at least 1 min and preferably 2. The longer period of exercise is also used when the brief exercise fails to alter the response to stimulation.

The period of exercise should be followed immediately with five or six stimuli at 2–3/sec to look for post-tetanic facilitation. Then, without further exercise, the same series of stimuli are repeated at 30-sec intervals for 3–5 min while watching for the appearance of or increase in decrement indicating postactivation exhaustion.

During this portion of the examination, there are two major causes of error. The first is movement of the stimulating or recording electrodes, which could lead to spurious tracings. It is important to check periodically during the course of the study to determine whether the stimulus has remained supramaximal. The second cause of error is coolness of the patient's limb. In order to be certain that a transmission defect will become manifest, the temperature of the muscle being investigated must remain above 33° C. The effect of temperature on myasthenic neuromuscular block has been amply demonstrated (6).

Step 8. Exercise Under Ischemia

If efforts to this point have been unsuccessful in revealing an abnormality of neuromuscular transmission, the combination of ischemia plus exercise will expose an occult defect in a significant number of patients who are suspected of having myasthenia gravis. Ischemia without exercise does not produce a decrement; the combination of ischemia plus exercise does not cause a significant decrement in normal subjects.

To perform the test, a sphygmomanometer cuff is placed on the arm and inflated above systolic pressure. Exercise followed by electrical stimulation is done as in Step 7 above. Because the ischemic limb becomes cold quickly, an infrared lamp should be used during the test to maintain warmth and avoid missing an abnormal response. Although ischemia limits the procedure to the distal limb muscles, a number of nerve-muscle combinations are possible and should be tried before reporting a negative result.

Summary of the Procedure for Repetitive Stimulation

If the patient has been taking drugs that affect neuromuscular transmission, these drugs should be discontinued for at least 3–6 hr and for 24 hr or more, if tolerated by the patient, prior to the examination. If necessary, several muscles must be evaluated, since it is common to find some muscles normal and others abnormal in the same patient. Both proximal and distal sites should be tested.

Recording and stimulating electrodes must be applied with great care to avoid movement during the procedure relative to the underlying structures. Whether using surface electrodes or subcutaneous needles or wires, the key is to avoid movement.

When a stimulus in the approximate range of 150% of maximal has been established, repetitive stimulation is initiated, usually at 2–3/sec before and after exercise, then repeated every 30 sec for 3–5 min. In the absence of abnormality, the procedure is repeated under ischemic conditions.

If a decrement is induced, an attempt to repair the defect can be attempted by a 10–15-sec period of exercise or by the intravenous injection of 2 mg of edrophonium chloride. The additional information gained in this step can add weight to the interpretation of results.

In selected cases, repetitive stimulation at 10–50/sec can be tried. This is useful primarily in disorders that respond to facilitation.

Diseases Affecting Neuromuscular Transmission

MYASTHENIA GRAVIS

In the past 4 or 5 years, increasing evidence has accumulated indicating a postsynaptic defect in myasthenia gravis, resulting in decreased sensitivity of the postsynaptic membrane to ACh (10–12). The typical electrophysiological defect is a progressive decrement at slow rates of stimulation. The defect is repaired immediately after exercise and after the injection of edrophonium chloride. In the few minutes following exercise, the defect is accentuated. Rapid repetitive stimulation may or may not induce an initial decrement but will often result in an incremental response that may be greater than 40–50%, the upper limits of normal.

It is important to note that atypical responses occur in patients with myasthenia gravis (13–15). Most commonly these responses simulate those of Eaton-Lambert syndrome. However, the more typical findings of myasthenia gravis are usually detectable in other muscles of these patients or in the same muscles at other times. It must be emphasized that several muscles of each patient, proximal and distal, should be examined.

MYASTHENIC SYNDROME (EATON-LAMBERT)

The characteristic defect (16) of this syndrome is a very low number of quanta being released by a nerve action potential. MEPP amplitude is normal but EPP amplitudes are abnormally low, often failing to exceed the threshold for initiating a propagated muscle action potential. However, available stores of ACh are normal.

Electrodiagnostically the initial evoked compound muscle action potential has a very low amplitude. At slow rates of stimulation, a minimal decrement may be seen, but immediately after exercise a marked facilitation is noted, usually greater than 200%. Two to 4 min later, the amplitude drops below the pre-exercise values. In this syndrome, as well as others that respond to facilitation, rapid rates of stimulation are useful in demonstrating the defect.

BOTULINUM INTOXICATION

The neuromuscular abnormality in botulism (17) is a defect of ACh release. In contradistinction to myasthenic syndrome, postactivation facilitation does not always occur, and when it does, it does not result in amplitudes that approach the normal range but tends to last much longer. Postactivation exhaustion does not occur. Rapid repetitive stimulation in the range of 20–40/sec seems to be of less value than 2/sec stimulation.

MYOTONIA

Electrical stimuli trigger repetitive myotonic bursts that result in refractoriness causing small decrements at slow rates of stimulation (18). Immediately after exercise, the decrement is accentuated, and within 2–3 min there is a return to the base line value.

NEUROGENIC ATROPHIES

Several diseases, including amyotrophic lateral sclerosis (19), poliomyelitis (20), and syringomyelia (21), have for sometime been known to produce EMG evidence of failure of neuromuscular transmission. They reveal similar electrodiagnostic abnormalities and sometimes show an observable electrophysiological response to edrophonium chloride.

NERVE TERMINAL DISORDERS

High rates of stimulation are known to produce intermittent failure of conduction in motor nerve terminals. When neuropathies occur that affect these terminals, the tendency for conduction block increases and slow rates of stimulation are found to produce variable decrements that are unaffected by exercise. In these cases, faster rates enhance the decrement.

DISEASES OF THE CENTRAL NERVOUS SYSTEM

Reports of progressive muscle weakness during exercise followed by recovery with rest in patients with encephalitis have recently been reviewed (22), but this phenomenon has not been systematically studied electrodiagnostically. Similar symptoms have long been recognized in some patients with multiple sclerosis. A recent study revealed a decremental response to rapid stimulation and a tendency for postactivation exhaustion with no facilitation, all of which showed improvement with the administration of edrophonium (8). The pathophysiologic mechanism remains unknown.

Special Studies

Since approximately 95% of all patients with myasthenia gravis (15) can be diagnosed with the standard techniques described above, and since most cases of myasthenic syndrome and other disorders of neuromuscular transmission can also usually be recognized by these techniques, it is evident that only in selected situations will it be necessary to proceed to additional methods of diagnosis. The performance of special studies adds to the discomfort of the patient, often requires considerably more time, and, in some cases, will increase risk factors. In addition, these tests tend to require special expertise, expensive equipment, or additional personnel beyond the scope of the routine electrodiagnostic laboratory.

CURARE TEST

For many years curare has been known to accentuate the symptoms of myasthenia gravis and has been used to reveal a decremental response to repetitive stimulation that could not otherwise be detected. Because patients suffering from this disease show an exquisite sensitivity to the drug, very small doses can sometimes lead to respiratory arrest. Arrangements for management of this situation must therefore be available during the testing period. To avoid systemic administration of the drug, a regional curare test (23) has been devised by which, after application of a sphygnomanometer cuff above systolic pressure, 0.2 mg d-Tubocurarine in 20 ml of 0.9% NaCl is injected intravenously into the forearm. This is followed by repetitive stimulation under ischemic conditions. The test is designed to produce decremental responses in patients with myasthenia gravis but not in normal subjects.

MECHANICAL RESPONSES

The well known phenomenon of progressive weakness during exercise in patients with myasthenia gravis can be recorded by simple ergometry, but more quantitative methods for recording mechanical responses to electrical stimulation have been described (24).

Forces produced during isometric contractions can be recorded in a number of ways using pressure transducers or strain gauge devices. During 61repetitive stimulation in normal subjects, there is a successive increase in force known as the staircase phenomenon. In patients with myasthenia gravis, the staircase potentiation tends to be diminished, although there is no serious discrepancy between amplitudes of compound muscle action potentials and simultaneously recorded forces of isometric contraction. Explanation of the staircase mechanism is still open to question, as is the possibility of abnormality of the contractile process in myasthenia gravis.

SINGLE FIBER EMG

The technique of single fiber EMG is described in detail elsewhere in this volume. Basically it is a method of measuring intervals between the occurrence of action potentials of two or more individual muscle fibers of the same motor unit resulting from a single nerve volley. There is a random variation of the interval of less than 50 μsec that occurs normally, but in disorders that affect the neuromuscular junction this interval, known as jitter, tends to increase. In addition, intermittent failure of transmission produces a phenomenon known as blocking. These abnormalities have been noted in myasthenia gravis (25) and myasthenic syndrome (26).

MICROELECTRODE STUDIES

Evaluation of the endplate region of the muscle fiber by microelectrodes has become a very fruitful method of analyzing pathophysiological mechanisms of neuromuscular transmission. The current state of the method was recently reviewed by Lambert (27).

A number of parameters can be monitored. The number of quanta released by a nerve impulse can be calculated, as well as the rate of random release and the rate at which quanta can be mobilized for release. The store of readily available quanta can be ascertained. The response of the postsynaptic membrane to a single quantum can be measured, and the sensitivity of the membrane to iontophoretically applied ACh can be estimated.

The typical microelectrode findings have been established for myasthenia gravis, myasthenic syndrome, and other better known disorders of the neuromuscular junction, such as botulinum intoxication. Microelectrode techniques, however, do not lend themselves to widespread use, and, in fact, are only available in a very limited number of laboratories. They seem likely to be most useful for research purposes and for illuminating previously unrecognized disorders of neuromuscular transmission.

REFERENCES

1. LAMBERT, E. H., EATON, L. M., AND ROOKE, E. D.: Defect of neuromuscular conduction associated with malignant neoplasm. *Amer. J. Physiol., 187:* 617, 1956.
2. ECCLES, J. C.: The mechanism of synaptic transmission. *Ergeb. Physiol., 51:* 299, 1961.
3. KATZ, B.: *Nerve, Muscle and Synapse.* New York: McGraw-Hill, 1966.
4. HARVEY, A. M., AND MASLAND, R. L.: A method for the study of neuromuscular transmission in human subjects. *Bull. Johns Hopkins Hosp., 68:* 81, 1941.
5. OZDEMIR, C., AND YOUNG, R. R.: Electrical testing in myasthenia gravis. *Ann. N.Y. Acad. Sci., 183:* 287, 1971.
6. BORENSTEIN, S., AND DESMEDT, J. E.: New diagnostic procedures in myasthenia gravis. In *New Developments in Electromyography and Clinical Neurophysiology,* vol. 1. pp 350–374, ed. by. J. E. Desmedt, Basel, Switzerland: S. Karger, 1973.
7. JOLLY, F.: Uber Myasthenia Gravis pseudoparalytica. *Berl. Klin. Wschr., 32:* 1, 1895.
8. OH, S. J., NICHIHIRA, T., AND SARALA, P. K.: The diagnostic value of the Jolly test: Reappraisal. Presented at the 23rd annual meeting of the American Association of Electromyography and Electrodiagnosis, San Diego, 1976.
9. DESMEDT, J. E. (Ed.): The neuromuscular disorder in myasthenia gravis, I. In *New Developments in Electromyography and Clinical Neurophysiology,* vol. 1, pp. 241–305, Basel, Switzerland: S. Karger, 1973.
10. ENGEL, A. G., LAMBERT, E. H., AND SANTA, T.: Study of long term anticholinesterase therapy. *Neurology, 23:* 1273, 1973.
11. FAMBROUGH, D. M., DRACHMAN, D. B., AND SATYAMURTI, S.: Neuromuscular junction in myasthenia gravis: Decreased acetylcholine receptors. *Science, 182:* 293, 1973.
12. LINDSTROM, J. M., LENNON, V. A., SEYBOLD, M. E., AND WHITTINGHAM, S.: Experimental autoimmune myasthenia gravis: Biochemical and immunochemical aspects. *Ann. N.Y. Acad. Sci., 274:* 254, 1976.
13. MAYER, R. F., AND WILLIAMS, I. R.: Incrementing responses in myasthenia gravis. *Arch. Neurol., 31:* 24, 1974.
14. MORI, M., AND TAKAMORI, M.: Hyperthyroidism and myasthenia gravis with features of Eaton-Lambert syndrome. *Neurology, 26:* 882, 1976.
15. OZDEMIR, C., AND YOUNG, R. R.: The results to be expected from electrical testing in the diagnosis of myasthenia gravis. *Ann. N.Y. Acad. Sci., 274:* 203, 1976.
16. ELMQVIST, D., AND LAMBERT, E. H.: Detailed analysis of neuromuscular transmission in a patient with the myasthenic syndrome sometimes associated with bronchogenic carcinoma. *Mayo Clin. Proc., 43:* 689, 1968.
17. GUTMANN, L., AND PRATT, L.: Pathophysiologic aspects of human botulism. *Arch. Neurol., 33:* 175, 1976.
18. DESMEDT, J. E.: Observations sur la réaction myotonique en stimulo-détection. *Rev. Neurol., 110:* 324, 1964.
19. LAMBERT, E. H., AND MULDER, D. W.: Electromyographic studies in amyotrophic lateral sclerosis. *Mayo Clin. Proc. 32:* 441, 1957.
20. HODES, R.: Electromyographic study of defects of neuromuscular transmission in human poliomyelitis. *Arch. Neurol. Psych., 60:* 457, 1948.
21. KUGELBERG, E., AND TAVERNER, D.: Comparison between voluntary and electrical activation of motor units in anterior horn cell diseases; on central synchronization of motor units. *Electroencephalogr. Clin. Neurophysiol., 2:* 125, 1950.

22. DESMEDT, J. E. (Ed.): The neuromuscular disorder in myasthenia gravis, II. In *New Developments in Electromyography and Clinical Neurophysiology*, vol. 1, pp. 305–342, Basel, Switzerland: S. Karger, 1973.

23. CENDROWSKI, W.: Multiple sclerosis associated with defective neuromuscular transmission. *N. Neurol., 209:* 297, 1975.

24. HOROWITZ, S. H., GENKINS, G., KORNFELD, P., AND PAPATESTAS, A. E.: Electrophysiologic diagnosis of myasthenia gravis and the regional curare test. *Neurology, 26:* 410, 1976.

25. SLOMIĆ, A., ROSENFALCK, A., AND BUCHTHAL, F.: Electrical and mechanical responses of normal and myasthenic muscle. *Brain Res., 10:* 1, 1968.

26. STÅLBERG, E., TRONTELJ, J. V., AND SCHWARTZ, M. S.: Single muscle-fiber recording of the jitter phenomenon in patients with myasthenia gravis and in members of their families. *Ann. N.Y. Acad. Sci., 274:* 189, 1976.

27. SCHWARTZ, M. S., AND STÅLBERG, E.: Myasthenic syndrome studied with single fiber electromyography. *Arch Neurol., 32:* 815, 1975.

28. LAMBERT, E. H.: Symposium on electrophysiologic studies in defects of neuromuscular transmission. Presented at the 23rd annual meeting of the American Association of Electromyography and Electrodiagnosis, San Diego, 1976.

5

Radiculopathies

HAROLD P. WEINGARDEN, M.D.
LYNN M. MIKOLICH, M.D.
ERNEST W. JOHNSON, M.D.

The plagues of low back and neck pain together comprise the greatest cause of musculoskeletal related disability. In 1934, when Mixter and Barr published their paper implicating the intervertebral disc as an etiologic factor in spinal cord compression (1), a reasonable cause for sciatica and brachialgia became apparent. Since that time, the diagnostic evaluation of the patient presenting with neck, mid, and low back pain has become increasingly important, with decisions of surgical intervention, immobilization, compensation, and life long disability based on these findings. EMG has become an especially important part of this evaluation in patients with these complaints. Among the advantages of the EMG are its availability as an outpatient study, the capability of differentiating mono- and polyneuropathies from radiculopathy, and possibly the avoidance of more hazardous diagnostic procedures, especially when evidence of "functional" disease is found.

In 1944, Weddell et al. (2) noted in a patient with sciatica the findings of fibrillations, "vigorous and prolonged motor unit action potentials" repeating rhythmically following insertion into a muscle at rest (positive waves), and a decrease in the number of motor unit action potentials on voluntary contraction. These findings were in a specific nerve root distribution. Shea et al. (3) and Crue et al. (4) presented a large series of patients with emphasis placed on findings of fibrillation potentials in a specific nerve root distribution for the diagnosis of radiculopathy. Brazier et al. (5), using an EEG type printout, described a method of localizing cervical nerve root compression by the use of surface electrodes for the detection of fasciculations within a nerve root distribution. A similar means of localizing lumbar radiculopathy has been described by Wise and Ardizzone (6).

In a comprehensive monograph by Knutsson (7), a comparison was made of EMG, myelographic examinations, and clinical examinations with operative findings in nerve root syndromes. It was noted that the EMG may show abnormalities without abnormal clinical neurologic findings. The EMG may localize the lesion to one level, whereas a clinical examination would indicate two levels. Also, the EMG may be abnormal with a normal myelogram.

More recently, the use of reflex study has been advocated, especially in the diagnosis of S1 nerve root lesions (8, 9). This has led to standardization of procedures for performing these reflex studies and a definition of normal latencies (10).

The degree of accuracy and sensitivity of the EMG has been evaluated in numerous studies (3, 4, 7, 11–13). In comparing the EMG with the myelogram, it was found that these tests had an essentially equal degree of accuracy and sensitivity, with EMG as the indicator of neurophysiologic dysfunction and myelography demonstrating anatomic abnormalities. Each of the studies did indicate the occurrence of instances of negative myelography, with positive EMG and nerve root compression found in the resultant surgery. Several studies noted the greater incidence of EMG abnormalities in L5,S1 disc herniations as compared to myelography, and, conversely, a greater number of abnormal myelograms in L4,5 disc disease. In a detailed breakdown of types of disc lesions at different levels, Knutsson (7) noted that with lumbosacral disc herniations, the EMG was abnormal in 80% of cases and the myelogram abnormal in 62%. For lumbosacral disc protrusion, the EMG was accurate in 82% and the myelogram in 36%. In L4,5 herniations, the myelogram was abnormal in 93% and the EMG in 76%, and in protrusions without herniation at this level, the EMG was correct in 79% and the myelogram in 64%. All of these cases showed nerve root abnormalities at surgery. Thus, even at the more easily detected L4,5 level, myelography is not reliable for disc lesion other than frank herniation, even though nerve root compression has occurred.

In comparing abnormalities of EMG findings to clinical neurologic findings in cervical radiculopathy, Honet and Puri (14) found that in 82 patients with definite clinical neurologic abnormalities, all showed evidence of muscle weakness. Deep tendon reflexes were diminished in 53 of the 82 patients (65%), with sensory changes in 48 (59%). An EMG was performed on 41 of the patients with abnormality noted in 35 (85%). The criterion for EMG diagnosis was the presence of positive waves and/or fibrillation potentials. Early in the course, a decreased number of motor unit action potentials was also accepted as an indication of abnormality.

The reliability of the EMG in the diagnosis of nerve root compression syndromes is reflected in a study by Johnson et al. (15), showing that radiculopathy is the most common clinical condition for which EMG examination is requested. Jebsen and Long (16) demonstrated the usefulness of the examination in patients where psychogenic factors cloud the objectivity of the physical examination. As early as 1951, Woods and Shea (17) stress the importance of the EMG for medical-legal purposes and emphasized the need for reproducible records. They stated, "evidence of this nature is of great legal importance in this era of litigious-minded patients."

Anatomy

As is the case in other areas of EMG diagnosis, a good knowledge of anatomy is required. The reader is referred to the excellent anatomic guides by Goodgold (18) and Delagi et al. (19) for specific location of needle electrode insertion. Evaluation of paraspinal muscles is especially important, as Johnson and Melvin (20) demonstrated that in one-third of patients with radiculopathy, EMG abnormalities were found solely in the paraspinals. These long muscle masses are composed of three layers, from superficial to deep: the erector spinae, semispinalis, and multifidi. These muscles are all innervated by the dorsal rami of the spinal nerve roots. In addition to innervating the paraspinal muscles, the dorsal ramus also supplies sensation to the skin of the back (Fig. 5.1).

There is marked anatomic segmental overlap in the superficial erector spinae and, to a lesser degree, in the semispinalis with concomitant myotomal overlap. This would explain the findings by Gough and Koepke (21) in patients with spinal cord injury, that active motor unit function was found two or more segments lower in the posterior myotome than would have been predicted by the sensory level. The multifidus layer has the least degree of overlap; thus, this area is most important in the paraspinal examination and is reached by advancing the needle electrode to a depth of 3–5 cm within the muscle mass. Abnormalities at this depth in patients with lesions of a single nerve root frequently are found at one level only (Fig. 5.2). When more diffuse abnormalities are found in the multifidi, a process other than compression of a single nerve root must be ruled out.

A problem encountered by many electromyographers has been the difficulty in obtaining complete relaxation of the paraspinal muscles for adequate evaluation of insertional activity. Relaxation can usually be obtained having the patient prone, with pillows placed underneath the abdomen and ankles for exploration of the lumbosacral paraspinals (Fig. 5.3), under the chest for

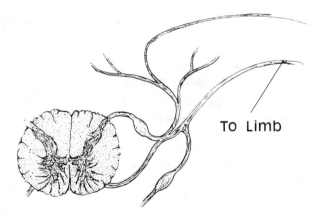

Fig. 5.1. Distribution of spinal nerve showing anterior primary ramus to limb and posterior primary ramus to paraspinal muscles and skin of back.

TABLE 5.1. *Cord Levels of Selective Muscles*

Upper Extremities	Lower Extremities
C5	L2, 3, 4
Rhomboids	Vastus lateralis
C5,6	Vastus medialis
Supraspinatus	Sartorius
Infraspinatus	Adductor longus
Teres major	Gracilis
Deltoid	L4,5-S1
Biceps brachii	Tensor fasciae latae
C5-7	Gluteus medius
Serratus anterior	L4,5
Pectoralis major	Anterior tibial
C5,6 (Clavicular)	Semimembranosus
C7-T1 (Sternal)	Semitendinosus
C6,7	L5-S1
Pronator teres	Bicep femoris
Extensor carpi radialis longus	Peroneus longus
C6-8	Extensor digitorum longus
Latissimus dorsi	Flexor digitorum longus
C7,8	Extensor hallucis longus
Triceps brachii	L5-S1, 2
Extensor carpi radialis brevis	Gastrocnemius
Extensor digitorum carpi	S1,2
Extensor pollicis longus	Soleus
Extensor pollicis brevis	Abductor hallucis
Abductor pollicis longus	Abductor digitus quint. ped.
Flexor digitorum superficialis	1st dorsal interosseus
Flexor carpi radialis	
Flexor digitorum profundus	
C8-T1	
Abductor pollicis brevis	
1st dorsal interosseous	
Abductor digitorum V	

(*NB:* Posterior tibialis is relatively inaccessible!)

the thoracic paraspinals, and beneath the upper chest and shoulders for the cervical paraspinals (Fig. 5.4).

EMG Findings

In acute nerve root compression, there is a usual sequence of EMG abnormalities. Initially, the axons would exhibit a conduction block which may be reversible. In the first 72 hr, only EMG abnormalities would reflect the conduction block in the involved portion of the nerve root axons. If there is a significant involvement, a decreased number of motor unit action potentials, as compared to the strength of muscle contraction, would be detected. With multilevel innervation in all peripheral muscles, aside from the rhomboids, it would take a nearly complete loss of a single nerve root to give recognizable reduction in the number of motor units early in the course.

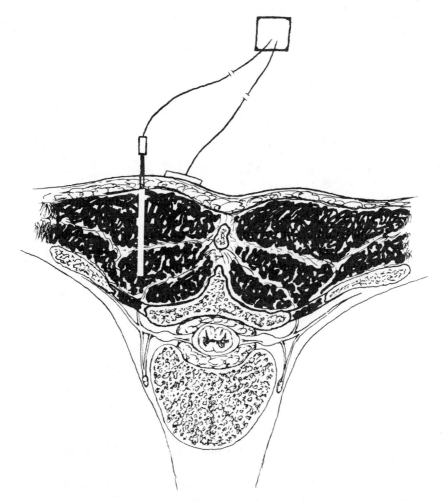

Fig. 5.2. EMG electrode inserted in the deep layers of paraspinal muscle.

During the initial few days following onset, the conduction block may be detected by means of reflex studies. Malcolm (9) found slowing of the latency, from the time of tap of the Achilles tendon to contraction of the gastrocnemius, of 1–4 msec in four of five patients with surgically proved S1 radiculopathy. In one patient with L4 radiculopathy, there was prolongation of the knee jerk. Only one patient with an L5 radiculopathy was studied and no slowing occurred in either the ankle or the knee jerk. Determination of the H reflex latency by stimulation of the I-a afferents may be useful in S1 radiculopathy. Magledary et al. (22) showed that in normals, the H reflex is obtainable in calf muscles consistently and never detected in the anterolateral leg muscles, forearm extensors, or hand intrinsics. Braddom and Johnson (10) found that the latency of the H reflex to the gastrocnemius can be

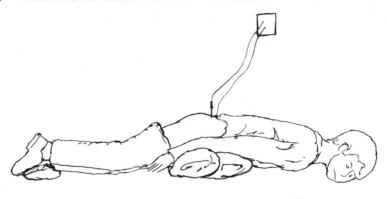

Prone

Fig. 5.3. Proper position for EMG exploration of lumbar paraspinal muscles.

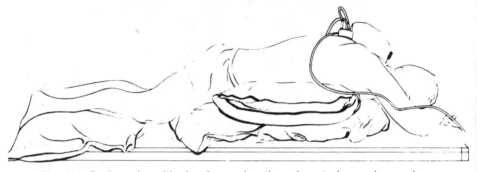

Fig. 5.4. Preferred positioning for exploration of posterior neck muscles.

predicted if the patient's height and age are taken into account and, that in normals, the difference between the two sides was less than 1.2 msec.

The method of determination of H reflex latency requires standardization for reproducible results. As described by Braddom and Johnson (10), the active electrode is placed over the medial gastrocnemius halfway between the popliteal crease and proximal medial malleolus. The reference electrode is placed over the Achilles tendon with the ground electrode being lateral to the active electrode. The tibial nerve is stimulated at the popliteal crease with the cathode proximal (Fig. 5.5). Use of a needle electrode for stimulation in this study has been advocated (23). It was found that the H latency value can be predicted from the following formula:

$$\text{H latency (msec)} = 9.14 + 0.46 \text{ leg length (cm)} + 0.1 \text{ age (years)} \pm 5.5 \text{ msec (2 S.D.)}$$

The predicted latency can also simply be determined from a nomogram (Fig. 5.6). When performing the study, the stimulus should be of short duration (0.05 msec), given at a frequency no greater than once every 2 sec

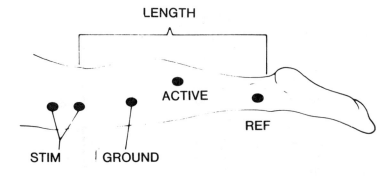

$$\text{PREDICTED LATENCY} = 9.14 + 0.46 \times L + 0.1 \times age$$

Fig. 5.5. Electrode placement for H latency determination in tibial nerve (S1 radiculopathy).

(Table 5.2). The H reflex will appear and become maximal with a stimulus that is submaximal, and amplitude will decrease as the strength increases to supramaximal. The measurement of latency is to the first deflection from the base line when a maximal response is obtained (Fig. 5.7).

Although the amplitude of the H wave will decrease in S1 radiculopathy, they found parameters, other than latency, to be highly variable and not as significant a finding. In 25 patients with clinical S1 radiculopathy, 9 had prolongation of the H reflex on the involved side and 16 had unilateral absence. The needle EMG showed abnormalities in only 20. Nine of these patients underwent surgery and all had unilateral S1 radiculopathy confirmed. In patients without L5 radiculopathy, none demonstrated prolongation of the H reflex to the gastrocnemius (24). This easily performed study is of value in the early stages of radiculopathy prior to the appearance of needle electromyographic findings. It is also helpful in localizing the level of lesion when the EMG findings are limited to the posterior rami (Table 5.3).

Approximately 72 hr after nerve injury, Wallerian degeneration usually begins to occur. Stimulation of peripheral nerves with recording of the area of the negative spike of the M response, compared to the contralateral M, could give an indication of the number of axons no longer excitable. Needle EMG at this time may show an increase in proportion of polyphasics within the nerve root distribution. At 7–10 days, the paraspinals may begin to show the presence of positive waves. At 2–3 weeks, positive waves in the anterior rami begin to occur with fibrillations occurring in the paraspinals (Table 5.4).

The most frequent abnormality found on an EMG for radiculopathy is the presence of positive waves. This is followed by an increased proportion of polyphasics and fibrillation potentials and a decreased number of motor units per strength of contraction (20). Knutsson (25) reported that in evaluating the mean duration of the action potentials, a 0–0.9 mesec duration difference existed between the normal and affected side. He concluded that

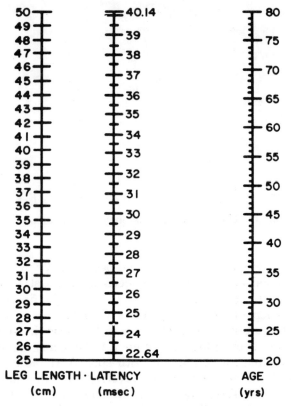

Fig. 5.6. Nomogram for H latency prediction (10).

TABLE 5.2. *Use of Predicted H Latency in L-S Radiculopathy*

1. Calculate predicted H latency (P).
2. Determine actual H latency (O).
3. If O > P, determine contralateral H latency.
4. Side-to-side difference > 1.0 msec suggests S1 radiculopathy.
5. If both H latencies > P, do tibial nerve conduction velocity.

this method of evaluation was time-consuming and added nothing beyond the evaluation of insertional activity in the relaxed muscle. In his study of 100 patients operated on for radiculopathy, in each case where nerve root compromise was surgically demonstrated, the preoperative EMG showed the presence of positive waves with or without fibrillation potentials. In cases where only polyphasic motor unit potentials and no positive waves or fibrillation potentials were found, no root compromise was grossly present at surgery.

Use of a multichannel ink writing oscillograph for detection of spontaneous fasciculation activity by means of surface electrodes has been used with reports of accurate determination of the presence of radiculopathy (5,

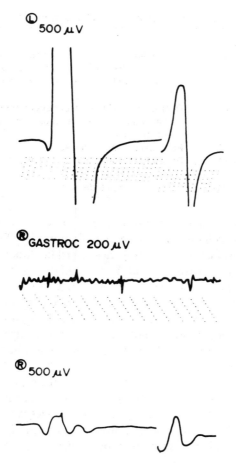

Fig. 5.7. H latency in S1 radiculopathy. *Top trace*, unaffected limb, normal H latency L ; *middle*, fibrillation potentials recorded in R gastrocnemius; *bottom*, prolonged H latency R .

TABLE 5.3. *Value of H Latency in S1 Radiculopathy*

1. Early in radiculopathy (0–10 days).
2. When needle EMG abnormalities limited to paraspinal.
3. If EMG findings are inconclusive, history and physical are suggesting.
4. EMG abnormalities do not separate L5 from S1.
5. Postlaminectomy if needle EMG abnormalities are widespread.

6). Unfortunately, this procedure is time-consuming and not sufficiently flexible for modification in response to unexpected findings. In another study in which only fibrillation potentials are considered to be evidence of abnormality, 50% of the patients also demonstrated the presence of fasciculations (3).

Alternative methods of studying the status of nerve roots are currently

TABLE 5.4. *Sequence of EMG Abnormalities*

Day	Finding
1–3	Prolongation of H reflex latency in S1 root compression; decrease number of motor units per strength of contraction.
4–7	Decrease amplitude on peripheral nerve stimulation; increase proportion of polyphasics.
7–10	Paraspinal positive waves.
17–21	Paraspinal fibrillation potentials; limb muscles positive waves.
60–240	Motor unit amplitude increase.

under investigation. The determination of F wave latency has not yet been demonstrated to be reliable or precise in radiculopathy. There has also been an attempt to demonstrate the presence of radiculopathy by intraspinal, extrathecal nerve root stimulations. In a small series it has been reported that there is slowing of conduction time (26). In a study of 32 nerve roots exposed at the time of surgery, stimulation above and below the level of the disc lesion showed no consistent finding regarding slowing or amplitude change. Those patients who did not show slowing or amplitude change had a better postoperative result than the patients who did show those abnormalities (27).

In general, findings in the paraspinals occur earlier and more consistently than in the limb muscles (2). Although the deeper paraspinal musculature shows only slight myotomal overlap, it is still necessary to correlate paraspinal findings with the history and physical examination or with H reflex study in order to localize the involved nerve root.

Clinical Correlation

The method of nerve root localization has been described (2, 3, 11, 17, 28). In essence, the presence of positive waves and/or fibrillation potentials should be found in a specific myotome without similar findings in muscles innervated by a different nerve root. Ideally, the abnormalities should be found both in the anterior and posterior rami of the nerve root. Of course, the electromyographer should be aware of possible anatomic variations and the possibility of multiple nerve root involvement (especially in the cauda equina).

In a C5 nerve root compression, the classic presentation is weakness of the deltoid and/or biceps, with a decrease in amplitude of the biceps tendon reflex. Electromyographically, positive waves and fibrillation potentials can be expected in the rhomboids, deltoid, supraspinatus, biceps, and serratus anterior. In the C6 radiculopathy, the clinical picture would be quite similar to the C5 but with the additional historical finding of paresthesias over the thumb. Electromyographically, these abnormal findings would be expected in the pronator teres and extensor carpi radialis longus in addition to the above C5, 6 muscles, with the exception of the C5 rhomboids only. C7 will frequently present with weakness of the triceps and pronators and decrease in the triceps tendon reflex. Paresthesias often are present over the index and middle fingers. EMG abnormalities are likely to be greatest in the triceps, pronator teres, flexor carpi radialis, and extensor digitorum communis. An interesting finding noted by Honet and Puri (14) was a greater incidence of EMG abnormalities in the pronator teres as compared to the triceps in patients with C7 radiculopathy, despite a greater frequency of clinical weakness in the triceps. In C8 radiculopathy, the patient is likely to have paresthesias over the medial two fingers with weakness of the hand intrinsics and possibly a decrease in the triceps tendon jerk. EMG abnormalities (positive waves and fibrillation potentials) would likely be greatest in the hand intrinsics, with additional involvement in the triceps and forearm muscles.

Reynolds et al. (29) studied a series of patients with "whiplash" injuries from auto accidents. The symptoms included stiffness of the neck, headaches, and radiation of pain to the occiput or upper back and shoulders, but not to the upper extremities. There were no objective clinical or radiologic abnormalities. The muscles evaluated were the trapezius, sternocleidomastoid, levator scapulae, and scaleni. The patients were examined 26 days to 5 years after the auto accident. Sixteen of the 17 patients had insertional abnormalities (positive waves) and increased proportion of polyphasic motor units in at least one of the muscles. The muscle most frequently showing abnormalities was the trapezius.

The nerve root most commonly involved in cervical radiculopathy is the C7 root secondary to herniation of the C6-7 disc. Of the remaining nerve roots, the most frequently abnormal is the C6, followed by C8 and C5 (30). The findings in chronic cervical radiculopathy have been reported to be more subtle than the acute findings. The most common abnormality noted was an increased proportion of polyphasics with prolonged insertional activity (31).

Among the differential diagnosis of cervical radiculopathy included are degenerative disc disease, thoracic outlet syndrome, neuralgic amyotrophy (brachial plexitis), pancoast tumor, ulnar nerve entrapment at the elbow, and carpal tunnel syndrome. In distinguishing a radiculopathy from these disorders, the major differential finding would be positive waves and fibrillation potentials in the paraspinals. Shoulder disorders may also mimic a cervical radiculopathy, in that there frequently is a radicular type of pain and clinical weakness, but the EMG will be negative. Reflex sympathetic dystrophy should be obvious on a clinical examination. In early syringomyelia, differentiation from cervical radiculopathy may be difficult; however, the EMG findings are usually bilateral, despite unilateral clinical findings.

Thoracic radiculopathy has been implicated as a possible etiology for abdominal complaints. This has been referred to as the pseudovisceral syndrome by Marinacci (30). In his series of patients with abdominal symptomology and negative workup for visceral cause, 5% had evidence of nerve root compression by electromyography. An alternative method of investigation for thoracic radiculopathy has been described with the use of intercostal nerve conduction studies. These studies were carried out by means of needle stimulation and pickup and performed under light anesthesia. There was an incidence of pneumothorax of 8.8%. Of 160 patients evaluated, 80 patients went to surgery. In 71, the surgical decision was based entirely on abnormal nerve conduction studies, and of these, 28 (39%) demonstrated no surgical abnormalities (32).

Diabetics with abdominal pain and signs of autonomic dysfunction may show diffuse paraspinal abnormalities. This may be evidence of multilevel radiculopathy (33). The differential diagnosis in thoracic radiculopathy is similar to lumbar and cervical radiculopathy, but finding of diffuse abnormality should cause a higher index of suspicion for intraspinal mass lesion, perispinal metastatic disease, or compression fracture. Herpes zoster may also give unilevel abnormalities.

In the lumbosacral radiculopathies, the EMG has the greatest sensitivity and reliability. In this region, complete relaxation of the paraspinals is easily obtained and EMG exploration is frequently rewarded. The standardization of the H reflex added an easily done study with reproducible results. For these reasons, EMG has great value in differentiating radiculopathy from the myriad of organic and functional disorders which result in back and lower extremity pain (Table 5.5).

In the L4 radiculopathy, the greatest weakness would be expected in the adductors, quadriceps, and anterior tibial. The patient would classically have difficulty in returning from a squat. The knee jerk would likely be decreased on the involved side. EMG abnormalities would follow the same pattern as the muscle weakness and include the paraspinals. Femoral neuropathy may give a picture similar to an L4 radiculopathy, but EMG abnormalities would not be expected in the adductors, anterior tibial, or paraspinals.

TABLE 5.5. *Possible Causes of Low Back Pain*

Intrinsic Back	Extrinsic Back
Mechanical	Vascular
Muscular	Visceral
Osteoarthritis	Prostate
Ankylosing spondylosis	Colon
Neoplasm	Pancreas
Infection	Peptic ulcer
Disk disease with or without root	Gynecologic
	Kidney
	CNS—Menningitic

Identification of muscles innervated by the L5 and S1 nerve root has been done by stimulation of the exposed nerve root at surgery (27). L5 stimulation caused contraction of the medial hamstrings, ankle dorsiflexors, and peroneals. Stimulation of the S1 root caused contraction of the lateral hamstrings and triceps surae. Clinically the patient with an L5 radiculopathy would have weakness of the hamstrings and toe extensors, with inability to walk on his heels. The Trendelenberg sign may also be present. The medial hamstring reflex may be reduced. In the S1 radiculopathy the patient would be unable to walk on his toes or would show easy fatigue when repeatedly coming up on to the toes. The ankle and biceps femoris reflexes may be decreased. EMG abnormalities in L5 radiculopathy would be in the anterior and lateral compartment muscles of the leg, the flexor digitorum longus, semimembranosus, gluteus medius, and paraspinals. The differentiation from peroneal nerve injury would be the finding of abnormalities in the latter mentioned muscle groups. S1 radiculopathy would most likely show abnormalities in the gluteus maximus, biceps femoris, gastrocnemius, and paraspinals. The addition of the H reflex is highly specific for S1 radiculopathy, assuming that sciatic and tibial nerve lesions are adequately ruled out. (Table 5.3)

In the differential diagnosis of low back pain, there are non-neurologic disorders which would not give EMG abnormalities. Muscle strains, ligamentous injury, and degenerative disc disease without nerve root compression should give a normal EMG. Metabolic disorders and, in particular, diabetes may give diffuse paraspinal abnormalities with no other evidence of radiculopathy. This abnormality appears to improve with control of the diabetes (34). Metastatic disease has also been shown to give localized paraspinal fibrillations and positive waves as well as a diffuse type of pattern (34, 35). In the syndrome of spinal stenosis, 77% of the patients had bilateral EMG abnormalities. An additional 20% had unilateral multilevel findings. One-third of the patients with stenotic canals will have only unilateral symptoms but will have bilateral EMG findings (36). Arachnoiditis gives a similar picture to spinal stenosis, and again the findings are more pronounced in the paraspinals than the anterior rami (4).

Special care in interpretation should be exercised when evaluating the extensor digitorum brevis. This muscle has been shown to be abnormal, both on histologic and EMG examinations in a significant number of control individuals with no apparent neurologic disorder (37). Sites of intramuscular injection should be avoided. Johnson et al. (38) demonstrated anatomic and physiologic disruption of muscle fibers at the site of intramuscular injection. EMG abnormalities included positive waves, fibrillation potentials, and reduced insertional activity. It was felt that abnormalities were due to local chemotoxicity of the drug, pressure, local hemorrhage, physical trauma by the needle, and inflammatory reaction. The drugs most likely to cause EMG abnormalities are Phenergan, Demerol and Compazine (38).

EMG and Management

Once the diagnosis of radiculopathy is established, management should be based primarily on the patient's symptoms and clinical findings. When there is reason to question the persistence of the findings, an EMG may be repeated. If there is evidence of clinical deterioration, serial peripheral nerve stimulation studies can be carried out to follow the course. In comparing the area of the negative spike of the evoked M response from the involved to the uninvolved side, an approximation may be made of the number of fibers undergoing Wallerian degeneration. Careful placement of recording electrodes is necessary, using the same location over the muscle belly on each side. In addition, it is important that the stimulation of the nerve be supramaximal. This study gives a more accurate picture of actual axonal loss than does the clinical examination, as there is no absolute correlation between degree of weakness and percentage of degenerating nerve fibers. Fibers which are neurapraxic will still function when stimulated distal to the site of the lesion. This evoked muscle action potential will be helpful in reassuring the patient and surgeon; in many cases, much of the weakness is neurapraxic and thus temporary. For L5 radiculopathy, stimulation of the peroneal nerve with recording over the extensor digitorum longus is used (Fig. 5.8). For the S1 nerve root, stimulation is of the tibial nerve, with

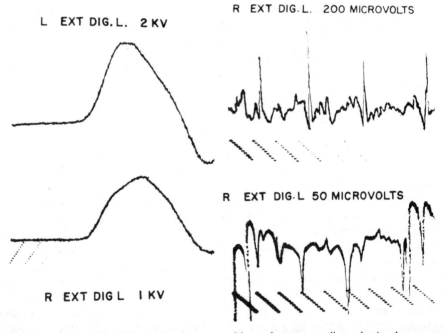

Fig. 5.8. Stimulation of peroneal nerve with surface recording electrodes over extensor digitorum longus in patient with severe L5 radiculopathy and dropped foot. Left—*top trace (L)*, uninvolved leg; *bottom trace (R)*, L5 radiculopathy dropped foot. Right—*top trace*, only one MUAP recorded in (*R*) Ext. Dig. L.; *bottom trace*, positive waves and fibrillation potentials recorded in Ext. Dig. L. (*R*).

recording over the medial gastrocnemius (20). In a series of patients with cervical radiculopathy with all patients initially treated conservatively, regardless of the severity of clinical and EMG abnormalities, there was no correlation of the degree of positive waves and fibrillation potentials to the patients that eventually came to surgery because of failure of conservative management (14). Thus, although neuronal function can be followed by serial stimulation studies, severity of EMG abnormalities on needle examination has not been shown as an indication for surgery.

EMG Postlaminectomy

The recurrence rate following surgery for lumbar disc disease has been reported from 0 to 24%. In a study of 900 patients, the occurrence rate was judged to be 4% (44). In another large series (7) in which all patients had preoperative evaluation to include a complete neurologic examination, an EMG, and a myelogram, recurrence rate was given for the various levels of disc herniation. Of patients with L5-S1 herniation, 15% had persistent sciatica, but less in severity, with no improvement in 1%. In L4,5 herniations, there was persistence of sciatica to a lesser extent than preoperatively in 15.5%, and 5.6% showed absolutely no improvement. An additional 20–30% of both the levels showed weakness of the back and continued back pain.

Knutsson (45) also demonstrated that EMG abnormalities tended to recede to a greater extent than do clinical findings. He found that sensory abnormalities depressed to absent reflexes are most likely to persist, with clinical weakness being a less common persistent abnormality. EMG abnormalities were the least likely to persist after surgery. Johnson et al. (39) found persistence of preoperative EMG abnormalities to be present as long as 3–4 years after surgery, when nerve root compromise by the herniated disc was severe.

In addition to difficulty in interpreting the clinical neurologic examination, in a postlaminectomy patient with persistence or recurrence of symptoms, the myelogram is also difficult to interpret. There is often postoperative scarrings which distort the myelogram. The EMG may show persistent abnormalities as previously noted, with the addition of the operative trauma obscuring the meaning of paraspinal findings. Weddell et al. (2) found that in 25 patients examined 3 weeks after surgery, fibrillations and lack of motor unit action potential were a consistent finding up to 3 cm from the scar. Three months after surgery, there was full motor unit recovery at 3 cm from the scar, with persistent fibrillation potentials at 1 cm from the scar. In all of these cases, self-retaining retractors were used. There was one additional case in which a hand-held retractor was used and no motor unit action potential loss was found, even in the early postoperative course. It was felt that the abnormalities were secondary to ischemia from the retractors. Mack (40) evaluated 18 patients with recurrence of low back pain 15–30 days following surgery. One-third of the patients had fibrillation potentials 5 cm lateral to the scar. He felt that the denervation may have been secondary to traction on the posterior ramus when the nerve root was retracted in removing the disc.

Blom and Lemperg (41) serially evaluated 51 patients postoperatively. At 6 weeks, all the patients had fibrillations and positive waves along the length of the scar. At 6 months, 40 of the 50 patients were examined. Seventeen of them showed no change from the 6-week examination, and 20 showed improvement, in that there was a decrease in fibrillation potentials and positive waves or there was less longitudinal extent of abnormalities. Three of the patients showed no abnormalities. At 1 year, 12 patients were examined. Ten of these showed persistent abnormalities, and in 3 there was no change from the 6-month examination. They found no correlation between the EMG paraspinal findings and the postoperative clinical course. They propose that the injury was to the posterior primary ramus, as it ran along the medial border of the paraspinals. They felt that injury occurred in all patients operated on, and more persistent abnormalities were present when the injury occurred more centrally (near the intervertebral joint). On the other hand, Aguilar (42) noted that in four patients who had postoperative symptoms of being unable to bend forward because of back weakness and having persistent back pain, there were positive waves and fibrillation potentials present at 3–4 cm lateral to the scar. Two of these patients recovered neurologically with abatement of their symptom and had a return to normal on the EMG. He evaluated seven asymptomatic patients, and in each case there was a return to normal on the EMG at 2 months postoperatively, with no abnormalities whatsoever at 3–4 cm lateral to the scar. A similar impression was reported by Johnson et al. (39) in evaluation of 60 patients with return of symptoms postoperatively. Significant findings of localized EMG abnormalities at 3 cm from the scar and 3–5 cm in depth occurred in 20 of the patients. These findings, when correlated with the clinical picture, were felt to support the diagnosis of a current radiculopathy. However, no conclusion can be based on the study of the paraspinals when diffuse abnormalities were found, even if present 3 cm from the scar (Fig. 5.9).

See and Kraft (43) described a postlaminectomy EMG in 20 asymptomatic patients. The studies were carried out from 3½ to 41 months postoperatively. Seventeen patients showed abnormalities. In four of the patients, the abnormalities were found 3 cm lateral to the scar at one level only. They determined that no conclusion may be inferred from paraspinal abnormalities in the postlaminectomy patient.

The differences in the literature regarding paraspinal findings in the postlaminectomy patients may be due to local differences in surgical technique. In any case, at this time, the electromyographer should be guided by the clinical presentation of the postlaminectomy patient and the correlation of paraspinal findings to the remainder of the EMG. If many positive waves and fibrillation potentials are found in the paraspinals with no motor unit activity present and no abnormalities present in the distribution of the

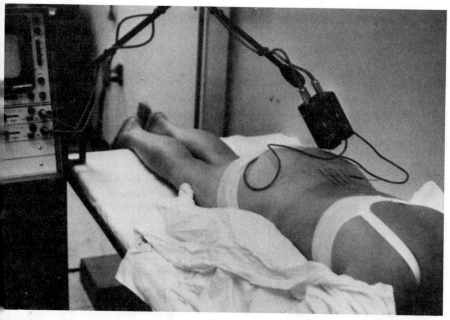

Fig. 5.9. Paraspinal area marked with lines at 1 cm and 3 cm from midline lumbar laminsectomy scar. Muscle is explored at least 3 cm lateral to scar and 4–5 cm deep.

anterior rami, it would be logical to conclude that the paraspinal findings are most likely due to the surgical trauma, even if the abnormalities are found at one level. On the other hand, in a patient with acute recurrence of symptomatology and localized paraspinal abnormalities, especially if found at a level different from a patient's previous episode of radiculopathy, this may well suggest the possibility of a new radiculopathy.

Summary

In EMG evaluation of radiculopathy, the hallmark is the finding of positive waves in a specific nerve root distribution. These abnormalities are likely to occur first in the paraspinals and may appear as early as 7 days. Prior to the occurrence of positive waves and fibrillations, polyphasic motor unit action potentials and a decreased number of motor unit action potenials may give early indication of nerve root compression. The H latency in he tibial nerve is specific for the S1 nerve root. In compression of this nerve root, there will be prolongation of the latency in the 1st day following onset.

In the management of patients with radiculopathy, the severity of abnormalities on needle EMG does not necessarily inversely correlate with the likelihood of successful conservative management. The degree of neuraraxia in patients with profound weakness can be estimated by the appropriate nerve stimulation studies. In the difficult clinical picture of a patient who has undergone a laminectomy and has recurrence of symptoms, the EMG may be the only reliable and objective method of evaluation.

REFERENCES

1. MIXTER, W. J., AND BARR, J. S.: Rupture of the intervertebral disc with involvement of the spinal canal. *N. Engl. J. Med., 211:* 210, 1934.
2. WEDDELL, G., FEINSTEIN, B., AND PATTEL, R. E.: The electrical activity of voluntary muscle in man under normal and pathological conditions. *Brain, 67:* 178, 1944.
3. SHEA, P. A., WOODS, W. W., AND WERDEN, D. H.: Electromyography in diagnosis of nerve root compression syndrome. *Arch. Neurol. Psychiat., 64:* 93, 1950.
4. CRUE, B. L., PUDENZ, R. H., AND SHELDON, C. H.: Observations on the value of clinical electromyography. *J. Bone Joint Surg., 39A:* 492, 1957.
5. BRAZIER, M. A. B., WATKINS, A. L., AND MICHELSEN, J. J.: Electromyography in differential diagnosis of ruptured cervical disc. *Arch. Neurol. Psychiat., 56:* 651, 1946.
6. WISE, C. S., AND ARDIZZONE, J.: Electromyography in intervertebral disc protrusions. *Arch. Phys. Med. Rehabil., 35:* 442, 1954.
7. KNUTSSON, B.: Comparative value of electromyographic, myelographic and clinical-neurological examinations in diagnosis of lumbar root compression syndrome. *Acta Orthop. Scand. Suppl., 49:* 1, 1961.
8. BRADDOM, R. L., AND JOHNSON, E. W.: H-Reflex: Review and classification with suggested clinical uses. *Arch. Phys. Med. Rehabil., 55:* 412, 1974.
9. MALCOLM, D. S.: A method of measuring reflex times applied in sciatica and other conditions due to nerve-root compression. *J. Neurosurg. Psychiat., 14:* 15, 1951.
10. BRADDOM, R. I., AND JOHNSON, E. W.: Standardization of "H" reflex and diagnostic use in S1 radiculopathy. *Arch. Phys. Med. Rehabil., 55:* 161, 1974.
11. BONNER, F. J., AND SCHMIDT, W. H.: Electromyography in disc disease. *Arch. Phys. Med. Rehabil., 38:* 689, 1957.
12. FLAX, H. J., BERRIOS, R., AND RIVERA, D.: Electromyography in the diagnosis of herniated lumbar disc. *Arch. Phys. Med. Rehabil., 45:* 520, 1964.
13. FLAX, H. J., BERRIOS, R., AND RIVERA, D.: Electromyographic diagnosis of herniated lumbar disc. *Bol. Asoc. Med. P. Ri., 57:* 1, 1965.
14. HONET, J. C., AND PURI, D.: Cervical radiculitis: Treatment and results in 82 patients. *Arch. Phys. Med. Rehabil., 57:* 12, 1976.
15. JOHNSON, E. W., STOCKLIN, R., AND LaRAN, M. M.: Use of electrodiagnostic examination in a university hospital. *Arch. Phys. Med. Rehabil., 46:* 573, 1965.
16. JEBSEN, R. H., AND LONG, E.: Radiculopathy and the electromyogram in disability applicants. *Arch. Phys. Med. Rehabil., 54:* 471, 1973.
17. WOODS, W. W., AND SHEA, P. A.: The value of electromyography in neurology and neurosurgery. *J. Neurosurg., 8:* 595, 1951.
18. GOODGOLD, J.: *Anatomical Correlates of Clinical Electromyography.* Baltimore: The Williams & Wilkins Co., 1974.
19. DELAGI, E. F., PEROTTO, A., IAZZETTI, J., AND MORRISON, D.: *Anatomic Guide for the Electromyographer.* Springfield, Ill.: Charles C Thomas, 1975.
20. JOHNSON, E. W. AND MELVIN, J. L.: Value of electromyography in lumbar radiculopathy. *Arch. Phys. Med Rehabil., 52:* 239, 1971.
21. GOUGH, J. G., AND KOEPKE, G. H.: Electromyographic determination of motor root levels in erector spinal muscles. *Arch. Phys. Med. Rehabil., 47:* 9, 1966.
22. MAGLADERY, J. W., TEASDALL, R. D., PARK, A. M., AND LANUGTH, H. W.: Electrophysiological studies of reflex activity in patients with lesions of the nervous system. *Bull. Johns Hopkins Hosp., 91:* 219, 1952.
23. JOHNSON, E. W., WEBER, R., AND MILLS, P.: Needle electrode stimulation in electromyography. *Arch. Phys. Med. Rehabil., 58:* 530, 1977.
24. SCHUCHMANN, J. A.: Evaluation of the H-reflex latency in radiculopathy. *Arch. Phys. Med Rehabil., 58:* 560, 1976.

25. KNUTSSON, B.: Aspects of the neurogenic electromyographic records of voluntary contraction in cases of nerve root compression. *Electromyography, 2:* 238, 1962.

26. PEIRIS, O. A.: Conduction in the fourth and fifth lumbar and first sacral nerve roots: Preliminary communication. *N. Z. Med. J., 80:* 502, 1974.

27. GRANGER, C. V., AND FLANIGAN, S.: Nerve root conduction studies during lumbar disc surgery. *J. Neurosurg., 28:* 439, 1968.

28. KNUTSSON, B.: Electromyographic studies in the diagnosis of lumbar disc herniations. *Acta Orthop. Scand., 28:* 290, 1959.

29. REYNOLDS, G. G., PAROT, A. P., AND KENRICK, M. M.: Electromyographic evaluation of patients with posttraumatic cervical pain. *Arch. Phys. Med. Rehabil., 49:* 170, 1968.

30. MARINACCI, A. A.: *Applied Electromyography.* Philadelphia: Lea & Febiger, 1968.

31. WAYLONIS, G. W.: Electromyographic findings in chronic cervical radicular syndromes. *Arch. Phys. Med. Rehabil., 49:* 407, 1968.

32. JOHNSON, E. R., POWELL, J., CALDWELL, J., AND CRANE, C.: Intercostal nerve conduction and posterior shizotomy in the diagnosis and treatment of thoracic radiculopathy. *J. Neurol. Neurosurg. Psychiat., 37:* 330, 1974.

33. LANGSTRETH, G. F., AND NEWCOMER, A. D.: Abdominal pain caused by diabetic radiculopathy. *Ann. Intern. Med., 86:* 166, 1977.

34. WATSON, R., AND WAYLONIS, G. W.: Paraspinal electromyographic abnormalities as a predictor of occult metastatic carcinoma. *Arch. Phys. Med. Rehabil., 56:* 216, 1975.

35. LA BAN, M. M., AND GRANT, A. E.: Occult spinal metastases—Early electromyographic manifestations. *Arch. Phys. Med. Rehabil., 52:* 223, 1971.

36. JACOBSON, R. E.: Lumbar stenosis—An electromyographic evaluation. *Clin. Orthop., 115:* 68, 1976.

37. WIECHERS, D., GUYTON, J. D., AND JOHNSON, E. W.; Electromyographic findings in the extensor digitorum brevis in a normal population. *Arch. Phys. Med. Rehabil., 57:* 84, 1976.

38. JOHNSON, E. W., BRADDOM, R., AND WATSON, R.: Electromyographic abnormalities after intramuscular injections. *Arch. Phys. Med. Rehabil., 52:* 250, 1971.

39. JOHNSON, E. W., BURKHART, J. A., AND EARL, W. C.: Electromyography in postlaminectomy patients. *Arch. Phys. Med. Rehabil., 53:* 407, 1972.

40. MACK, E. W.: Electromyographic observations on the postoperative disc patient. *Neurosurgery, 8:* 469, 1951.

41. BLOM, S., AND LEMPERG, R.: Electromyographic analysis of the lumbar musculature in patients operated on for lumbar rhizopathy. *J. Neurosurg., 26:* 25, 1967.

42. AGUILAR, J. A.: Denervation of the sacrospinalis muscle after laminectomy. *Am. Surg., 29:* 740, 1963.

43. SEE, D. H., AND KRAFT, G. H.: Electromyography in paraspinal muscles following surgery for root compression. *Arch. Phys. Med. Rehabil., 56:* 80, 1975.

44. EPSTEIN, J. A., LAVINE, L. S., AND EPSTEIN, B. S.: Recurrent herniation of the lumbar intervertebral disc. *Clin. Orthop., 52:* 169, 1967.

45. KNUTSSON, B.: How often do the neurological signs disappear after the operation of a herniated disc? *Acta Orthop. Scand., 32:* 352, 1962.

6

Myopathies

JOHN R. WARMOLTS, M.D.
DAVID O. WIECHERS, M.D.

Electromyographic changes in diseases regarded by custom as being myopathic result from changes in muscle fibers and surrounding connective tissue. These muscle fiber changes can be separated into five categories:

1. Muscle fiber degeneration and regeneration (e.g., as in Duchenne muscular dystrophy and polymyositis).
2. Muscle fiber enlargement and splitting (e.g., as in limb-girdle and Duchenne muscular dystrophy).

Increase in endomysial connective tissue is most prominent in conditions having these two categories of muscle fiber change.

3. Atrophy of muscle fibers with little or no fiber degeneration, excluding ordinary denervation (e.g., as in early myotonic dystrophy, type II muscle fiber atrophy).
4. Faulty muscle fiber formation or maturation (e.g., as in congenital myopathies).
5. Impaired muscle membrane excitability (e.g., as in periodic paralysis).

It is to be realized that while the conditions in which they occur are termed myopathies, the changes within muscle fibers may prove to be determined by external influences, as for example, vascular injury in polymyositis or faulty trophic neuronal influences in the congenital myopathies, or be part of a wider disturbance as in certain endocrinopathies. More than one type of change may be found within the same condition.

In this chapter, how these categories of muscle fiber and connective tissue change affect the EMG will be developed along with discussion of the clinical disease states in which they occur. As background, the first part of the chapter will develop the electrophysiologic basis of normal and abnormal motor unit potentials and patterns of motor unit discharge and recruitment and will discuss muscle fiber histochemistry and its correlation with motor unit functional behavior.

Normal Motor Unit Potential Activity

A motor unit is defined as an alpha motoneuron, its axon, and the muscle fibers it innervates and is the basic functional unit of muscle. To initiate voluntary contraction, motoneurons discharge. Each impulse rapidly sweeps down the individual axon and into its distal arborizations, where, after brief synaptic delay at the neuromuscular junctions, it triggers a self-propagating impulse in each muscle fiber that spreads from endplate in both directions to tendonous insertion. An extracellular exploratory needle tip situated in the muscle records the volume conducted electrical currents accompanying muscle fiber depolarization and repolarization as they advance upon, pass by, and recede from the probe tip. Those currents from activated muscle fibers sufficiently close to allow detection by the electrode summate algebraically to form a motor unit action potential. Depolarization of the muscle fiber membrane is followed by a twitch which contributes no electrical activity. The contractile response of each muscle fiber lasts longer than its action potential. Repetitive discharge of motoneurons permits summation of contractions if the contractile elements are reactivated before having completely relaxed. Thus, fusion of mechanical contractions produces increased tension.

Most motor unit action potentials are triphasic in configuration, with an initial positive phase, followed by a negative spike, and a terminal positive wave. Roughly 10–12% of motor unit potentials may have over three phases in normal limb muscle. Potentials from different motor units vary considerably in the relative size of each phase and in their overall amplitude, duration, and configuration (Fig. 6.1). However, the action potential of each individual motor unit is recognized by its consistency of shape and configuration on repetitive discharge, changing only when the exploratory tip is moved (Fig. 6.2).

Motor unit action potentials vary in size according to the strength of contraction, the muscle recorded from, and age of the individual. Motor unit potential measurements also depend upon the type of electrode, mode of recording and time constant of the amplifier (1). Factors influencing motor unit potential amplitude, duration, and configuration are complex and include the size of the motor neuron cell soma; scatter in conduction

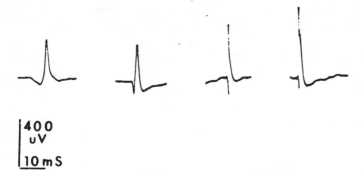

400
uV

10 mS

Fig. 6.1. Variation in size and configuration of normal motor unit potentials recorded on minimal effort from biceps.

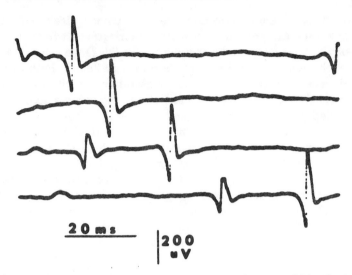

Fig. 6.2. Action potentials of different motor units are of identical shape and configuration on consecutive discharge.

velocities and lengths of arborized terminal branches of its axon; the three-dimensional expanse over which its terminal arborizations distribute; neuromuscular junction transmission time; the number, density, diameter, and propagation velocity of activated muscle fibers; conduction properties of the extracellular medium; and the distance from and geometric relationship of the exploratory tip to the fibers contributing to the composite potential (2).

Because of small delays stemming from differences in terminal branch lengths or conduction velocity and neuromuscular transmission time, muscle fibers within a motor unit are not excited simultaneously. This disparity by which membrane potentials propagate sooner down some muscle fibers may be enhanced where the neuromuscular junction lies somewhat further toward the poles of some muscle fibers than others. The net effect is that waves of current are received by the electrode tip for several milliseconds longer than from a single muscle fiber, increasing the duration of the motor unit action potential to several-fold that of a single muscle fiber action potential.

Experiments in animals have shown that muscle fibers of one motor unit do not lie grouped side by side but rather are randomly scattered over a wider area of muscle (3–5). In limb muscles, they are spread over many muscle fascicles. Fibers of the same motor unit which may lie side by side or in a small group do not exceed that expected from distribution by random chance (4). Motor units vary in their number and density of muscle fibers and in the histochemical properties of their muscle fibers (3–5). Because the amplitude of electrical signals in a conducting medium declines with increasing radial distance, a restricted number of muscle fibers in close proximity to the exploratory electrode tip are the primary contributors to the main negative spike of the motor unit potential, whereas more distant fibers contribute heavily to the lower voltage initial and terminal phases (6). Minute changes in needle tip position relative to nearby action muscle fibers especially alters the shape and complexity of the negative spike. Potentials from distant motor units have round-topped lower voltage main negative deflections.

If the needle tip is situated on the same transverse plane as the zone of endplates, the initial deflection of the motor unit potential is negative, because muscle fiber depolarization currents travel away from the recording electrode. Thus, the electrode does not "see" an advancing positive current wavefront. The terminal positive phase, however, is recorded.

Three mechanisms exist by which the force of voluntary contraction can be increased: (a) increase number of active motor units (recruitment), (b) increase discharge frequency of already active units (rate coding), and (c) activate motor units that generate greater force in preference to those that generate lesser force.

Motor units are recruited in an orderly programmed, not random, manner (7, 8). However, flexibility permits different motor units to be selected for activation according to the task. For example, smooth, low tension contraction is accomplished with different motor units than those used to initiate a sudden, large force contraction (9).

Customarily, an EMG analysis of voluntary activity begins with observing motor unit potentials activated on sustained minimal effort. During inactivity, electrical silence is maintained in normal muscle (except for "endplate noise"). During least effort, action potentials of one or more units are recorded, the number of motor units activated depending upon the closeness in firing level of the motoneurons. Each motor unit discharges at an independent frequency, reaching a relatively rhythmic, stable discharge (their action potentials may even be observed to continue firing should the subject fall asleep) (10). The asynchronous discharge of different motor units at low discharge frequencies allows a smoother summed tension to develop.

Generation of further smooth stepwise force of contraction is accomplished by an increase in firing rate of already discharging motor units and recruitment of different motor units activated at next higher thresholds. During isometric voluntary contraction in humans and laboratory animals, the order in which different motor units are sequentially recruited is fixed; the order of recruitment is reproduced on successive contractions (7). Motor unit potentials successively recruited with increasing voluntary activity tend to be of increasing amplitude, presumably reflecting an increasing number and density of muscle fibers per motor unit (8). Single motor units generating less tension are recruited at a lower threshold than those generating higher tension (11). With full effort, potentials from up to six or eight rhythmically discharging different motor units may be recorded from a single exploratory tip position in large limb muscles (10). On maximum voluntary effort, the base line is continuously interrupted by motor unit action potentials, and individual motor unit potentials can no longer be identified.

Abnormal Motor Unit Potential Activity

Motor unit action potentials may be pathologically reduced in size when (a) there is a reduction in the number and density of activated muscle fibers in a motor unit, or (b) there is a reduction in the cross-sectional area of individual muscle fibers within a motor unit. Examples of the former would be a failure of activation of a fraction of muscle fibers in a motor unit due to impaired conduction in distal neuronal arborizations within a motor unit distal axonopathy), impaired neuromuscular transmission (as in botulism, curare intoxication and myasthenia gravis), muscle membrane inexcitability (paralytic phase of periodic paralysis), and muscle fiber necrosis (pseudo-hypertrophic muscular dystrophy). Examples of pathological reduction in motor unit potential size due to smallness of viable muscle fibers include "type I fiber" smallness in myotonic atrophy, type I hypotrophy, and myotubular myopathy. Motor unit potentials are reduced in size because the amplitude of potentials of individual muscle fibers is related to the circumference of the fiber (12). Smaller potentials contributed by smaller fibers summate to smaller motor unit potentials. Proliferated fat and connective tissue and inert muscle fibers might reduce motor unit potential size by acting as intervening filters between active fibers and an exploratory electrode tip.

Because of normal variation of motor unit potentials even within the same muscle, motor unit potentials must be studied in several different areas of a given muscle before a composite estimate of mean motor unit potential size can be made. Further difficulty is introduced through the observation that pathological changes may not be uniform throughout muscle in many disease states. For example, in Duchenne dystrophy, a 5-mm cross-sectional diameter muscle biopsy may demonstrate widespread muscle fiber degeneration, whereas an immediately adjacent 5-mm diameter biopsy specimen may be comparatively uninvolved.

When the number of size of active muscle fibers in motor units is reduced, either those motor units must compensatorily fire more rapidly in order to achieve a desired tension or other motor units need to be recruited.

Conversely, motor unit potentials may be pathologically increased in size when (a) there is an increase in the number and density of muscle fibers in a motor unit, or (b) with an increase in the cross-sectional area of individual muscle fibers within a motor unit. The former may follow reinnervation through collateral sprouting. When muscle fibers become denervated through disease of their parent motor neuron, they undergo atrophy but may attract twigs from adjacent surviving motor neurons to reinnervate them. Thus, the surviving motor unit comes to contain an increased complement of more closely packed muscle fibers, contributing to a larger composite motor unit potential.

Normal motor unit potentials, as mentioned, tend to be of increasing size according to their order to recruitment. When, in a neuropathy, the motor units normally expected to be the first recruited have dropped out, recruitment of the next higher threshold, normally larger motor units in their place, may contribute a picture of enlargement of earliest recruited motor unit potentials, in this instance not due to collateral sprouting. A motor unit potential may clearly be considered pathologically large when its amplitude and/or duration exceed the topmost limits of normal for that muscle and the age of the patient. Lower degrees of enlargement may be more difficult to recognize.

Surviving muscle fibers in subjects with neuropathy may hypertrophy up to several times their normal diameter (10). Whether these fibers have retained their original innervation or have been reinnervated is unknown. Nonetheless, they may contribute larger single fiber spikes to the composite motor unit potential and thus may increase its amplitude.

An absolute increase in amplitude of the main positive-negative motor unit potential spike alone or an absolute increase in motor unit potential duration alone does not allow the conclusion, a priori, of conventional neuropathy with reinnervation. For example, muscle fibers in Duchenne dystrophy and limb-girdle dystrophy may also hypertrophy several-fold in diameter, contributing high amplitude, rapid rise time, and brief duration spikes. Conversely, in Duchenne dystrophy, muscle fiber segments presumably separated from their nerve supply by segmental necrosis of the muscle fiber may be reinnervated by slow conducting embryonic neuronal twigs, resulting in late occurring action potentials causing pathological prolongation of the motor unit potential.

As motor units drop out in neuropathies, either surviving motor units must discharge more rapidly or additional next higher threshold motor units must be recruited to achieve the desired tension. With reinnervation, this compensatory need may be in part offset.

Muscle Histochemistry

Physiological and histological (and in particular histochemical) studies have shown that motor units and their muscle fibers differ in histochemical, physiological, and biochemical properties and in their involvement by disease. Of special importance is recognition that certain neuromuscular diseases can cause changes in size or numerical preponderance in muscle fibers of one or more histochemical types without causing necrosis or phagocytosis of muscle fibers. Because conceptual analysis of EMG alterations in these diseases must take these changes into account, muscle histochemistry will be briefly reviewed.

When stained histochemically, individual muscle fibers show different degrees of coloration, but each are histochemically uniform throughout their length. A number of animal studies have demonstrated that all muscle fibers within a given motor unit are of the same histochemical type and that the histochemical characteristics are influenced by the lower motor neuron (3–5, 13).

In humans, two basic muscle fiber types are distinguished by the myofibrillar adenosine triphosphatase (ATPase) reaction at pH 9.4 (14). Fibers termed type I stain more lightly with the myofibrillar ATPase reaction and with reactions associated with glycolysis and glycogenolysis but stain more deeply with many mitochondrial oxidative enzyme reactions. Conversely, type II fibers stain more darkly with myofibrillar ATPase reaction and reactions connected to glycolysis and glycogenolysis, while staining more deeply with many mitochondrial enzyme reactions. Muscle fibers of opposite histochemical type belonging to different motor units interdigitate, giving a mosaic of histochemically staining fiber types (Fig. 6.3).

A composite of animal (8, 12, 13, 15, 16) studies and limited studies in humans (9) support a close relationship of histochemical and physiological specialization of muscle fibers to the functional role of their motor unit (13). While sufficient differences exist between species and muscles to create difficulties in extrapolation, broad assessments can be cautiously advanced.

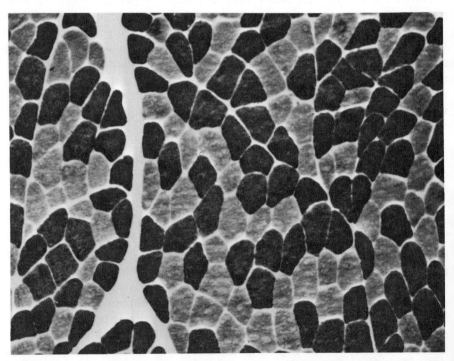

Fig. 6.3. Cross section of normal muscle showing close interdigitation of type I (light) and type II (dark) muscle fibers. Myofibrillar ATPase, pH 9.4.

Motor units containing type I fibers (Figs. 6.4 and 6.5) are discharged at lower thresholds; are capable of prolonged, slow, relatively rhythmic discharge; develop slower twitch contraction and smaller tension; and rely upon aerobic metabolism. Motor units containing type II fibers (Figs. 6.6

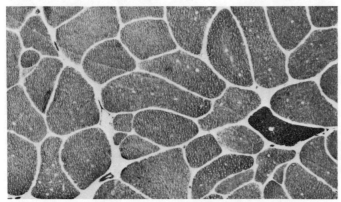

Fig. 6.4. Massive preponderance of light type I muscle fibers as the presumed consequence of collateral reinnervation in a patient with chronic low-grade motor neuropathy. Muscle fibers reinnervated by a new parent motor neuron have converted their histochemical properties to that of the original muscle fibers innervated by the motor neuron. Myofibrillar ATPase, pH 9.4.

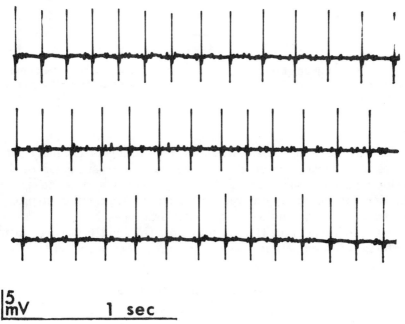

Fig. 6.5. Low frequency, rhythmic motor unit potential activated during minimal effort. Recorded by open biopsy EMG from biopsy shown in Figure 6.4.

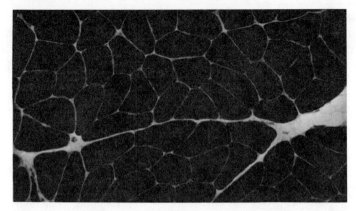

Fig. 6.6. Biopsy containing massive preponderance of dark type II muscle fibers as the presumed consequence of collateral reinnervation in a patient with chronic, low-grade neuropathy. Myofibrillar ATPase, pH 9.4.

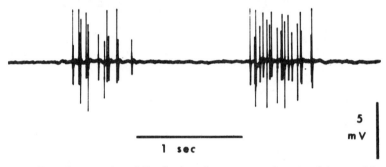

5
m V

1 sec

Fig. 6.7. Brief bursts of rapidly discharging motor unit potentials requiring maximum effort of contraction for activation. Recorded by open biopsy EMG from biopsy shown in Figure 6.6.

and 6.7) discharge at higher thresholds, require higher discharge rates to achieve stable firing frequency, are less capable of sustained discharge, develop higher tetanus fusion, fatigue more readily, and are anaerobically dependent. Motor units with overlapping mixes and gradations in properties are inferred to bridge the two basic motor unit types.

The subdivision of type II fibers into types IIA and IIB has been matched with further differentiation of physiologic properties in the cat (13), but not as yet in man.

Duchenne Muscular Dystrophy

Duchenne muscular dystrophy is both the commonest and most severe form of muscular dystrophy. It is usually transmitted as an x-linked character, with expression in males as pseudohypertrophy (particularly of calves) in 80% of cases, progressive painless proximal lower limb muscle weakness and atrophy appearing in the first 3 years of life and, later, proximal upper extremity weakness (17). Steady progression leads to wheelchair confinement by age 10; death is usually from pneumonia.

The earliest formulation of a "myopathic EMG" was drawn from this illness. In patients with disease of several years duration, EMG exploration found motor unit potentials of diminished duration and amplitude and increased polyphasicity, with a compensatory increase in discharge frequency and recruitment to achieve the effort desired (18, 19). Random loss of spike contributions from degenerating fibers near the exploratory electrode tip was considered to reduce the amplitude and fullness of the main negative spike. Loss of distant fibers subtracted from the low voltage initial and terminal positive phases; as their amplitudes decreased, their slow departure from and return to the base line became hidden in the base line, resulting in estimation of shorter motor unit potential duration (20).

Histologically, the earliest muscle changes are fibers undergoing degeneration and small groups of regenerating muscle fibers scattered through fields of normal fibers (21). A significant increase in endomysial connective tissue occurs early in the illness (22). In mildly involved muscles, statistical measurement of deviation from the norm of the duration of motor unit potentials recorded from several areas within the same muscle may be required for first recognition of EMG abnormality.

Fibers undergoing degeneration and small groups of fibers undergoing regeneration become more prominent as the illness progresses (Fig. 6.8), and the abnormal EMG pattern becomes more pervasive and easily recognized. In addition to changes following additional muscle fiber degeneration, complex alterations in motor unit action potential size and configuration are likely introduced by abnormal enlargement of some muscle fibers, by muscle fiber splitting, by reinnervation of regenerating fibers, and by con-

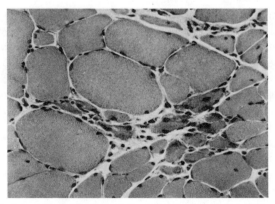

Fig. 6.8. Duchenne muscular dystrophy. Trichrome stain ×190. Abnormal variation in size of muscle fibers and a central group of small regenerating fibers. (Courtesy of Dr. Jerry R. Mendell.)

mild contraction

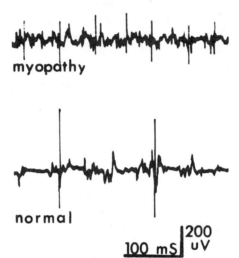

Fig. 6.9. *Upper trace*, Duchenne muscular dystrophy. Motor unit potentials of diminished size and increased discharge frequency activated during mild effort. *Lower trace*, for comparison, motor unit potentials of normal size and discharge frequency activated during minimal effort.

nective tissue proliferation. The net effect is production of shorter duration, polyphasic, lower amplitude potentials, not only of low threshold units (Fig. 6.9) but also of higher threshold units (Fig. 6.10) (although this effect becomes more difficult to judge because of overlapping potentials). However, components of motor unit potentials occurring at latencies of up to 50 msec after the main motor unit potential have been identified in Duchenne dystrophy patients using delay line techniques. These are the presumed consequences of slowly conducting collateral neuronal sprouts to sections of muscle fibers separated from their initial nerve supply by segmental necrosis or axonal sprouts innervating fibers formed from myoblasts (23). In addition, very high voltage, short duration spikes having single fiber characteristics may tower out from some motor unit potentials, probably derived from close-by hypertrophied fibers.

In far advanced disease, areas are encountered in which distal potentials only are detected, presumably conforming to areas in which only widely scattered fibers are found on biopsy, separated by markedly proliferated endomysial connective tissue and fat.

With diligent search, fibrillation potentials and positive waves may be found in at least half of Duchenne dystrophy patients. Bizzare high frequency discharges may be encountered.

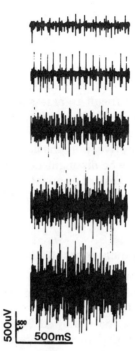

Fig. 6.10. Duchenne muscular dystrophy. Motor unit potentials activated on mild, moderate, and full effort are reduced in amplitude.

Female Duchenne dystrophy carriers may be asymptomatic or have varying degrees of proximal muscle weakness appearing from their teens to 30s. Several authors have found the presence of short duration polyphasic motor unit potentials useful in carrier detection (24–27).

Limb-Girdle Dystrophy

The term limb-girdle dystrophy encompasses a "rag-bag" group of patients who have the appearance in childhood or adult life of shoulder girdle or pelvic girdle weakness which varies greatly in severity, rate of progression, and degree of spread to other muscles. The condition may be transmitted as an autosomal recessive or appear sporadically.

The extent of findings on muscle biopsy also varies. The most striking changes are considerable variation in the size of muscle fibers, with some fibers enlarged and split and others small; frequent fibers with a motheaten or whorled internal appearance on cross section; and variable connective tissue proliferation. Necrotic and regenerating muscle fibers are a lesser feature, as compared with Duchenne dystrophy (22). Predominance of one histochemical muscle fiber type is common (22).

EMG findings are as variable as the clinical and histological features of the condition and reflect the complicated relative effect on motor unit potentials of fiber hypertrophy (contributing larger fiber spikes), smallness (contributing smaller fiber spikes), and connective tissue proliferation. Because fiber necrosis is a less dominant histological feature, it may be that loss of action potentials from necrotic fibers is a less significant factor in diminishing motor unit potential size and configuration. In mildly weak muscles of some patients, a difficult-to-assess increase in polyphasicity may be the only notable feature, and mean motor unit potential duration may remain normal. In others, and especially in weaker muscles, a focal or widespread pattern of diminutive, polyphasic, excessively rapidly discharging motor unit potentials may be distinguished. However, single or multiple higher voltage single fiber spikes are frequently encountered in medium and higher threshold motor unit potentials (10). Fibrillation, positive sharp wave, and bizzare frequency discharges are found far less commonly than in Duchenne dystrophy.

Facioscapulohumeral (FSH) Dystrophy

This less common form of muscular dystrophy is transmitted usually as an autosomal-dominant character with complete penetrance but highly variable expression. In its classical form, there is the onset in childhood or adult life of facial weakness first, followed by trapezius muscle weakness, with frequent subsequent appearance of anterior tibial weakness, and in some cases, even proximal lower extremity weakness. The disease is very slowly progressive, sometimes, however, punctuated by brief periods of rapid progression. Life span is not usually shortened. In many patients, weakness is quite mild and remains restricted to one or more muscle groups for years (17). Asymmetrical involvement is common. Modest serum muscle enzyme elevation is found in half of patients.

Biopsy abnormalities vary but are less prominent than in Duchenne or limb-girdle dystrophy. In some patients, scattered necrotic or regenerating fibers are found in mildly affected muscles. In other patients occasional scattered atrophic dark angular fibers (resembling denervated fibers) are found, at times in addition to the necrotic fibers, or at other times by themselves (22, 28). Type grouping is not observed.

In clinically weak muscles, EMG abnormalities may sometimes be meager. When the composite pattern is sufficiently abnormal to be recognized, it is on the basis of motor unit potentials of decreased duration, diminished amplitude, and increased polyphasicity. Despite the distribution of abnormality implied in the name of the disease, patients may have the most prominent EMG abnormality in anterior tibial muscle. Fibrillation and positive sharp waves have been described (29). The presence and degree of EMG abnormalities can vary considerably within different areas or different heads of the same muscle and between homologous muscles.

Because weakness in an FSH distribution may indeed be the result of differing pathogeneses, the term FSH syndrome may be preferable (30).

Polymyositis and Dermatomyositis

Polymyositis and dermatomyositis may appear at any age, most typically with symmetrical proximal limb weakness, which is often accompanied by muscle pain, tenderness, and swelling. Weakness may extend to involve facial muscles, muscles of deglutition, and distal limb muscles. Deep tendon reflexes are preserved relative to weakness; sensation remains uninvolved. The disease may be mild and evolve slowly or follow a rapidly progressive tempo. Associated skin manifestations in dermatomyositis are violaceous discoloration of the eyelids, telangiectasis over knuckles, and erythema over knees, elbows, and at times over face, neck, and chest.

Histologically, degeneration and phagocytosis of muscle fibers and regenerating muscle fibers are expected in polymyositis and dermatomyositis (22). In addition, "perifascicular atrophy" (Fig. 6.11), which consists of large numbers of small, probably regenerating, neighboring fibers confined to the periphery of muscle bundles or fascicles (felt to follow ischemic changes in muscle secondary to disease in blood vessels (31, 32), may be found, particularly in dermatomyositis. Muscle fiber hypertrophy is not commonly found.

On an EMG recording in resting muscle, fibrillation potentials, positive sharp waves, and bizzare high frequency discharges may be found, typically with ease, and at times in profusion.

On voluntary contraction in mildly affected patients, motor unit potentials of variably diminished amplitude and duration and increased polyphasia may be identified focally in muscle, while 5–10 m transversely the voluntary record may be quite normal. With more advanced involvement, the finding of polyphasic potentials of reduced size and increased discharge frequency becomes more widespread and uniform (Fig. 6.12). The increased motor unit

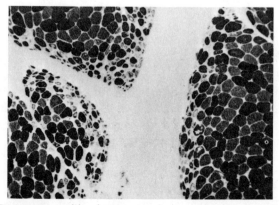

Fig. 6.11. Dermatomyositis. Large numbers of small, probably regenerating, muscle fibers confined to the periphery of muscle fascicles. Myofibrillar ATPase stain, pH 9.4, ×65. (Courtesy of Dr. Jerry R. Mendell.)

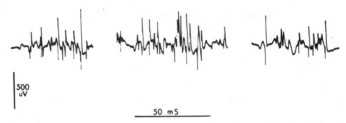

500
uV

50 mS

Fig. 6.12. Polymyositis. Excessively recruited motor unit potentials of abnormally short duration activated during mild contraction of moderately severely involved muscle.

potential discharge frequency and polyphasia contribute a richer pattern of spikes that may lead to full interference on less than full effort.

Degeneration of muscle fibers at random within motor units would subtract distant and near single fiber spike contributions, diminishing the size and increasing polyphasicity of composite motor unit potentials. Conversely, what role the presumably regenerating adjacent muscle fibers at the periphery of muscle fascicles or bundles might have in shaping motor unit potentials cannot be forecast at this time. For example, it is not known whether they are even under neural control. Subsequent connective tissue proliferation might further alter the motor unit potentials.

In far advanced involvement, a reduced number of motor unit potentials relative to effort may be recorded, presumably reflecting depopulation of muscle fibers within motor units to the point where their motor unit potentials cannot be distinguished. Improvement in clinical strength, either spontaneously or with corticosteroid therapy, may not be accompanied by improvement in the EMG record. The EMG in patients with polymyositis and dermatomyositis in association with cancer does not differ in its essentials from (dermato) polymyositis without cancer (10).

Myotonic Dystrophy

Myotonic dystrophy is a dominantly inherited multisystem disease, two features of which are (a) slowly progressive weakness and wasting of masseter, temporalis, sternocleidomastoid, and distal greater than proximal extremity muscles, and (b) delayed muscle relaxation following stimulation or voluntary contraction. Frontal balding, ptosis, early cataracts, gonadal atrophy, abnormal glucose and gamma-globulin metabolism (33), abnormal endocrine functions, and cardiac conduction defects are commonly present. Although typically presenting in adolescent or adult life, the condition may be present in infancy or childhood (34).

Characteristic early biopsy changes, particularly conspicuous in biceps brachii, are atrophy of type I muscle fibers (Fig. 6.13) and hypertrophy of type II fibers, with little evidence of degeneration in fibers of either type (9, 35).

In early stage myotonic dystrophy, numerous motor unit potentials acti-

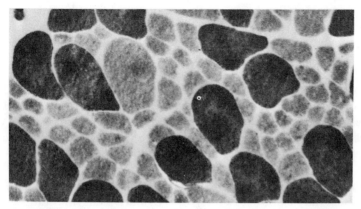

Fig. 6.13. Myotonic dystrophy. Atrophy selectively involving light type I fibers in biceps muscle. Myofibrillar ATPase, pH 9.4, ×160.

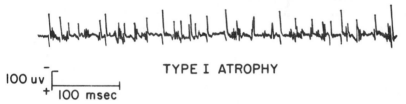

TYPE I ATROPHY

100 uv ⌐
⌐
+ 100 msec

Fig. 6.14. Motor unit potentials of diminutive size recorded during mild effort by open biopsy EMG from biopsy shown in Figure 6.13.

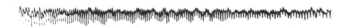

Fig. 6.15. Myotonia. Decline in frequency and amplitude of potentials of muscle fiber origin. 500 ms.

vated on mild effort may be pathologically diminutive even in normal strength muscles. By open biopsy EMG, motor unit potentials of very low voltage and short duration (Fig. 6.14) have been consistently recorded in vivo during mild contraction from biopsies demonstrating type I atrophy without fiber degeneration (9). In patients with early myotonic dystrophy where open biopsy EMG has failed to disclose pathologically small, low threshold motor unit potentials, type I fibers have been of normal size (9).

Myotonic discharges can be electrically recorded in numerous muscles, including facial, tongue, and intercostal, as well as proximal and distal limb muscles. The discharges are most exuberant in hand muscles. Myotonic discharges are made up of repetitive wave forms of similar configuration on consecutive discharge that may resemble fibrillation, positive sharp (Fig. 6.15), or even larger, sometimes bizzare, shaped potentials. These are evoked by needle movement, muscle percussion, or repetitive nerve stimulation.

An individual volley begins with a sputtering of potentials of like form which increase rapidly in frequency then trail off in a gradual clear decline in frequency and decrease in amplitude. Their muscle fiber origin is shown by persistence despite curarization. Microelectrode recording of prepotentials before each spike of the myotonic volley demonstrates that the discharge arises at the electrode tip and provides evidence for local muscle membrane hyperexcitability to mechanical stimulation (36). Several different crescendo-decrescendo volleys of potentials may overlap, some creasing their discharge before others. The intensity of myotonia is enhanced by cold exposure and diminished after a "warm-up" of repeated voluntary contractions of the muscle.

In muscle biopsies from more advanced cases, groups of small angular fibers, which may stain excessively with oxidative enzyme stains, clumps of pyknotic nuclei, and mild endomysial connective tissue increase are found, still with meager fiber necrosis and phagocytosis. These changes are reminiscent of those found in conventional neuropathy (2). With advance in illness, the EMG finding of lowered amplitude, shortened duration potentials becomes more florid. Open biopsy EMG correlation studies on such cases have not been published.

Myotonia Congenita

Myotonia congenita is an inherited neuromuscular disorder (either antosomal dominant or autosomal recessive), featuring myotonia of a more burdening degree than in myotonic dystrophy and overgrowth of musculature. The muscle weakness and atrophy and multisystem abnormalities seen in myotonic dystrophy are not present. Changes on muscle biopsy are limited to occasional small angulated fibers (22).

By EMG, myotonia is usually more exuberant and in wider distribution than in myotonic dystrophy. Repetitive contraction or warming of muscle lessens the myotonia and permits better analysis of the voluntary record. Unless obscured by myotonic discharges, voluntary motor unit potentials are of normal size and configuration and are normally recruited on graduated effort.

Congenital Myopathies

Within recent years a group of uncommon neuromuscular disorders which are present at birth, frequently inherited, and nonprogressive or slowly progressive have been identified through the use of muscle biopsy. Specifically lacking necrosis or phagocytosis in muscle fibers on one hand and changes resembling ordinary neuropathy on the other, the conditions were regarded as being "myopathic" on the basis of distinguishing histologic pecularities within muscle fibers. The finding of myopathic EMG patterns lent substantiation.

The group of congenital myopathies for which EMG findings have been delineated include central core disease, nemaline (rod) disease, and myotubular myopathy. These conditions are regarded as resulting from faulty muscle fiber maturation in utero. Increasing appreciation of the role of neural influence of muscle fiber maturation has focused recent attention on the potential pathogenetic role of faulty trophic influence of nerve on muscle in these conditions (37). To facilitate communication, however, these conditions will be discussed under their historical designation as myopathies.

CENTRAL CORE DISEASE

This dominantly inherited condition features a mild, generally nonprogressive proximal weakness that is present from infancy (38). Histologically, muscle fibers contain cores characterized histochemically by the lack of phosphorylase and mitochondrial oxidative enzyme activity (39) and which stain poorly with the myofibrillar ATPase reaction at pH 9.4 when unstructured or deeply when structured (40). Cores are usually confined to type I fibers, which may be of normal or reduced diameter (Figure 6.16). In some biopsies, core fibers have been interspersed among normal size type II fibers. Other biopsies have demonstrated a predominance of type I fibers (22).

In two patients we have studied, motor unit potentials were normal in size and configuration, even in mildly weak muscles, but were recruited in increased number and had an increased discharge frequency per effort exerted (10). In a third patient, the motor unit potentials were abnormal only in being highly polyphasic and excessively, richly recruited. To explain this, it is plausible to consider that these patients had low threshold motor units containing normal sized fibers in normal distribution permitting motor unit potentials to be normal size and shape. However, their muscle fiber cores being mechanically inert would thus develop less tension, requiring compensatory excessive recruitment and discharge rates to achieve desired tensions.

In cases where type I fibers with cores are diminished in size, diminished size of low threshold motor unit potentials, with further excessive recruitment and discharge rates, would be anticipated. Fibrillation, sharp poten-

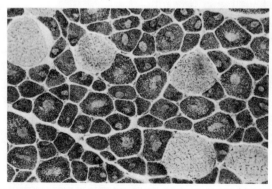

Fig. 6.16. Central core disease. NADH-trichrome stain. Cores are present in small dark staining type I fibers. ×140. (Courtesy of Dr. Jerry R. Mendell.)

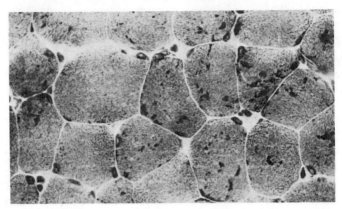

Fig. 6.17. Rod disease. Rod-like structures in muscle fibers. Trichrome stain.

tials, and other types of abnormal discharges at rest have not been found in central core disease.

ROD DISEASE

Rod disease is characterized by aggregations of rod-like structures in muscle fibers (41–43) (Fig. 6.17). Rod disease may be congenital with nonprogressive or slowly progressive weakness or severe weakness and atrophy. Rod disease has had a late onset in two cases (44, 45). Both sporadic and probably dominantly inherited cases are reported (22). Histochemically, rods may selectively be present in type I fibers (43, 46) or in type II fibers (42) or both without preference. In many cases there has been a marked, sometimes almost universal presence of type I fibers (9). Type I fibers may be of small or of normal diameter and configuration (9, 46). In other cases type II fibers have been found to be either small or large (46). The rod-like structures do not stain with histochemical enzyme reactions or the ATPase reaction, appearing as clear areas in the fibers (42). Muscle fiber degeneration is usually not present.

EMG findings vary as well. Silence is maintained during inactivity. Motor unit action potentials recruited on low threshold effort were found in one patient to be normal in size, configuration, recruitment, and discharge frequency (Fig. 6.18) when recorded from the biopsy site (by open biopsy EMG) of a normal strength limb muscle containing massive preponderance of type I muscle fibers (Fig. 6.19), many containing rods (9). In another case, motor unit potentials of diminutive duration, amplitude, and increased discharge frequency per effort were recorded in weak muscles (10). It is considered likely that the low threshold motor unit potentials of reduced size, where seen, reflect either a small diameter of type I muscle fibers within those motor units, or, alternately, fewer muscle fibers present in type I motor units due to faulty motor unit development (30).

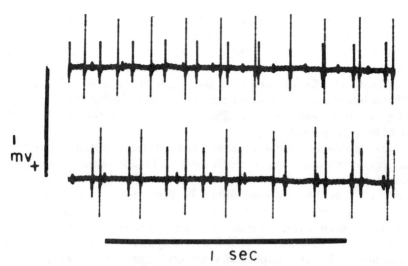

Fig. 6.18. Rod disease. Massive preponderance of light type I muscle fibers, which are of normal size. Myofibrillar ATPase stain, pH 9.4.

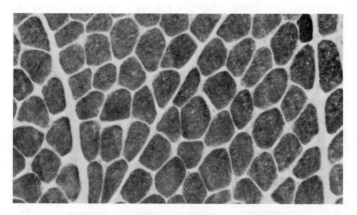

Fig. 6.19. Rod disease. Motor unit potentials of normal size, discharge frequency, and recruitment recorded on mild effort by open biopsy EMG from biopsy pictured in Figure 6.18.

MYOTUBULAR MYOPATHY

Myotubular myopathy presents a varied clinical disorder, either with nonprogressive or slowly progressive weakness, rarely proving fatal, appearing in infancy, late childhood, or adult life (47–51). Ptosis and external ophthalmoparesis are often present.

Muscle biopsy reveals from one to several centrally placed nuclei in muscle fibers of either histochemical fiber type. In the zones around nuclei, oxidative enzyme activity may be heightened or diminished (Fig. 6.20) and myofibrillar ATPase staining absent (47). In some cases, fibers have been predominantly type I, and type I fibers may be small.

Electromyographically, fibrillation and positive sharp potentials and myotonic discharges have been reported in proximal and distal muscles in several cases (47, 51). Motor unit potentials of short duration and low amplitude have been reported in a greater number of cases. The presence of activity in resting muscle distinguishes this entity from the other described types of congenital myopathy.

By open biopsy EMG, we have recorded fibrillation potentials in myotubular myopathy from a biopsy which contained predominantly type I fibers which were of reduced diameter but had no conventional evidence of denervation (angular, atrophic fibers) or fiber necrosis, and we wonder whether these fibrillation potentials originated from a fraction of muscle fibers that never received innervation during development. From this biopsy, motor unit potentials, many of which were polyphasic, and all of which were reduced in duration and amplitude, were discharging excessively rapidly for the degree of effort exerted (Fig. 6.21) Small diameter fibers contributing small single fiber spikes to the composite motor unit potential and generating less tension per fiber (therefore requiring more rapid motor unit discharge to increase summated tension), and perhaps a developmentally depleted number of fibers per motor unit, are considered to account for these findings (52).

Type II Atrophy

Preferential atrophy of type II muscle fibers is found in diverse conditions as disuse, inanition, and chronic steroid intoxication and occurs as an early systemic manifestation of malignancy (Fig. 6.22). Open biopsy EMG studies on strong limb muscles in patients with nonmetastatic malignancy and anorexia nervosa have consistently shown that mild to moderately severe diffuse type II atrophy in the biopsy specimen may be accompanied by no

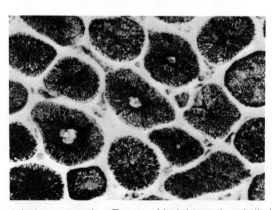

Fig. 6.20. Myotubular myopathy. Zones of heightened and diminished oxidative enzyme activity around central nuclei. NADH-trichrome stain, ×340.

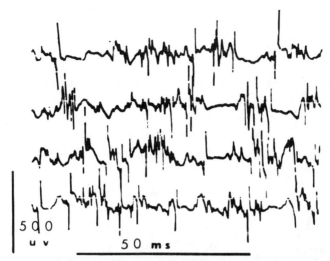

Fig. 6.21. Myotubular myopathy. Excessively rapidly discharging polyphasic motor unit potentials of reduced duration and amplitude. Recorded by open biopsy EMG from biopsy containing predominantly type I fibers which were of reduced diameter.

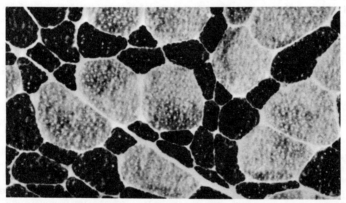

Fig. 6.22. Atrophy preferentially involving dark type II fibers. Myofibrillar ATPase, pH 9.4.

recognizable abnormality or only failure to achieve full interference on maximal voluntary effort. Specifically the first, second and third recruited motor unit potentials remain unaltered in size and configuration, recruitment, and discharge frequency as a function of effort (9, 52, 53). These are considered reflect normal first recruited type I motor units.

Hypokalemic Periodic Paralysis

During evolution of weakness in an attack, muscle fiber external membranes become electrically inexcitable on a seemingly random distribution within motor units. Attacks may be induced by administration of carbohydrate and insulin and followed electromyographically. Before eventually disappearing, motor unit action potentials become increasingly briefer in duration, lower in amplitude, and polyphasic. The potentials of some motor units decrease in size or disappear before others. With increasing weakness, the compound muscle action potential evoked by stimulating the nerve trunk to the muscle diminishes in size (54).

REFERENCES

1. GULD, C., ROSENFALCK, A., AND WILLISON, R. G.: Technical factors in recording electrical activity of muscle and nerve in man. *Electroencephalogr. Clin. Neurophysiol., 28:* 399, 1970.
2. WARMOLTS, J. R., AND ENGEL, W. K.: A critique of the "Myopathic" electromyogram. *Trans. Am. Neurol. Assoc., 95:* 173, 1970.
3. EDSTROM, L., AND KUGELBERG, E.: Histochemical composition, distribution of fibers and fatigability of single motor units. *J. Neurol. Neurosurg. Psychiat., 31:* 424, 1969.
4. BRANSTATER, M. E., AND LAMBERT, E. H.: A histological study of the spatial arrangement of muscle fibers in single motor units within rat tibialis anterior muscle. *Bull. Am. Assoc. Electromyogr. Electrodiag., 15–16:* 82, 1969.
5. DOYLE, A. M., AND MAYER, R. F.: Studies of the motor unit in the cat. *Bull. Sch. Med. Univ. Md., 54:* 11, 1969.
6. ROSENFALCK, P.: *Intra and Extracellular Potential Fields to Active Nerve and Muscle Fibers*, Copenhagen: Akadmisk Forlag, 1969.
7. GRIMBY, L., AND HANNERZ, J.: Recruitment order of motor units on voluntary contraction: Changes induced by afferent activity. *J. Neurol. Neurosurg. Psychiat., 21:* 565, 1968.
8. OLSON, C. R., CARPENTER, D. O., AND HENNEMAN, E.: Orderly recruitment of muscle action potentials, motor unit threshold and EMG amplitude. *Arch. Neurol., 19:* 591, 1968.
9. WARMOLTS, J. R., AND ENGEL, W. K.: Open-biopsy electromyography. 1. Correlation of motor unit behaviour with histochemical muscle fiber type in human limb muscle. *Arch. Neurol., 27:* 512, 1972.
10. WARMOLTS, J. R.: Unpublished data.
11. MILNER-BROWN, H. S., STEIN, R. B. AND YEMMA, R.: The orderly recruitment of human motor units during voluntary isometric contractions. *J. Physiol., 230:* 359, 1973.
12. HAKANNSON, C. H.: Conduction velocity are amplitude of the action potential as related to circumference in the isolated fiber of frog muscle. *Acta Physiol. Scand., 37:* 14, 1956.
13. BURKE, R. E., AND TSAIRIS, P.: The correlation of physiological propertes with histochemical characteristics in single motor units. *Ann. N.Y. Acad. Sci., 228:* 145, 1974.
14. ENGEL, W. K.: The essentiality of histo- and cytochemical studies of skeletal muscle in the investigation of neuromuscular disease. *Neurology, 12:* 778, 1962.
15. HENNEMAN, E., AND OLSON, C. B.: Relations between structure and function in the design of skeletal muscle. *J. Neurophysiol. 28:* 581, 1965.
16. WUERKER, R. B., McPHEDRAN, A. M., AND HENNEMAN, E.: Properties of motor units in a heterogeneous pale muscle (M. gastrocnemics of the cat.). *J. Neurophysiol., 28:* 85, 1965.
17. WALTON, J. N.: Muscular dystrophy (clinical, genetic, and pathological aspects). In *Biochemical Aspects of Neurological Disorders*, pp. 1–27, ed. by John N. Cummings and Michael Kremer. Philadelphia: F. A. Davis Co., 1965.
18. KUGELBERG, E.: Electromyography in muscular dystrophies. *J. Neurol. Neurosurg. Psychiat., 12:* 129, 1949.
19. PINELLI, P., AND BUCHTHAL, F.: Muscle action potentials in myopathies with special regard to progressive muscular dystrophy. *Neurology, 3:* 347, 1952.
20. BUCTHAL, F., ROSENFALCK, P., AND ERMINIO, F.: Motor unit territory and fiber density in myopathies. *Neurology, 10:* 398, 1960.

21. MENDELL, J. R., ENGEL, W. K., AND DERRER, E. C.: Duchenne muscular dystrophy. Functional ischemic reproduces its characteristic lesion. *Science, 172:* 1143, 1971.
22. DUBOWITZ, V., AND BROOKE, M. H.: *Muscle Biopsy: A Modern Approach.* Philadelphia: W. B. Saunders Co., 1973.
23. DESMEDT, J. E., AND BORENSTEIN, S.: Regeneration in Duchenne muscular dystrophy: Electromyographic evidence. *Arch. Neurol., 33:* 642, 1976.
24. DESMEDT, J. E., AND BORENSTEIN, S.: Spontaneous fibrillation potentials in human muscular dystrophy: Relation to muscle fiber segmentation. *Nature, 258:* 531, 1975.
25. VAN DEN BOSCH, J., GARDNER-MEDWIN, D., AND HAUSMANOWA-PETRUSEWICZ, I.: Investigation of the carrier state in the Duchenne type of dystrophy. *Proceedings, 2nd Symp. Research in Muscular Disease,* pp. 23–30, London: Pittman Medical Publishers, 1963.
26. HAUSMANOWA-PETRUSEWICZ, I., PROT, J., MJEBROJ-DOBOSZ, I., EMERY, B., WASOWICZ, B., SLUCKA, C., HETNARAKA, L., BONDARZEWAKA, B., AND PUZEK, Z.: Investigations of healthy relatives of patients with Duchenne type dystrophy. *Excerpta Med. Int. Congr. Ser.,* No. 94, Abstract 210, pp. 635–637, 1965.
27. GARDNER-MEDWIN, D.: Studies of the carrier state in the Duchenne type of muscular dystrophy. 2. Quantitatlve electromyography as a method of carrier detection. *J. Neurol. Neurosurg. Psychiat., 31:* 124, 1968.
28. ENGEL, W. K., AND WARMOLTS, J. R.: Multiplicity of muscle changes postulated from motoneuron abnormalities. In *Muscle Biology,* pp. 229–253, ed. by R. G. Cassens, New York: Marcel Decker, Inc., 1972.
29. MUNSAT, T. L., PIPER, P., CANCILLA, P., AND MEDNICK, J.: Inflammatory myopathy with facio-scapulo-humeral distribution. *Neurology, 22:* 335, 1973.
30. ENGEL, W. K., AND WARMOLTS, J. R.: The motor unit: Diseases affecting it in toto or in portio. In *New Developments in EMG and Clinical Neurophysiology,* vol. 1, pp. 144–177, ed. by J. E. Desmedt, Basel, Switzerland: S. Karger, 1973.
31. BANKER, B. Q.: Dermatomyositis of childhood. *Trans. Am. Neurol. Assoc., 87:* 11, 1962.
32. WHITAKER, J. N., AND ENGEL, W. K.: Vascular deposits of immunoglobulin and complement in idiopathic inflammatory myopathy. *N. Engl. J. Med., 286:* 333, 1971.
33. ENGEL, W. K., McFARLIN, D. E., DREWS, G. A., AND WOCHNER, R. D.: Protein abnormalities in neuromuscular disease—Part 1. *J. A. M. A., 195:* 754, 1966.
34. DODGE, P. R., GAMSTORP, I., BYERS, R. K., AND RUSSEL, P.: Myotonic dystrophy in infancy and childhood. *Pediatrics, 35:* 3, 1965.
35. BROOKE, M. K., AND ENGEL, W. K.: The histographic analysis of human muscle biopsies with regard to fiber types. 3. Myotonias, myasthenia gravis, and hypokalemic periodic paralysis. *Neurology, 19:* 469, 1969.
36. McCOMAS, A. J., AND MROZEK, K.: The electrical properties of muscle fiber membranes in dystrophica myotonia or myotonia congenita, *J. Neurol. Neurosurg. Psychiat., 31:* 441, 1968.
37. ENGEL, W. K., AND WARMOLTS, J. R.: New concepts on the possible role of motoneuron abnormalities in neuromuscular disorder not usually considered neurogenic. In *Proceedings 2nd Journees Int. De Marseille,* pp. 19–34, ed. by Sarratice & Roux, Expansion Scientifique Francais, Paris, 1971.
38. SHY, G. M., AND MAGEE, K. R.: A new congenital nonprogressive myopathy. *Brain, 79:* 610, 1956.
39. DUBOWITZ, V., AND PEARCH, A. G. E.: Oxidative enzymes and phosphorylase in central core disease of muscle. *Lancet, 20:* 23, 1960.
40. NEVILLE, H. E., AND BROOKE, M. H.: Central core fibers: Structured and unstructured. International Congress on Muscle Diseases, Perth, Australia. *Excepta Med. Int. Congr. Ser. 237.* (Abstract), 1971.
41. SHY, G. M., ENGEL, W. K., SOMERS, J. E., AND WANKO, T.: Nemaline myopathy. A new congenital myopathy. *Brain, 86:* 793, 1963.
42. ENGEL, W. K., WANKO, T., AND FENICHEL, G. M.: Nemaline myopathy, a second case. *Arch. Neurol., 1:* 22, 1964.

43. GONATAS, J. G., SHY, G. M., AND GODFREY, E. H.: Nemaline myopathy. *N. Engl. J. Med.,* *274:* 535, 1966.
44. ENGEL, A. J.: Late onset rod myopathy. (A new syndrome?) Light and electronmicroscopic observations in 2 cases. *Mayo Clin. Proc., 41:* 713, 1966.
45. ENGEL, W. K., AND RESNICK, J. S.: Late onset rod myopathy. A newly recognized, acquired, & progressive disease. *Neurology, 16:* 308, 1966.
46. ENGEL, W. K.: Selective and nonselective susceptibility of muscle fiber types: A new approach to human neuromuscular diseases. *Arch. Neurol. 22:* 97, 1970.
47. SPIRO, A. J., SHY, C. M., AND GONATAS, N. K.: Myotubular myopathy, *Arch. Neurol., 14:* 1, 1966.
48. BETHLEM, J., MEIJER, A. E. F. H., SCHELLENS, J. P. M., AND VROOM, J. J.: Centronuclear myopathy. *Eur. Neurol., 1:* 325, 1968.
49. VAN WIJNGAARDEN, G. K., FLEURY, P., BETHLEM, J., AND MEIJER, A. E. F. H.: Familial "myotubular" myopathy. *Neurology, 19:* 901, 1969.
50. CAMPBELL, J. J., REBEIZ, J. J., AND WALTON, J. N.: Myotubular, centronuclear, or pericentronuclear myopathy? *J. Neurol. Sci., 8:* 425, 1969.
51. MUNSAT, T. L., THOMPSON, L. R., AND COLEMAN, R. F.: Centronuclear ("myotubular") myopathy. *Arch. Neurol., 20:* 120, 1969.
52. WARMOLTS, J. R., AND MENDELL, J. R.: Unpublished data.
53. WARMOLTS, J. R., RE, P. K., LEWIS, R. J., AND ENGEL, W. K.: Type II atrophy: An early systemic manifestation of cancer. *Neurology, 25:* 374, 1975.
54. SHY, M. G., WANKO, T., ROWLEY, P. T., AND ENGEL, A. G.: Studies in familial periodic paralysis. *Exp. Neurol., 3:* 53, 1961.

7

Anterior Horn Cell Diseases

DAVID O. WIECHERS, M.D.
JOHN R. WARMOLTS, M.D.

Neurophysiology and Pathophysiology

Motor neuropathies refer to any disorder directly affecting the motor unit, excluding those disorders which specifically are believed to be the result of muscle fiber abnormalities. Neuropathies may affect principally the motor neuron, the axon and/or its nerve sheath, the terminal nerve branches to specific muscle fibers, or the myoneural junction. If the motor neuron or axon is sufficiently affected by the disease state, a shutdown of the entire motor unit occurs. With involvement of the myelin sheath, slowing in conduction and possibly complete blockage of impulse conduction results. If the disease process attacks the terminal nerve branches, a dropout of individual muscle fibers is seen that may make EMG differentiation from a myopathy difficult. Abnormalities of the myoneural junction result in difficulty in transmitting the impulse from a distal neuron to the individual muscle fibers. In this chapter, the focus will be principally on those conditions that are felt to affect primarily the motor neuron, or anterior horn cell.

Many different types of disorders affect the motor neuron, or anterior horn cell. The motor neuron can be compromised by a vascular insult, infection, mechanical compression, direct trauma, and/or injury. There are disease states or syndromes that preferentially affect the motor neuron, some of which follow genetic patterns. The EMG findings in these disorders affecting the motor neuron, or anterior horn cell, are all essentially identical. There are no specific EMG findings or pathonomonic potentials that are diagnostic of any disorder affecting the motor neuron, or anterior horn cell.

When the motor neuron is sufficiently affected, its physiologic functions are lost and the cell becomes unexcitable. As a result of motor neuron inexcitability, there is a dropout of individual motor units. If the number of motor neurons, and therefore motor units, affected in a muscle is significant, clinically muscle weakness is detected. The location and number of motor neurons affected determine the clinical presentation of the motor neuron disease. Since usually there is no sensory nerve involvement, the early hallmark of motor neuron disease is painless weakness. With a basic understanding of some of the concepts of neurophysiology and pathophysiology of the motor unit in these disorders, the classical EMG findings listed below are better understood:

1. Decreased number of recruited motor unit action potentials per strength of contraction.
2. Fasciculation potentials.
3. Positive sharp waves and fibrillation potentials.
4. Motor unit action potentials of increased amplitude and duration and phasicity.

Anatomically, all motor neurons are not alike (1, 2). Variations in size have been noted. Smaller anterior horn cells have been shown to have smaller diameter axons and are presumed to subsequently innervate fewer individual muscle fibers than do larger motor neurons.

Physiologically, the motor neuron is not completely understood. Motor neurons are known to have different physiologic properties (2, 3). Smaller anterior horn cells have smaller diameter axons, innervate a fewer number of muscle fibers, and are felt to have a lower threshold of excitation (4). Larger motor neurons have larger diameter axons and innervate a larger number of muscle fibers. These larger-sized motor neurons are felt to have a higher threshold of excitation. This variation in excitability is demonstrated clinically by the gradation in recruitment of normal motor units with increasing strength of contraction.

In man, there are currently felt to be two basic histochemical muscle fiber types determined by ATPase staining at pH 9.4 and, therefore, two basic motor neuron types (5). Animal studies suggest that all muscle fibers belonging to a specific motor neuron are of the same histochemical type. Type I muscle fibers are rich in oxidative enzymes; their motor units contract at slower rates with less tension produced than do type II units (6). Type I units are resistant to fatigue. Type I units are recorded electromyographically under minimal to moderate contraction strength. Type II units fire in rapid bursts and fatigue rapidly. They are recorded electromyographically when a maximum or sudden vigorous contraction is produced.

Early in some disease processes, there may be indiscriminate involvement of low or high threshold motor units. If high threshold motor units are first affected, normal firing and recruitment of lower threshold motor units with a dropout of higher threshold units under increasing strengths of contraction are recorded. If only low threshold motor units of low amplitude are affected, with increasing strength of contraction, a rapid recruitment of larger, higher threshold motor units are those first observed. Therefore, if first recruited motor unit potentials are larger than expected, it does not necessarily represent reinnervation by collateral sprouting.

Fasciculation potentials are the spontaneous synchronous discharges of some or of all muscle fibers of a motor unit. They almost always accompany disorders affecting the motor neuron, such that one is reluctant to accept the diagnosis in their absence. Fasciculations are classified by their shape—simple or complex. Complex fasciculation potentials may be highly polyphasic, long duration, and low amplitude and may be seen in reinnervative states; repetitive discharge types (iterative) seen in alkalotic states; and the large amplitude, increased polyphasic potentials often seen in anterior horn cell diseases. Simple fasciculation potentials may be normal appearing motor unit potentials or so-called "malignant" fasciculations which are tiny, short, duration-simple fasciculation potentials thought by some to be more frequent in amyotrophic lateral sclerosis.

In motor unit diseases, the fasciculation potentials may vary in amplitude and shape, since myoneural junctional transmission failure or blocking at terminal axon sprouting sites may occur on repeated activation.

Fasciculations occur normally, especially in anxious medical students who are studying motor neuron disease for the first time. The differentiation of benign fasciculations from those associated with disease of the motor neuron is best determined by the history, the physical, and associated EMG findings.

The occurrence of fasciculation potentials following spinal anesthesia, nerve section, and nerve block has led to the belief that they are mainly of peripheral motor nerve origin (7–9). The size of the fasciculation potential reflects the size of the motor unit from which it is generated. They may possibly represent the retrograde firing of a motor unit with the generator potential arising from the terminal axon. With the advancement of motor neuron disease, the occurrence of extremely large polyphasic fasciculation potentials has led many investigators to believe that these potentials were characteristic. An extensive study of polyphasic fasciculation potentials by Trojaborg and Buchthal (10) in pathologic and benign conditions disproved their specificity. They did, however, report that the frequency of firing of fasciculation potentials in motor neuron disease was decreased, as compared to benign conditions. They reported a firing frequency of 3/10 sec in motor neuron disease as compared to 1/sec in benign conditions. Other electromyographers have noted that the fasciculation potentials occurring in motor disease cannot be voluntarily controlled as they sometimes can be in other conditions (11).

When a motor neuron is destroyed, a process of degeneration progresses all along the motor unit. Each individual muscle fiber has one point of nerve attachment, the myoneural junction. This junction is the only place on the muscle cell membrane where the normal cell is chemically excitable by acetylcholine (ACh). With the loss of motor neuron influence, the presynaptic myoneural junction also undergoes degradation. Endplate receptor sites to ACh remain intact and new receptor sites to ACh develop along the muscle cell membrane. The muscle cells of a motor unit are interspersed among the fibers from other motor units (12). The denervated muscle fibers may be in nearby contact with the myoneural junctions of other normally functioning motor units. ACh then released by the nerve terminal of a functioning motor unit may come in contact with the nearby newly formed receptor site on the denervated muscle fiber and result in spontaneous depolarization of individual muscle fibers. The spontaneous depolarizations of individual muscle fibers are called fibrillation potentials. Thesleff and Ward (13) have recently demonstrated another possible mechanism for the production of fibrillation potentials. Recording from denervated muscle fibers, they found spontaneous action potentials initiated by spontaneous biphasic membrane oscillations of increasing amplitude.

Besides being chemically more sensitive to ACh, the muscle cell membrane, being somewhat unstable, can be rapidly triggered by mechanical stimulation. Thus, electrode insertion or mechanical stimulation of denervated muscle fibers can result in the production of spontaneous electrical activity recorded as positive sharp waves and irregular bursts of fibrillation potentials.

Denervated muscle fibers probably send out a distress signal. This is received by functioning neighboring motor units. A sprouting of distal axon terminals of functioning neighboring motor units occurs. With continued growth, these rescuing nerve sprouts contact the denervated muscle fibers (14, 16). A new myoneural junction then develops at the site of nerve contact. The muscle cell, upon being reinnervated, will change its fiber type if different from that of the rescuing motor neuron (16) (Fig. 7.1). The early result of this reinnervation process is that the functioning motor neuron has obtained by immature nerve twigs a greater total number of individual muscle fibers. These immature nerve twigs, until they mature, cannot conduct impulses at maximum speed. The site of the newly formed myoneural junctions on rescued muscle fibers may also be a long distance away from the site of the nerve attachment of the original muscle fibers.

The amplitude and shape of the motor unit action potential reflects the composite electrical depolarization of all the individual muscle fibers belonging to that motor unit that are within the pickup area of the recording electrode (17). Excitation of the new parent motor neuron results in coordinated depolarization of its original muscle fibers plus a depolarization of its newly rescued muscle fibers. Depolarization of these newly acquired muscle fibers innervated by immature nerve twigs changes the size and shape of the original composite motor unit action potential. This may result early in the production of the polyphasic motor unit action potentials, some of increased duration and amplitude. With maturation of these new reinnervating nerve twigs, their conduction velocity does increase, such that the composite action potential increases in amplitude and decreases somewhat in duration and polyphasicity.

The cause of this resultant motor unit action potential increase in amplitude, duration, and polyphasicity is no doubt complex. It is mainly the result of the new increased number of muscle fibers and their anatomical positions in the enlarged motor unit. Where the endplate region develops along the

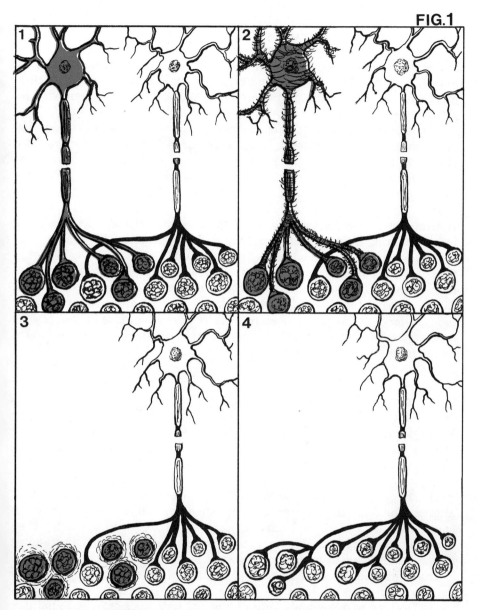

Fig. 7.1. Reinnervation. *Upper right,* anterior horn cell death and Wallerian degeneration in type I motor unit. *Upper left,* normal type I and type II motor units. *Lower left,* fibrillating type I muscle fibers. *Lower right,* axon sprouting from type II motor unit captures fibrillating muscle fiber. Captured muscle fibers change type to correspond to new parent anterior horn cell.

rescued muscle fiber is also a factor, since conduction speed along the muscle fiber is much slower than along the nerve terminals. The conduction time through the newly formed nerve terminals and delays at the newly formed myoneural junctions probably are also of significance in the production of alteration in motor unit action potentials, size, and shape. Blocking at branching sites of reinnervating nerve sprouts and at immature myoneural junctions can explain the decrementing response frequently seen with repetitive stimulation.

Synchronous firing of neighboring motor units as a means of producing large motor unit action potentials in motor neuron disease has been proposed (18–20). Although no definite proof has been forwarded to prove that synchronous firing does indeed occur, it is one additional way of explaining the changes observed in the EMG recording of motor units in this disease process.

As motor neuron disease progresses, the denervation and reinnervation of free fibrillating muscle fibers probably occurs repeatedly. The motor unit density and territory can become extremely large (19). Histologically, entire fields of many fascicles of muscle fibers are present that are of the same histochemical fiber type and possibly belong to a single motor neuron. Electromyographically, motor unit action potentials are seen with amplitudes as large as 25–30 mV peak-to-peak. The overall duration can also be markedly increased, especially the initial and terminal positive portions of single, large triphasic or polyphasic motor unit action potentials (21).

With a long-standing motor neuron disease, the recruitment pattern of the remaining functioning motor units may be altered. Smaller functioning type I motor units may have reinnervated a significant number of the denervated muscle fibers to become extremely large. Differentiation of type I motor units from high threshold motor units normally of a large size may become difficult. Many times only one or two motor units can be recorded in an area under examination, even for muscles with preservation of normal strength.

The frequency of firing of individual motor units may or may not be altered. The few remaining motor units, when requested to provide maximal contraction in a weakened muscle, may fire at frequencies greater than normally encountered. We have recorded motor units in long-standing neuropathies firing at frequencies as great as 100 Hz.

The consequences of the above pathophysiology explain why in motor neuron disease one observes:

1. Dropout of individual motor unit action potentials or reduced number of firing motor units per strength of contraction.
2. Fasciculation potentials.
3. Positive sharp waves and fibrillation potentials.
4. Increased incidence of polyphasic motor unit action potentials.
5. Motor unit action potentials of increased amplitude and duration.
6. Alterations in the recruitment pattern of motor unit action potentials

as strength of contraction increases. Larger amplitude motor unit action potentials recruited early.

7. Possible abnormal increase in frequency of firing of the remaining motor unit action potentials without recruitment of additional motor units.

8. Essentially normal motor and sensory nerve conduction studies.

Variations from the classical EMG presentation of motor unit disease frequently occurs. If reinnervation does not occur, for whatever reason, we may not see a significant increase in the size and shape of motor unit action potentials. The EMG findings may then demonstrate only a reduction in the number of motor unit action potentials recruited per strength of contraction. Findings of motor unit dropout with normal or increased firing frequency of remaining units and abnormal spontaneous activity may be the only EMG abnormalities.

If, on the other hand, the disease process is very slow and of a chronic low grade nature, or if reinnervation is extremely rapid, there may be very few or essentially no free fibrillating muscle fibers. In this situation, no abnormal spontaneous activity may be provoked in areas examined. Thus, a neuropathy without positive sharp waves and fibrillation potentials can occur. Electromyographically, one records voluntary motor units of increased amplitude and duration with a reduction in number recruited per strength of contraction.

Other variations from the classical EMG pictures of neuropathy surely exist. The historical approach to the EMG criteria of neuropathy and other diseases is retrospective. Electromyography today is prospective, and EMG findings need to be viewed objectively. These EMG findings must be with the history and physical examination, as well as with the biopsy and laboratory data.

Motor Neuron Disease

Disorders clinically and neurophysiologically affecting motor neurons can be divided into two broad categories: those with motor neuron involvement only and those in which motor neuron involvement is part of a more generalized neurological disturbance. Those disorders whose major manifestation primarily affects the motor neuron will be discussed in this section. Those disorders where motor neuron involvement is only a minor part of a generalized neurological disturbance, such as Familial Ataxias, etc., will be discussed elsewhere in this book (22). Disorders primarily affecting motor neurons can be of a hereditary or sporadic nature.

The most common disorder primarily affecting the motor neuron is amyotrophic lateral sclerosis with its clinical variants of progressive bulbar palsy, progressive muscular atrophy, pseudobular palsy, and primary lateral sclerosis. The term "motor neuron disease" is gaining wide acceptance for describing these sporadic syndromes of muscle weakness and atrophy without sensory loss or automonomic and sphincter dysfunction. The specific classification of the variants of motor neuron diseases is clinical, and the EMG differences are related to location and extent of abnormal findings.

The etiology of motor neuron disease remains unknown. A possible genetic transmission or a common toxic origin has been queried in an amyotrophic lateral sclerosis-like syndrome that occurs with high frequency among Chamorro Indians (23–25). The presence of a similar clinical syndrome with an apparent autosomal dominant pattern of inheritance in some families with other minor neurological abnormalities has raised the possibility of an enzyme defect (26). Intoxication by heavy metals and other organic compounds have been implicated but never proven as the cause of the disease. The etiologic possibilities of a slow or latent virus or immunologic abnormalities directly affecting motor neurons or accelerating the aging process have all been suggested as possible etiologies (27). Others have suggested that the disease or syndrome may be the result of multiple different etiologies that are entirely unrelated.

The condition is not rare and occurs worldwide. The incidence of the disease is felt to be approximately 1/100,000 per year. The male to female ratio is approximately 2:1. The disease is relatively rare before the age of 35, with the highest incidence in the fifth and sixth decades.

Motor neuron disease is progressive and usually begins as a painless asymmetric weakness and amyotrophy occurring in either proximal or distal limb muscles, in bulbar muscles, or in the form of upper motor neuron symptoms. The disease progresses at a variable tempo and in variable distribution. Symptomatic lower motor neuron involvement of the opposite extremity is common before becoming generalized. Weeks to months transpire before the patient seeks medical attention, depending on the rapidity of involvement. Fasciculations are frequent in affected muscles but may vary from being completely unnoticed by the patient to being exuberant and more of a complaint than a weakness. Muscle cramps are frequent and may be painful. The bulbar musculature may be involved early with an inability to talk loudly or to articulate clearly. Weakness of tongue and palate can result in problems of speech and, more importantly, of the handling of foods and fluid in the mouth and of swallowing. A feeding esophagostomy or gastrostomy is many times helpful and the need for one indicated early.

The patient continues to become progressively weak and loses weight. He fatigues easily, and cold may reduce his endurance. The patient does maintain bowel and bladder control. Eventually the muscles of respiration become involved. Associated respiratory problems are usually the cause of death.

Laboratory examinations, including a search for etiologies known to produce mimicking syndromes which include heavy metal intoxication, CNS syphilis, diabetic amyotrophy, and spondylosis, are normal. The EMG examination usually confirms the diagnosis in light of the history and physical and laboratory examinations. Early in the course of the disease, the EMG demonstrates a decreased number of voluntarily activated motor unit action potentials per strength of contraction. Fasciculation potentials, positive sharp waves, and fibrillation potentials are present not only in clinically affected muscles, but often in clinically unaffected opposite or distant limbs before other evidence of neuropathy is electromyographically apparent. Search for EMG involvement in clinically unaffected parts is invaluable. Occasionally one sees a bizarre high frequency discharge.

EMG demonstration of neuropathic involvement of tongue precludes the need for a myelography in diagnostic workup. The EMG examination of the tongue is simple and fairly painless (Fig. 7.2). The protruded tongue is grasped with a gauze sponge, and the electrode is inserted in the long axis, either along the lateral surface or underneath. The patient relaxes his tongue, carrying the inserted electrode back into his mouth. The tongue musculature is examined for fasciculations, positive sharp waves, and fibrillation potentials, taking care to ensure that the muscles are relaxed. Insertional activity can be examined by grasping the electrode, with the tongue relaxed in the floor of the mouth or held with a gauze sponge by the examiner's hand. One should be sure to hold the electrode throughout the study of insertional activity so that tongue movements will not be confused with provokable positive sharp waves due to pathologic abnormalities.

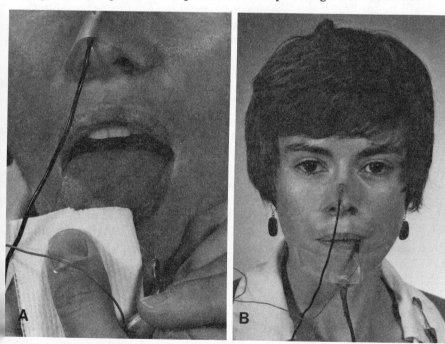

Fig. 7.2. Examination of the tongue. The tongue is held with a gauge sponge and the electrode inserted along the lateral margin. The patient relaxes the tongue musculature and it can be examined in this position. The patient can also retract the tongue and electrode into the mouth for examination at rest.

Repeated EMG examinations throughout the course of the disease may be helpful to the managing physician in following the activity of the disease process. The number and location of affected muscles, their number of active motor units, the presence or absence of reinnervation, and the number of positive sharp waves and fibrillation potentials are helpful indicators. They can be correlated with the clinical picture in determining the total course of rehabilitation and for alerting the physician to the development of possible complications. The number of motor units dropped out of a maximal contraction can give some indication as to the extent of muscle involvement. The maintenance of normal strength, in light of EMG evidence of fibrillation potentials and positive sharp waves and with motor unit action potentials of increased amplitude and duration, implies that, in spite of active disease, reinnervation is occurring. If the motor units remain of normal amplitude and duration over a period of several months, and if there is an abundance of fibrillation and positive sharp wave potentials with a marked reduction in number of voluntarily recruited motor units, there is no current evidence of reinnervation. Without reinnervation, the patient's progression of weakness and limitations of functional capacities may be expected to progress at a faster rate.

With relatively few or no fibrillation potentials and positive sharp waves, and with motor unit action potentials of increased amplitude and duration and apparently no dropout of motor units, electromyographically the disease process appears to be progressing slowly in this muscle. If this is seen throughout all muscles, this patient will most likely have a more chronic form of the motor neuron disease, especially in the absence of bulbar findings. With marked and progressive bulbar and respiratory muscle involvement, in spite of good extremity function, the prognosis remains quite poor, and the physician should be alerted to possible early respiratory compromise and difficulty in handling solid foods and liquids in the mouth.

In most cases, as the disease progresses, fewer active motor units are available for recruitment. The remaining motor units may become extremely large. Amplitudes as high as 20–30 mV with long durations are not uncommon (Fig. 7.3).

Nerve conduction studies, both sensory and motor, demonstrate the fastest fibers to be conducting within normal limits. Some observers have noted mild reduction in motor conduction velocities, but not lower than 70% of the normal value (28).

Single fiber EMG can be an adjunct to the routine EMG studies in revealing information about the continuous process of the deinnervation and reinnervation (29). Fiber density, or the number of single muscle fibers belonging to the same motor unit within the pickup area of the single fiber electrode (200 mm), is increased. The increase in fiber density then relates that reinnervation of the deinnervated muscle fibers is occurring. With reinnervation, immature distal axons and newly developed motor endplates are conducting impulses to reinnervated muscle fibers. As a result of their

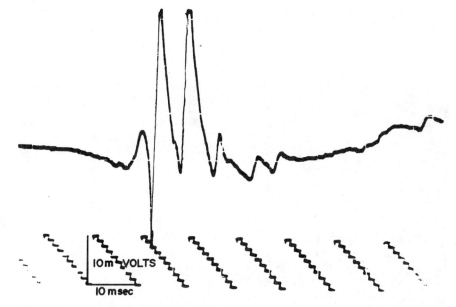

Fig. 7.3. Increased amplitude long duration, polyphasic motor unit action potential recorded in progressive spinal muscular atrophy.

immaturity or their inability to develop to a completely normal state, an increase in the time of conducting the impulses to these reinnervated muscle fibers now added to the composite motor unit results in alterations in size and shape. This represents an increase in jitter.

Occasionally an impulse will fail to be conducted and a block or dropout of a specific muscle fiber from the motor unit complexes is recorded. If blocking becomes significant, a decremental response to repetitive stimulation may be seen. With maturation of reinnervated distal axons and newly developed motor endplates, a reduction in jitter and impulse blocking will occur.

Histologically there are no pathognomonic changes (Fig. 7.4). The muscle biopsy demonstrates a fairly typical neuropathic picture. The presence of small angulated fibers with atrophy of both type I and type II muscle fibers is seen in most patients. Some type II muscle fiber hypertrophy may be seen early in the disease process. Variably-sized groups of fibers of the same histochemical type suggest collateral reinnervation. Nonspecific nuclear changes with an occasional targetoid fiber are common.

Teased fiber preparations from peripheral nerve reveal an axonal degeneration with normal peripheral nerve myelin. This explains why nerve conduction velocities remain essentially within normal limits, even in later stages of the disease process.

Treatment of the patient is like treatment of most medical problems, that of strict management. Although there is no pharmacological cure for the

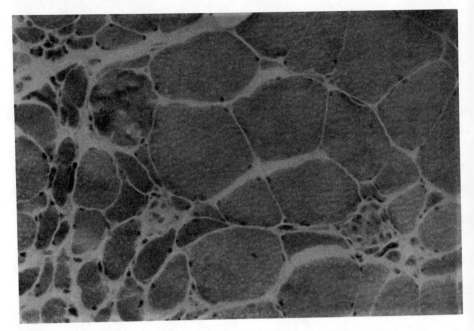

Fig. 7.4. Muscle biopsy amyotrophic lateral sclerosis with the presence of small angulated fibers next to normal fibers.

disease, a total and comprehensive rehabilitation program needs to be continuously maintained to allow the patient to function independently as long as possible. Mechanical ventilation assistance is now being requested and discussed freely by more families, and it can provide continuous human interaction and exchange in the proper family situations.

Post-Polio Amyotrophic Lateral Sclerosis Syndrome

The presence of progressive muscle atrophy occurring many years after an acute episode of poliomyelitis has been noted (30, 31). Those patients who have had severe degrees of motor neuron involvement secondary to poliomyelitis at an early age suddenly, in later years, develop a progression of symptoms in a syndrome resembling amyotrophic lateral sclerosis. In our experience and that of others, this progression is usually of a less rapid nature than motor neuron disease (32). Whether this syndrome is a result of reactivation of a now mutated latent virus, a primary motor neuron disease by chance affecting a patient who previously had polio, or just the aging process of a limited number of functioning or previously physiologically compromised motor neurons is open to debate. The EMG picture is again nonspecific and shows all the characteristics of classical motor neuron disease. The differentiation between acute and chronic disease by EMG alone may be most difficult if prior EMG reports are not available.

Hereditary Motor Neuron Disease

The remaining primary motor neuron disorders are of hereditary nature. They may be of either autosomal recessive or dominant inheritance and vary in age of onset, severity, and rate of progression. They involve primarily the motor neurons of the spinal cord, often the bulbar motor nuclei, but rarely the pyramidal tracts. Weakness is proximal at onset, and clinical differentiation from myopathies must be made. In most cases, there are no clear demarcations between the various forms of hereditary motor neuropathies. For the purpose of this text and since they are electromyographically nondescript, these disorders will be considered as varying degrees of Spinal Muscular Atrophy.

The most common of these disorders is the autosomal recessive transmitted Werdnig-Hoffmann disease of acute infantile progressive spinal muscular atrophy. The disease may occur in utero, and has been associated with a decrease in fetal movements. Approximately one-third of the cases are diagnosable at birth. Most cases have commenced prior to the 1st year of life. In general, the earlier the presentation of weakness, the more rapid the course and the poorer the prognosis. The more severely affected infant is hypotonic, inactive, and areflexic. Paradoxical respiratory movements due to severe intercostal weakness are frequent. Fasciculations may be visible only in the tongue because of the thick layer of subcutaneous fat. The cry is weak. The infant, however, is alert and appears to have normal intellectual functions. If the infant does not succumb to respiratory complications early, some motor skills such as hand control and sitting in a forward, leaning position are possible. Paralysis of the trunk muscles leads to chest wall deformity and scoliosis and may even lead to cardiac decompensation through mechanical deformation on the heart. If the disease has its onset later in the 1st year, a less acute form of the disease is observed. The patient may even develop the capacity to scoot about in the sitting position using the upper extremities. With the passage of time, the motor skills are lost, and the patient's demise is usually secondary to respiratory infection and failure.

On muscle biopsy, the histologic pattern is diagnostic (Fig. 7.5). Large seas of round atrophic fibers of both histochemical fiber types are seen in proximity to groups of normal-sized or hypertrophied fibers. Fibrosis is seen in bands surrounding the fascicles.

Emg examination demonstrates positive sharp waves and fibrillation potentials. Voluntary activated movements, or movements produced by cutaneous stimulation, demonstrate a reduced number of motor units per strength of contraction.

In the first days of life, these findings associated with normal (for age) nerve conduction velocities may be the most significant finding, since it may be difficult to get the infant to provide voluntary activation sufficient to allow specific motor unit potential analysis. With time and increasing age,

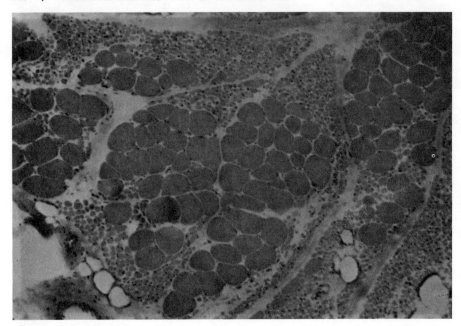

Fig. 7.5. Muscle biopsy of Werdnig-Hoffmann disease with large areas of round atrophic fibers in proximity to groups of normal-sized or hypertrophied fibers.

all the classical findings of motor neuron disease can be demonstrated: (a) decrease in number of voluntarily recruited motor unit action potentials per strength of contraction, (b) fasciculation potentials, (c) abnormal spontaneous insertional activity in the form of positive sharp waves and fibrillation potentials, (d) increase in polyphasicity, (e) motor unit action potentials of increased amplitude and duration, (f) alterations in the recruitment pattern of motor unit action potentials as strength of contraction increases, (g) frequency of firing of remaining motor unit action potentials may be abnormally increased, and (h) essentially normal motor and sensory nerve conduction studies.

The other forms of spinal musculature atrophy are extremely variable in their age of onset, severity, and rate of progression. There are no sharp lines of demarcation clinically or electromyographically. The clinical picture as a whole represents a more benign disease with a slower course.

A more chronic form of Werdnig-Hoffmann disease has been described to encompass those infants whose onset it is felt occurs before the age of 2 and whose mean survival is approximately 10 years (33, 34). This group of children seem to have a more chronic form of the disease with less severe bulbar involvement. Some learn to sit independently. Few learn to stand and reciprocate with assistance.

Kugelberg and Welander in 1956 (35) described 12 cases of a more chronic but progressive proximal spinal muscular atrophy occurring between the ages of 2 and 17 years. The majority of these cases had an autosomal recessive inheritance. Wolhfart in 1942 (36) and 1949 (37) described two similar cases. Weakness characteristically occurs in the proximal musculature of the lower extremities. The presence of fasciculations and the typical EMG picture of motor neuron disease help to differentiate this process from a myopathy.

Many other chronic forms of spinal muscular atrophy are described with onset in later life. Their differentiation from amyotrophic lateral sclerosis or motor neuron disease is based on their inheritance pattern, symmetry, more proximal involvement, and a more benign and less rapid progression. Some of these forms have been described initially with distal weakness and differentiation from the neuronal form of Charcot-Marie-Tooth may be difficult.

There are many reports of families in which the severity of the disease is greatly variable in the affected sibs. One child may be severely affected while the other has only mild symptoms. One child in the family may have a more classical form of Werdnig-Hoffmann disease while another child may have a Kugelberg-Welander type picture.

Histologically, the milder forms of spinal muscular atrophy differ somewhat from the more severe Werdnig-Hoffmann disease. The atrophic fibers are variable in shape. They tend to be more angular (as seen in amyotrophic lateral sclerosis), then rounded (as seen in Werdnig-Hoffmann). Fiber type grouping with fiber type predominance is common. The differentiation of the various forms of spinal muscular atrophy is then determined mainly by the history and physical examination.

The EMG findings in these various forms of spinal muscular atrophy are nonspecific, and the classical findings of motor neuron disorders are found in varying distributions and to a varying degree (Fig. 7.6). Single muscle fiber EMG may be helpful as an adjunct to routine EMG in following the activity of the disease process by monitoring the amount of reinnervation. Single fiber EMG will demonstrate a reduction in jitter and blocking with the maturation of the reinnervated sprouted distal axons and their newly developing motor endplates. With activation of the disease or further degeneration and reinnervation, an increase in jitter and blocking is demonstrated. Fiber density is increased due to the process of reinnervation. In more chronic forms of progressive spinal muscular atrophy, single fiber EMG has demonstrated some of the largest number of component spikes to the compound motor unit action potentials.

Myelopathies Affecting Motor Neurons

Disorders affecting the spinal cord as a whole may have their primary effect on the ventral horn. Infections, lesions from direct trauma, and pressure or infiltration from tumors, radiation, and vascular insults may have more a selective effect on the anterior horn or motor neurons, producing an EMG picture that can be identical with motor neuron disease. The

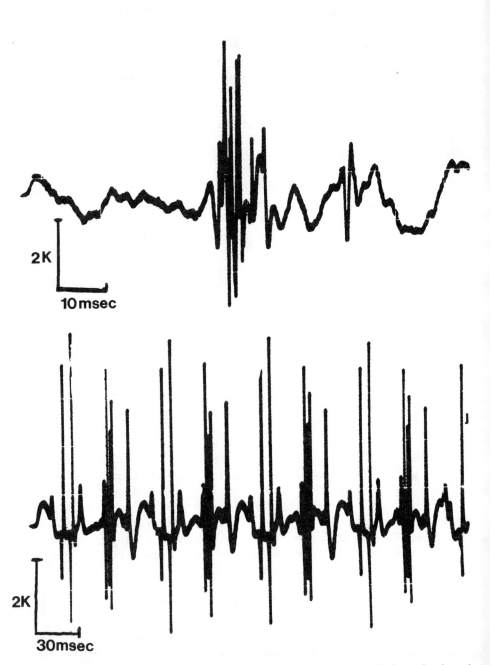

Fig. 7.6. *Top*, polyphasic fasciculation potential in amyotrophic lateral sclerosis, (ALS). *Bottom*, "neuropathic" interference pattern in ALS.

clinical impression must then be confirmed in light of the history, physical examination, and clinical course, as well as other laboratory methods.

Poliomyelitis, fortunately, is today in almost all countries a disease of historic interest. The authors did, however, have an example last year in a mother whose infant son had been immunized 3 weeks prior to the onset of her symptoms. The disease is caused by an enterovirus. Not everyone exposed to the virus will develop symptoms (38). Only one-third to one-half with symptoms will develop paralysis.The paralytic phase of the disease is heralded by malaise, fever, and vague gastrointestinal complaints. These symptoms usually resolve slowly, only to be followed by an increased fever, stiffness, pain, and later paralysis.

The virus attacks the motor neurons preferentially. There is no segmental distribution, and weakness is a matter of where and how many motor neurons lose their physiological function. Old polio patients are not immune to other disorders and are frequently referred for neurophysiological testing to detect new neurological lesions or abnormalities overlying their residuals from prior polio. An appreciation for EMG findings of old anterior horn cell disease is necessary to evaluate acute changes. The EMG in polio shows reinnervation. Very large and complex motor unit action potentials exist. Usually large complex fasciculation are present. Positive sharp waves and fibrillation potentials initially present have been demonstrated to persist for greater than 20 years in some patients. Recruitment patterns may demonstrate only large motor units with a reduction in the total number of motor units recruited per strength of contraction. In all, varying degrees of the eight more classical findings of motor neuropathy are seen in affected muscles.

There are many other pathogenic organisms that can and do intermittently attack the spinal cord. They usually present, however, with a clinical picture of transverse myelitis, with evidence of upper motor neuron disease. Rarely are they selective in affecting only the motor neurons. One should, however, always consider the possibility of tertiary syphilis as the cause of the myelopathy.

One other virus, however, is becoming more common in its selective attack on the motor neurons. Herpes zoster myelitis is being seen in increasing frequency due to an increased population of persons on immunologic compromising pharmacologic agents (39). Most of these patients do, however, develop, with time, a full picture of transverse myelitis.

Direct segmental trauma to the spinal cord, such as a knife wound, could produce the familiarly discussed Brown-Séquard syndrome. Few spinal cord injuries give only localized or segmental neurological defects and are usually easily diagnosed. EMG of muscles below the spinal cord lesion have been reported by several observers to demonstrate positive sharp waves and fibrillations (40). The etiology of this abnormal spontaneous electrical activity is unknown and is discussed in another chapter of this text.

Cervical spondylosis can frequently result in a myelopathy. With the development of degenerative joint disease and osteophyte formation, the cervical canal can become markedly narrowed. Flexion or extension of the neck can result in the anterior compression of the spinal cord over anteriorly developed osteophytic bars. Extension, on the other hand, can result in a buckling of the ligamenta flava and again result in trauma to the ventral spinal cord. Clinically, the patient may present with a myelopathy, and differentiation from motor neuron disease may require myelography. More frequently, the patient will also demonstrate clinical evidence of an associated cervical radiculopathy and spastic paraparesis. The EMG, then, presents abnormalities of both radiculopathy and motor neuron disease and thus is helpful in localizing the neurologic lesions.

Compression of the spinal cord and/or infiltration by both primary and secondary tumors can produce a myelopathy. Direct metasteses to the spinal cord is rare. However, the cord can frequently be compressed by tumor invasion of surrounding areas. Primary tumors of the spinal cord are also relatively rare, but most commonly of glial tissue origin. Associated neurologic abnormalities, sensory loss, spastic paraparesis, and bowel and bladder incontinence rarely make the differentiation from motor neuropathy difficult, except early in cases where tumor growth may be centrally located or limited solely to the anterior horn. More commonly, treatment of tumors by radiation may result in a delayed (as long as several years) myelopathy. The onset may be slow and progressive, but the whole cord is most frequently involved with sensory abnormalities, spastic paraparesis, and bowel and bladder incontinence.

Vascular insults to the spinal cord are being recognized with increasing frequency. Arterial insufficiency secondary to generalized arterial sclerosis is the most common vascular insult and can result in acute onset of a rapidly progressive loss of motor function. The thoracic area of the cord is most susceptible due to its poor arterial supply. The patient usually rapidly develops paraplegia. Associated pain, dysesthesias at a segmental level due to involvement of the spinothalamic and corticospinal tracts, is common and aids in the diagnosis. Venous thrombosis, though infrequent, rarely produces selective involvement of the motor neurons.

It may take 10–14 days for the EMG to demonstrate abnormal spontaneous activity in the form of provoked positive sharp waves and fibrillation potentials and weeks for the sign of reinnervation to appear. The early finding of a reduced number of voluntary recruited motor unit action potentials per strength of contraction, which solely is always difficult to evaluate, initially may be the only EMG clue in a developing vascular insult to the spinal cord.

Developmental abnormalities of the spinal cord can produce a myelopathy. Syringomyelia and hematomyelia, because of their central location, can produce a significant motor neuropathy. The associated findings of segmental pain and temperature loss due to compromise of crossing fibers is a major clue to the diagnosis. Many patients have presented, however, with pure motor symptoms. The EMG may demonstrate a classical neuropathic picture, and myelography will usually confirm the clinical impression.

REFERENCES

1. CAJAL, RAMON Y. S.: Histologie du systeme nerveux de l'homne et des vertebres. Paris, Maloine, Vol. 1, 1909.
2. HENNEMAN, E., SOMJIN, G., AND CARPENTER, D.: Functional significance of cell size in spinal motor neurons. *J. Neurophysiol., 28:* 560, 1965.
3. HENNEMAN, E., AND OLSON, C. B.: Relations between structure and function in the design of skeletal muscle. *J. Neurophysiol., 28:* 581, 1965.
4. HENNEMAN, E.: Relation between size of neurons and their susceptibility to discharge. *Science, 126:* 1345, 1957.
5. ENGEL, W. K.: The essentiality of Histo- and cytochemical studies of skeletal muscle in the investigation of neuromuscular disease. *Neurology, 12:* 778, 1962.
6. WARMOLTS, J. R., AND ENGEL, W. K.: Open biopsy electromyography. *Arch. Neurol., 27:* 512, 1972.
7. SWANK, R. L., AND PRICE, J.: Fascicular muscle twitching in amyotrophic lateral sclerosis. *Arch. Neurol. Psychiat., 49:* 22, 1943.
8. FORSTER, F., AND ALPERS, B.: Site of origin of fasciculations in voluntary muscle. *Arch. Neurol. Psychiat., 51:* 264, 1944.
9. FORSTER, F., BORKOWSKI, W., AND ALPERS, B.: Effects of denervation on fasciculations in human muscle. *Arch. Neurol. Psychiat., 56:* 276, 1946.
10. TROJABORG, W., AND BUCHTHAL, F.: Malignant and benign fasciculations. *Acta Neurol. Scand. 41, Suppl. 13:* 251, 1965.
11. BUCHTHAL, F., AND TROJABORG, W.: Fasciculation in anterior horn cell disease (Abstract). International EMG Meeting, Copenhagen, pp. 62–64, 1963.
12. AXELSSON, J., AND THESLEFF, S.: A study of supersensitivity in denervated mammalian skeletal muscle. *J. Physiol., 149:* 178, 1963.
13. THESLEFF, S., AND WARD, M. R.: Studies on the mechanism of fibrillation potentials in denervated muscle. *J. Physiol., 244:* 313, 1975.
14. VAN HARREUELD, A.: Reinnervation of denervated muscle fibers by adjacent functioning motor units. *Am. J. Physiol., 144:* 477, 1945.
15. WOHLFART, G.: Collateral regeneration from residule motor nerve fibers in amyotrophic lateral sclerosis. *Neurology, 7:* 124, 1957.
16. KARPATI, G., AND ENGEL, W. K.: "Type grouping" in skeletal muscles after experimental reinnervation. *Neurology, 18:* 447, 1968.
17. BUCHTHAL, F.: The general concept of the motor unit. *Res. Publ. Assoc. Nerv. Ment. Dis., 38:* 1, 1961.
18. BUCHTHAL, F., AND MADSEN, A.: Synchronous activity in normal and atrophic muscle. *Electroencephalogr. Clin. Neurophysiol., 2:* 425, 1950.
19. ERMINIO, F., BUCHTHAL, F., AND ROSENFALCK, P.: Motor unit territory and muscle fiber concentration in paresis due to peripheral nerve injury and anterior horn cell involvement. *Neurology, 9:* 657, 1959.
20. DENNY-BROWN, D.: Interpretation of the electromyogram. *Arch. Neurol. Psychiat., 61:* 99, 1949.
21. BUCHTHAL, F., AND PINELLI, P.: Action potentials in muscular atrophy of neurogenic origin. *Neurology, 3:* 591, 1953.
22. ROWLAND, L. P., AND LAYZER, R. B.: Muscular dystrophies, atrophies, and related disease. In *Clinical Neurology*, 3rd ed., vol. 3, pp. 1–100, ed. by A. B. Baker, New York: Harper & Row, 1971.
23. KURKLAND, L. T., AND MULDER, D. W.: Epidemologic investigations of amyotrophic lateral sclerosis II. *Neurology, 5:* 182, 1955.
24. MULDER, D. W.: The clinical syndrome of amyotrophic lateral sclerosis. *Mayo Clin. Proc., 32:* 427, 1957.

25. KURKLAND, L. T., CHOI, N. W., AND SAYRE, G. P.: Implications of incidence and geographic patterns on the classification of amyotrophic lateral sclerosis. In *Motor Neuron Disease*, p. 22, ed. by F. H. Norris and L. T. Kurkland, New York: Greene and Stratton, 1969.
26. PRATT, R. T. C.: *Genetics of Neurological Disorders*, London: Oxford University Press, 1967.
27. BORDY, J. A., HIRANO, A., AND SCOTT, R. M.: Recent neuropathologic observations in amyotrophic lateral sclerosis and parkinsonism dementia of Guam. *Neurology, 21:* 528, 1971.
28. LAMBERT, E. H.: Diagnostic value of electrical stimulation of motor nerves. *Electroencephalogr. Clin. Neurophysiol. Suppl., 22:* 9, 1962.
29. STALBERG, E., SCHWARTZ, M. S., AND TRONTELJ, J. V.: Single fiber electromyography in various processes affecting the anterior horn cell. *J. Neurol. Sci., 24:* 403, 1975.
30. POTTS, C. S.: A case of progressive muscular atrophy occurring in a man who had had acute poliomyelitis nineteen years previously: With a review of the literature bearing upon the relations of infantile spinal paralysis to the spinal diseases of later life. *Univ. Pa. Med. Bull., 16:* 31, 1903.
31. CAMPBELL, A. M. G., WILLIAMS, E. R., AND PEARCE, J.: Late motor neuron degeneration following poliomyelitis. *Neurology, 19:* 1101, 1969.
32. MULDER, D. W., ROSENBRUM, R. A., AND LAYTON, D. D.: Late progression of poliomyelitis or forme fruste amyotrophic lateral sclerosis. *Mayo Clin. Proc., 47:* 756, 1972.
33. DUBOWITY, V.: Infantile muscular atrophy. A prospective study with particular reference to a slowly progressive variety. *Brain, 87:* 707, 1964.
34. GAMSTORP, I.: Progressive spinal muscular atrophy with onset in infancy or early childhood. *Acta Paediat. Scand., 56:* 408, 1967.
35. KUGELBERG, E., AND WELANDER, L.: Heredofamilial juvenile muscular atrophy simulating muscular dystrophy. *Arch. Neurol. Psychiat., 75:* 500, 1956.
36. WOHLFART, G.: Zwei falle von dystrophia musculorum progressiva mit fibrillaren zuchungen and atypischen muskelbefund. *Deutsch Z. Nervenheilk, 153:* 189, 1942.
37. WOHLFART, G.: Muscular atrophy in diseases of the lower motor neuron. *Arch. Neurol. Psychiat., 61:* 599, 1949.
38. RUSSELL, W. R.: *Poliomyelitis*, 2nd ed., London: Edward Arnold Ltd., 1956.
39. Paralysis in herpes zoster. *Br. Med. J., 2:* 379, 1970.
40. TAYLOR, R. G., KEWALRAMANI, L. S., AND FOWLER, W. F.: Electromyographic findings in lower extremities of patients with high spinal cord injury. *Arch. Phys. Med. Rehabil., 55:* 16, 1974.

8

Peripheral Neuropathies

GEORGE H. KRAFT, M.D.

Peripheral neuropathies are diseases causing dysfunction of peripheral nerve axons, their myelin sheaths, or both. Usually they are generalized and affect many nerves. They tend to be most severe in distal portions of extremities, especially in lower legs and feet. Clinically, peripheral neuropathies generally produce motor weakness, impaired sensation, and hyporeflexia.

The purpose of this chapter is to outline nerve conduction and EMG abnormalities seen in various peripheral neuropathies. It should be emphasized that an electroneuromyographic examination does *not* give a diagnosis. However, electrophysiologic information about peripheral nerve function will help the electromyographer sort through the large number of conditions which can cause peripheral neuropathies and identify the most likely causes of a neuropathy in a particular patient. Not only is EMG important for making a diagnosis, it is also necessary for an accurate prognosis and determination of appropriate treatment.

Types of Peripheral Neuropathies

There are two general categories of peripheral neuropathies: (a) diseases producing primary axonal degeneration, usually also causing secondary demyelination, and (b) diseases causing segmental demyelination, which, if severe enough, may cause secondary axonal changes. In addition, some investigators have speculated that some diseases may cause primary degeneration of both axon and myelin.

Different peripheral neuropathies may also selectively affect different nerves or certain segments of nerves. For example, lead toxicity in adults classically produces greatest damage to the radial nerve. Some neuropathies have a predilection for motor nerves, others for sensory nerves. Although peripheral neuropathies generally produce the greatest dysfunction in distal portions of a nerve, some neuropathies (e.g., Guillain-Barré polyneuritis) may preferentially affect other segments during certain stages of disease.

Nerve Conduction Changes in Peripheral Neuropathy

In the clinical recording of motor nerve conduction velocity, conduction velocity of the fastest conducting fibers (A, alpha) is measured. There is a linear relationship between the diameter of a myelinated fiber and its conduction velocity; as the diameter decreases, the conduction velocity decreases (1). Thus, in diseases in which there is loss of large diameter myelinated fibers, or in diseases in which there is a reduction in diameter of all myelinated fibers, conduction velocity is generally mildly to moderately reduced. Amplitudes of evoked potentials are usually decreased, but temporal dispersion may be only minimal (Fig. 8.1C).

Disorders of myelin are thought to reduce nerve conduction velocity in two ways. First, thinning of myelin will itself slow conduction. Conduction remains saltatory until there is a conduction block, but the loss of current

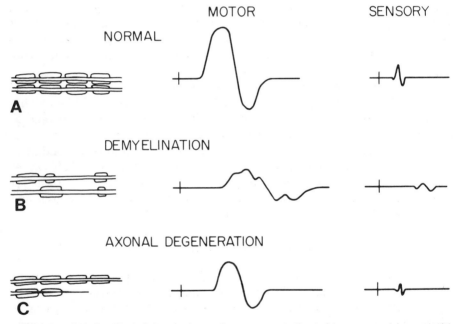

Fig. 8.1. (A) On the left is a schematic representation of two normal axons with normal myelin sheaths. Normal evoked motor and sensory action potentials are demonstrated. (B) In segmental demyelination, axis cylinders are preserved with random loss and attenuation of myelin internodes. In the diagram of the evoked muscle action potential, the stimulus artifact is represented by the vertical line; it will be noted that there is an increased latency between the stimulus and the action potential. The action potential shows temporal dispersion and decreased amplitude. The sensory potential also shows prolonged latency, temporal dispersion and attenuation of amplitude. (C) In axonal degeneration, reduction in the diameter of the intact upper axis cylinder and "dying back" of the lower axis cylinder are demonstrated; myelin may be unaffected except on the discontinuous axis cylinder. The motor and sensory nerve responses show slightly prolonged latencies with reduction in action potential amplitudes.

through a damaged internode increases the time required for the next internode to reach threshold, causing some fall in conduction velocity (2). Second, conduction block can occur in severely demyelinated fibers as a result of the failure of an impulse to excite a node adjacent to a severely demyelinated internode (Fig. 8.*1B*) (3). With loss of myelin, conduction velocity is moderately to markedly reduced, and temporal dispersion can be quite marked (Fig. 8.2) (4, 5).

In diseases in which both axonal degeneration and demyelination occur, a combination of the above findings will be noted. Primary axonal diseases produce nerve dysfunction and slowing of conduction either throughout the length of the nerve or in the most distal portions; the exact pattern depends on the type of nerve dysfunction. Because of the great distance from the metabolic factory of the nerve cell body, nerve dysfunction and slowing of nerve conduction in neuronal atrophy is most pronounced in the distal portion of the lower extremity.

Demyelinating diseases, on the other hand, may result in slowing of proximal nerve conduction during certain stages of disease, causing conduction abnormalities even in the nerve roots. Because there is generally variation in the demyelination of different axons, the difference in conduction velocity between the fastest and the slowest fibers will be greater the

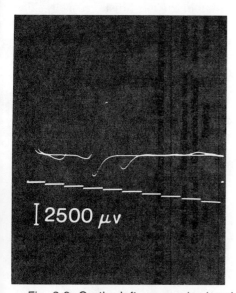
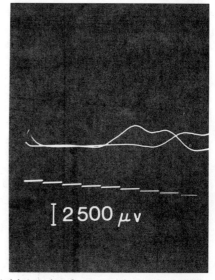

Fig. 8.2. On the left are proximal and distal latencies from a guinea pig sciatic nerve 5 days after receiving peripheral nerve antigen. Conduction velocity was 59 m/sec. On the right is the response in the same nerve 22 days after receiving antigen. Note the marked prolongation of both proximal and distal latencies, the loss of amplitude and the quite striking temporal dispersion. Nerve conduction velocity was calculated to be 22 m/sec. The vertical bar indicates 2500 μV. Each horizontal step represents 1 msec.

longer the distance over which the impulse is transmitted; consequently, temporal dispersion is more pronounced on proximal stimulation.

Certain nerve conduction techniques can be used to obtain information about conduction changes in a peripheral neuropathy. Conduction in the most proximal segments can be studied by means of the F wave and H reflex. Nerve conduction velocity can be determined in proximal and distal segments of an extremity by using conventional techniques. Terminal latency measurements over a standard distance are useful, and residual latency determinations can give specific information about unique conduction characteristics in the most distal segments of nerve (6). It is helpful to be able to record averaged nerve potentials to obtain information on sensory and mixed nerve conduction velocities; cerebral-evoked potential recording permits the determination of proximal sensory nerve conduction values (7). Quantification of the evoked muscle response is also useful (8).

Motor nerve conduction studies should be done using surface recording electrodes where possible, but in severe peripheral neuropathies, a coaxial needle may be preferred for recording the muscle response (9).

EMG Changes in Peripheral Neuropathies

In mild peripheral neuropathies, very little in the way of abnormalities may be seen on EMG examination. The most pronounced findings in peripheral neuropathy will generally be seen in the most distal muscles. The most subtle changes are an increase in polyphasicity of motor unit action potentials and a slight increase in amplitude and duration of the action potentials. In more severe axonal neuropathies, fibrillation potentials and positive sharp waves may be seen, and motor unit action potentials will be increased in amplitude and duration and will be fewer in number. In severe acute axonal neuropathic conditions, positive sharp waves may occur as much as 10 days before fibrillations can be noted. In diseases producing segmental demyelination, fibrillation potentials will generally be rare, although some positive sharp waves may be noted (4) (Fig. 8.3).

Peripheral Neuropathies (Table 8.1)

HEREDITARY NEUROPATHIES (Table 8.2)

Charcot-Marie-Tooth Disease (Peroneal Muscular Atrophy, Hereditary Motor Sensory Neuropathy I)

This autosomal dominant disorder, which is probably more common than appreciated, is now considered to be a neuronal atrophy with secondary demyelination (10). Recent studies by Brimijoin et al. (11) have demonstrated that there is an abnormality of axonal flow; they support the hypothesis that there is an inborn metabolic derangement in peripheral neurons which prevents substances essential for the development and maintenance of the cell from being properly synthesized, packaged, or trans-

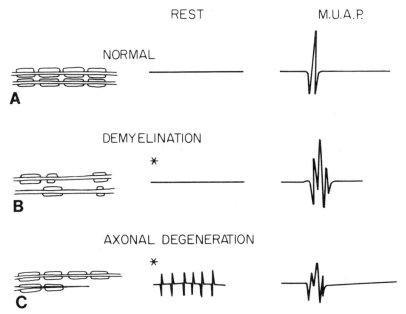

Fig. 8.3. (A) Schematic representation of two axons and their myelin sheaths is at the left. At rest, no electrical activity is seen. (B) Segmental demyelination is schematically represented. No fibrillation potentials are seen at rest and voluntary motor unit action potentials are polyphasic and have prolonged duration. (C) Schematic axonal degeneration is shown at left. At rest, spontaneous fibrillation potentials will be seen, and voluntary motor unit action potentials initially will be decreased in amplitude, be polyphasic, and have prolonged duration. On needle movement, positive sharp waves will be seen in axonal degeneration. Muscle may be irritable in demyelinating diseases and, under some circumstances, positive sharp waves seen.

TABLE 8.1. *Categories of Peripheral Neuropathies*

1. Hereditary neuropathies
2. Toxic neuropathies
   a. Heavy metals
   b. Organic compounds
   c. Drugs
3. Neuropathies associated with diseases
4. Idiopathic neuropathies

ported. The cycle of demyelination and remyelination of atrophic fibers leads to onion-bulb formation.

Presenting symptoms usually begin in the second decade or later and consist of high-arched feet and weakness of foot and lower leg muscles. Sensation is either generally not affected or only minimally diminished. Peripheral nerves, especially the greater auricular nerve, are often large and palpable. Sporadic cases probably represent dominant inheritance with poor

TABLE 8.2. *Hereditary Neuropathies*

1. Charcot-Marie-Tooth disease
2. Hereditary motor sensory neuropathy II
3. Déjèrine-Sottas disease
4. Roussy-Levy syndrome
5. Hereditary sensory neuropathy
   a. Autosomal dominant
   b. Autosomal recessive
6. Hereditary compression neuropathy
7. Riley-Day syndrome
8. Infantile neural axonal dystrophy
9. Friedreich's ataxia
10. Spinocerebellar degenerations of adulthood
11. Familial spastic paraplegia
12. Pelizaeus-Merzbacher disease
13. Refsum's disease
14. Fabry's disease
15. Metachromatic leukodystrophy
16. Krabbe's leukodystrophy
17. Tangier disease
18. Abetalipoproteinemia
19. Primary amyloidosis
20. Myotonic dystrophy
21. Acute intermittent porphyria

expressivity in one of the parents. Histologically, many nerve fibers disappear, especially at the periphery.

Conduction velocities of myelinated fibers are generally strikingly low, depending on the age of the patient and severity of the disease. (Penetrance can vary.) However, *in vitro* conduction in unmyelinated fibers is normal. Dyck and Lambert (12) reported distal motor latencies to average almost three times longer than normal, conduction velocities less than half normal, and evoked muscle amplitudes less than half. In reviewing our recent experience with Charcot-Marie-Tooth disease, we found residual latencies in the upper extremities to be approximately 2 S.D. above the mean. We also studied the evoked muscle response and found a highly significant difference between the integrated M response of normal adult males and those with Charcot-Marie-Tooth disease ($P < 0.001$) (8). Humberstone (13) states that the earliest conduction changes are a decrease in sensory nerve action potential amplitude and prolongation of sensory latency. Studies of F wave conduction velocity of the median and ulnar nerves show that proximal nerve segments are affected but not as greatly as the more distal segments (14).

EMG changes may be widespread but are especially marked in distal muscles of hands and feet. They consist of fibrillation potentials and positive sharp waves as well as increased amplitude, duration and polyphasicity of motor unit action potentials firing in reduced number. In long-standing cases, complete neurogenic atrophy may have been present in the feet for so long that the muscles are electrically silent and show decreased insertional activity on needle movement.

Thus, the characteristic electrodiagnostic findings are strikingly reduced motor and sensory nerve conduction velocities, with conduction slowing greatest in distal segments of nerve and with greatly prolonged residual latencies. One of the slowest motor nerve conduction velocities I have seen (7.8 m/sec in the ulnar nerve) was in a patient with Charcot-Marie-Tooth disease; most of his affected family members also had motor conduction velocities below 15 m/sec (Fig. 8.4).

Hereditary Motor Sensory Neuropathy II

This is perhaps the best term for this dominantly inherited rare peripheral neuropathy which is clinically similar to Charcot-Marie-Tooth disease. It

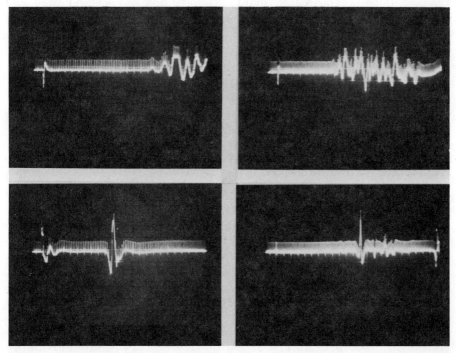

Fig. 8.4. Motor nerve conduction latencies in the ulnar nerve of a patient with Charcot-Marie-Tooth disease. The upper photographs show proximal latencies recorded with surface electrodes. Each vertical marking represents 0.5 msec. In the photograph in the upper right hand corner, sweep speed was reduced to demonstrate the striking temporal dispersion. The bottom photographs show latencies recorded with a needle recording electrode. On the left is the distal latency, on the right the proximal latency. Sensitivity of the upper photographs is five times that of the lower photographs and had to be increased that amount to demonstrate the take-off point of the action potential. Each vertical grid marking represents 1000 μV in upper photos, 200 μV in lower photos.

differs primarily in that symptoms occur at a somewhat later age and peripheral nerves are not enlarged. Electrodiagnostically, it differs strikingly because in this disorder, peripheral nerve conduction velocities are in the normal range. In more severely affected individuals, it may not be possible to obtain sensory nerve action potentials, although, if obtained, distal latencies are normal (15).

Déjerine-Sottas Disease (Hypertrophic Interstitial Neuropathy)

This recessively inherited disorder usually begins in infancy and is associated with marked onion-bulb formation caused by repeated demyelination and remyelination (16). Nerve conduction velocities are some of the lowest reported, being as low as 3–5 m/sec in the upper extremity. Distal latencies are often more than four times normal, with the amplitude of the evoked motor response often ¹⁄₁₀ or ¹⁄₂₀ of normal. Frequently, no sensory potential can be obtained (17). An abnormality of axonal flow has been reported, and it is considered that the disease is a neuronal atrophy. Primary dysfunction of the Schwann cells may be present as well (15).

Roussy-Levy Syndrome

In the peripheral nervous system, this disorder appears to be identical to Charcot-Marie-Tooth disease. However, essential tremor also occurs as part of the clinical syndrome (15). Nerve conduction and EMG findings are identical with those seen in Charcot-Marie-Tooth disease (18).

Hereditary Sensory Neuropathy (Autosomal Dominant and Autosomal Recessive Types)

The autosomal dominant disease has its onset in the second or third decade, with lower extremity sensory deficit the major clinical symptom. Motor nerve conduction velocities are in the low normal range and sensory nerve action potentials are generally not obtainable. The autosomal recessive disease is generally more severe and present at birth or shortly thereafter. Motor conduction velocities are in the low normal range, but amplitude of the muscle response is abnormally low. Sensory conductions are unobtainable. EMG of distal muscles may show a few fibrillation potentials and signs of chronic denervation (19).

Hereditary Compression Neuropathy (Hereditary Mononeuropathy Multiplex)

Patients with this disorder have an autosomal dominant inheritance of a propensity to develop multiple entrapment neuropathies of peripheral nerves. Frequently, a history of minor trauma to the nerve coincides with the onset of paresis. Partial or complete return is common but not invariable. Motor conduction velocity in most nerves is in the low normal range in segments not affected, but nerves which have been repeatedly affected show slowing of conduction. Nerve conduction through areas of entrapment is slow. Needle EMG reveals the residuals of neurogenic damage in distal muscles of the affected extremities (20).

Riley-Day Syndrome (Familial Dysautonomia)

In this rare, recessively inherited disorder of autonomic function in Jewish children presenting with insensitivity to pain, absence of tears, postural hypotension and other autonomic signs and symptoms, motor nerve conduction velocity hovers around the lower limits of normal. Sensory conduction velocities may be unobtainable but, when they can be obtained, are in the normal range (21).

Infantile Neuroaxonal Dystrophy

This is most likely an autosomal recessive disorder, producing the infantile onset of motor and corticospinal symptoms (hyperactive reflexes and Babinski sign). Axonal degeneration is most likely a primary occurrence. The condition clinically resembles metachromatic leukodystrophy, and conduction studies of the peripheral nerves can be most helpful in separating these two disorders. Motor nerve conduction velocity is normal in the early stages and mildly reduced in the later stages, in striking contrast to the dramatic nerve conduction velocity slowing in metachromatic leukodystrophy. EMG, even when conduction velocities are normal, shows the characteristic findings of distal denervation (22).

Friedreich's Ataxia

This is perhaps the most common variety of spinocerebellar degeneration and it is inherited in an autosomally recessive manner. Sensory nerve conduction is either unobtainable or shows a strikingly diminished nerve action potential. Motor nerve conduction velocity and amplitude of evoked muscle action potential are either low normal or mildly reduced (23).

Spinocerebellar Degenerations of Adulthood

A number of kinship studies in this category have been reported (23). In the extensive autosomal dominant kinship reported by Ziegler et al. (24), nerve conduction studies showed mild slowing of both sensory and motor conduction velocity. EMG showed fibrillations and positive sharp waves in distal muscles in most patients.

Familial Spastic Paraplegia

This autosomal dominant disease has been reported by Dyck (15) to produce borderline low motor nerve conduction velocities and diminished sensory action potentials and by McLeod and Morgan (25) to produce normal motor and sensory nerve conduction velocities. Needle electrode examination of the distal leg and foot muscles may show fibrillations and increased size of the voluntary action potentials (15).

Pelizaeus-Merzbacher Disease

This rare, sex-linked central nervous system demyelinating disease affecting male children can produce moderately slow motor and sensory nerve conductions with low amplitude responses. EMG may show denervation (26).

Refsum's Disease (Heredopathia Atactica Polyneuritiformis)

This rare, autosomal recessive disorder generally has, as its initial clinical presentation, night blindness; the age of onset is from childhood to early adult years. The clinical manifestations are pigmentary retinal degeneration, chronic polyneuropathy, and ataxia; the diagnosis is made by identifying elevated serum levels of phytanic acid. The pathology is an inborn error of metabolism causing an accumulation of phytanic acid. Accurate early diagnosis is mandatory since phytanic acid stems exclusively from exogenous sources and the disease can be controlled and degeneration prevented by dietary modification. Both motor and sensory nerve conduction velocities are reduced, with the reduction sometimes very marked. The EMG examination may show evidence of denervation (27).

Fabry's Disease (Angiokeratoma Corporis Diffusum)

This is a sex-linked recessive disease of boys and young men who present with painful burning sensations of the feet and legs. It is a storage disease in which stored glycolipid produces a reddish-purple maculopapular rash, renal impairment, and symptoms of neuropathy. Diagnosis is made by assaying serum alpha-galactosidase and finding it reduced. Both motor and sensory nerve conduction studies and EMG studies are normal, even though there is a loss of small peripheral sensory axons (28).

Metachromatic Leukodystrophy

This autosomal recessive disease begins in infancy with progressive central and peripheral nervous system symptoms starting as hypotonia. A variety also exists in which symptoms do not begin until early adult life. This is a disease of myelin lipids, and diffuse demyelination in the central and peripheral nervous system occurs.

Motor nerve conduction velocity is markedly reduced, especially in the infantile form, and is frequently below 20 m/sec (29). Occasionally, patients with this disorder may be misdiagnosed as having "cerebral palsy"; nerve conduction velocity studies are useful in separating the two diseases.

Krabbe's (Globoid) Leukodystrophy

This is a very rapidly progressive form of leukodystrophy starting in early infancy. Both central and peripheral nervous system symptoms are prominent. Nerve conduction studies show motor conduction velocities to be only about one-half of what would be expected and distal latencies to be about double. EMG may show an increase in the number of polyphasic motor unit potentials with a few fibrillation potentials (30).

Tangier Disease

This is an extremely rare autosomal recessive storage disease producing tonsillar hypertrophy, hepatosplenomegaly, and severe motor and sensory peripheral neuropathy. Fibrillation potentials are seen on EMG and nerve conduction velocities show either mild slowing or normal conduction. Patients with this disorder have an extremely low concentration of high density lipoprotein, which causes cholesterol and cholesterol ester to accumulate in the reticuloendothelial system and in other tissues, including the peripheral nerve (31).

Abetalipoproteinemia

Patients with this autosomal recessive disease do not synthesize the precursor for the development of very low density lipoprotein, low density lipoprotein, and chylomicrons. The earliest symptoms are gastrointestinal and begin in infancy. Stocking-glove hypesthesia occurs. Nerve conduction velocities are moderately reduced (31).

Primary Amyloidosis

Electrophysiologic changes in peripheral nerve, except for possible entrapment neuropathies, are very rare in sporadic primary amyloidosis or in secondary amyloidosis. However, in autosomal dominant primary amyloidosis, conduction velocities in peripheral motor nerves frequently show borderline low nerve conduction velocities. Needle EMG may show typical changes of a mild peripheral neuropathy (32).

Myotonic Dystrophy Neuropathy

It is still controversial whether there is a peripheral neuropathy associated with myotonic dystrophy. However, recent studies suggest that, in a significant portion of patients with myotonic dystrophy, there is some motor nerve conduction velocity slowing which cannot be explained on any other basis (33).

Acute Intermittent Porphyria

Peripheral neuropathy is a symptom in almost 20% of patients with this disease; the majority of the neuropathies are either motor or mixed sensory and motor. Motor conduction velocities are moderately decreased in both upper and lower extremities with reduction in amplitude of the evoked muscle potentials. Distal motor latencies are normal or only slightly prolonged. EMG shows fibrillation potentials in the acute stage (34). The EMG data suggest an axonal neuropathy with abnormal findings first occurring proximally.

TOXIC NEUROPATHIES (Table 8.3)

1. Heavy Metals

Lead

Lead toxicity classically occurs in children in the form of encephalopathy and in adults as a radial neuropathy. Children with lead toxicity generally live in the poorer neighborhoods of large cities, while adults with lead toxicity generally work in occupations where they come in contact with lead-containing compounds. The incidence of lead toxicity in children is considerably less since the removal of lead from paints. Occasionally, there are still reports of lead toxicity in painters, workers in the lead industry, persons eating food stored in ceramic containers, and persons drinking lead-contaminated illicit alcohol (35). Diagnosis should be confirmed by finding elevated levels of lead in blood or urine and the presence of lead lines in x-rays of long bones.

Lead neuropathy produces primarily motor symptoms. It can produce a

TABLE 8.3. *Toxic Neuropathies*

Heavy Metals
1. Lead
2. Arsenic
3. Thallium
4. Mercury
5. Antimony
6. Gold

Drugs
1. Nitrofurantoin (Furadantin)
2. Diphenylhydantoin (Dilantin)
3. Vincristine
4. Isoniazide
5. Dapsone
6. Corticosteroids
7. Sodium cyanate
8. Halogenated oxyquinoline derivatives
9. Thalidomide
10. Hydralazine
11. Chloramphenical
12. Disulfiram (Antabuse)
13. Sulfonamides
14. Heroin
15. LSD

Organic Compounds
1. *N*-Hexane
2. Acrylamide
3. Tri-ortho-cresyl phosphate
4. Methyl-butyl-ketone
5. Carbon disulfide
6. Carbon monoxide
7. Dichlorophenoxyacetic acid

more severe neuropathy in the upper extremities than in the lower, and it is not always symmetrical. In children, encephalopathy may be related to the acute ingestion of large amounts of lead, whereas the peripheral neuropathy appears to be related to prolonged ingestion of small amounts. Motor nerve conduction velocities in children with chronic lead neuropathy are mildly reduced (36). Fibrillations and positive sharp waves may be found in the weakest muscles.

In the adult with acute lead toxicity, slowing of nerve conduction takes several weeks to become maximal. Distal motor latencies appear to be prolonged more than conduction velocity is slowed; residual latencies are prolonged (35). Although slowing of nerve conduction velocity is not marked, there can be a striking reduction in the amplitude of the evoked muscle action potential (35). Sensory conduction studies appear to be the most sensitive in detecting subclinical chronic lead toxicity (37). Thus, lead neuropathy in humans is probably an axonal degeneration rather than a demyelinating neuropathy as seen in experimental animals given large amounts of lead orally (38).

Arsenic

Arsenic poisoning can result from household and agricultural accidents as well as industrial contact or poisoning. Survival from severe arsenic poisoning is rare but now possible with supportive medical care and the use of British anti-Lewisite.

We have followed a patient for almost 3 years following arsenic ingestion and found maximal nerve conduction slowing to occur several weeks after ingestion. Slowing in the elbow-to-wrist and knee-to-ankle segments paralleled slowing of the distal latencies; residual latencies never become strikingly prolonged. Therefore, the toxic effect appears to be on all segments of nerve with the longer nerves of the lower extremities most severely affected. Conduction was lost in the peroneal nerves at 3 weeks, although it was present at 2 weeks.

The lowest conduction velocities in the upper extremities that we obtained were between one-half and two-thirds of normal. There was a marked decrease in the amplitude of the evoked muscle response. At 146 weeks, the ulnar and median motor nerve conduction velocities returned to normal, but conduction never returned in the distal segments of the peroneal nerves. EMG revealed profuse fibrillation and positive sharp wave potentials in the affected distal muscles (39).

Thallium

Toxicity from this metal is very rare. If seen, it is probably the result of ingestion of insecticides or rodenticides. The symptoms of toxicity are paresthesias, arthralgias, and alopecia. Thallium neuropathy is mainly sensory, and the pathology is primarily axonal degeneration (40). Therefore, it would be expected that conduction velocities would be only slightly decreased but the amplitude of the sensory action potential markedly diminished (41). In severe cases, fibrillation potentials might be seen.

Mercury

Generally, the toxicity of mercury is industrially related. Neuropathy is rare, but when it occurs it tends to be mainly sensory. Limited data indicate motor conduction velocities are normal but that there are mild abnormalities of sensory nerve conduction (40).

Antimony

Antimony intoxication can result in alopecia and weakness but, although it has been considered to cause a peripheral neuropathy, it has not been determined for certain if the weakness is due to central or peripheral nerve dysfunction (40).

Gold

It is uncertain whether observed gold neuropathy is due to a direct toxic effect of the drug, an allergic reaction, or the underlying disease. Axonal degeneration is the predominant pathologic change in nerves (42, 43). Conduction velocities might be expected to be only minimally reduced with attenuated sensory nerve action potentials and fibrillation potentials on EMG.

2. Drugs

Nitrofurantoin (Furadantin)

As of 1973, 137 cases of peripheral neuropathy attributed to Furadantin had been reported in the world's literature. Symptoms are sensory and motor, and recovery relates to the severity of symptoms and not to the dosage. Symptoms start, in most cases, within a month and a half following institution of treatment (44).

The first report of electrophysiologic studies in Furadantin neuropathy was by Honet (45), who reported generalized denervation potentials on EMG of both proximal and distal muscles of upper and lower extremities. He found it impossible to obtain motor nerve conduction in the peroneal, tibial, and median nerves of his patient but was able to obtain moderately reduced ulnar and radial conduction velocities by using a needle recording electrode. In Furadantin neuropathy, the amplitude of the evoked muscle response is also diminished (46).

The effect on peripheral nerve is due to toxicity by the drug rather than to underlying renal disease. Tool and Parrish (47) gave the usual therapeutic Furadantin dose and course (400 mg daily for 14 days) to 14 healthy volunteers. They reported very slight slowing of motor nerve conduction velocities (especially noticeable in some subjects) as well as slowing of mean sensory conduction velocity and slight prolongation of distal sensory latencies.

Diphenylhydantoin (Dilantin)

Long-term use of Dilantin can result in the development of peripheral neuropathy. Clinically, the syndrome presents with a striking loss of deep tendon reflexes in the lower extremities. The toxic effects of Dilantin appear to be cumulative and are more likely to occur in patients who have been on therapy more than 10 years.

Conduction velocities in areflexic patients are mildly slowed in the lower extremities and may be low normal in the upper extremities. EMG shows fibrillations and reduced numbers of voluntary action potentials in affected muscles (48). In patients who have been on Dilantin for more than 10 years but who have no clinical signs of neuropathy, some subtle electrical abnormalities may be present. Eisen et al. (49) found that slightly under 20% of these asymptomatic patients showed conduction slowing in peroneal motor nerves, distal median motor nerves, or distal median sensory fibers.* In general, motor findings predominated over sensory. They also tested the H reflex and found it to be minimally prolonged in patients who had the most severe distal slowing. This suggests that the pathology which was present tended to be most marked in the distal portion of nerve.

Vincristine

Vincristine can cause peripheral neuropathy which produces a minimal reduction in motor nerve conduction velocity. However, the amplitude of both the evoked motor response and the sensory response can fall dramatically to only 10 or 20% of normal (42). Distal latencies are essentially unchanged (50). Needle EMG shows fibrillation potentials in affected muscles with reduced numbers of voluntary action potentials. As would be expected from the electrodiagnostic studies, Vincristine produces primary axonal degeneration.

Isoniazide (INH, Isonicotinic Acid Hydrazide)

Isoniazide clinically produces more severe sensory symptoms than motor symptoms which are limited almost exclusively to the legs. Isoniazide toxicity is predominately axonal (46). It first affects the distal portions of the longest nerve fibers, then slowly spreads centripetally, producing a so-called "dying back" disease (51). EMG would be expected to show evidence of denervation in severely affected muscles; nerve conduction should be only mildly reduced, if altered at all, but amplitudes of the evoked responses should be decreased.

Dapsone

Dapsone is a sulfone which has, in recent years, come to be used for dermatologic conditions other than leprosy. Recently there have been cases

* Caution is advised in using motor or sensory conduction velocities from distal portions of the median nerve, especially in a chronic neuropathic disease, as criteria for the presence of a peripheral neuropathy because of the frequency of conduction slowing at points of pressure in chronic neuropathies.

of axonal disease reported, presumably produced by this drug. Motor and sensory conduction velocities and latencies were normal, but the amplitude of the M response was reduced. EMG showed fibrillations and a neuropathic pattern of action potentials in affected muscles (52).

Corticosteroids

It is not commonly recognized that corticosteroids can produce disease of the peripheral nerves. Administration of high doses of prednisone in rabbits has been reported to produce segmental demyelination in peripheral nerves. A study in humans with chronic obstructive lung disease showed motor nerve conduction velocity in both upper and lower extremities to be reduced approximately 10% when compared to controls with the same clinical disorder but who were not receiving steroids (53). The severity was proportional to the dose and duration of steroid therapy.

Sodium Cyanate

Since the early part of the 1970s, when it was first noted that sodium cyanate inhibits sickling of erythrocytes *in vitro* with no toxicity to the erythrocyte, this compound has received increasing attention as a possible treatment for sickle cell disease. Early studies showed relative lack of toxicity, and the compound has recently been tried clinically. In 1974, two patients undergoing this treatment were identified as having developed motor and sensory peripheral neuropathies while on the drug. The severity of the neuropathy appeared to be related to the duration of treatment as well as the dosage. In patients in whom the neuropathy developed, some improvement was noted several weeks following cessation of sodium cyanate. Slowing of nerve conduction was more pronounced in sensory fibers than in motor nerves and more pronounced in the lower extremities than in the upper. Slowing appeared to affect the nerve in a rather diffuse manner so that the abnormal prolongation of the distal latency was about equal to the slowing of nerve conduction velocity in more proximal nerve segments. In addition to the two patients who presented obvious clinical signs of neuropathy, some electrodiagnostic evidence of alteration of peripheral nerve function was seen in 16 out of 27 asymptomatic patients receiving the drug (54).

Needle EMG of muscles in affected patients showed fibrillation potentials and reduced voluntary motor unit action potentials, indicating the presence of axonal degeneration. It appears prudent that any patient who receives the drug during future clinical studies should be evaluated with periodic nerve conduction velocity determinations to detect early reversible neuropathy (54).

Halogenated Oxyquinoline Derivatives

A variety of case reports have suggested that this class of drugs is potentially neurotoxic when given in high doses over an extended period of time. Symptoms of neurotoxicity are optic nerve atrophy and/or polyneuropathy. The drugs appears to produce axonal degeneration (55).

Thalidomide

Although this drug is no longer available, it is thought to have produced irreversible axonal degeneration in some cases. Conduction studies have shown motor nerve conduction velocities to be unaffected and sensory nerve action potentials to be reduced in amplitude or absent (42).

Hydralazine (Apresoline)

Whether the sensory neuropathy produced by this drug is a direct effect of the medication or due to the pyridoxine deficiency produced by the drug is unclear (42). The amplitude of the sensory action potential might be expected to be reduced.

Chloramphenicol (Chloromycetin)

Relatively mild sensory symptoms in the feet, preceded by optic neuritis, have been reported. This has been seen only in patients with impaired renal function who have been taking the drug and is most likely due to impaired drug excretion (42). Sensory nerve potential amplitude might be expected to be diminished.

Disulfiram (Antabuse)

This drug is used in the treatment of chronic alcoholism. Even though peripheral neuropathy is associated with chronic alcoholism, it is likely that Disulfiram is itself neurotoxic, since the neuropathy appears to be dose-related. Motor nerve studies show very slight reduction in conduction velocity, and the amplitude of the sensory potential is decreased. EMG shows signs of denervation (42).

Sulfonamides

Although mentioned as a cause of peripheral neuropathy, it is not certain that they are directly neurotoxic (51).

Heroin

DiBenedetto (56) recently reported motor and sensory nerve conduction velocities to be normal and sensory potential amplitudes to average only half normal in a group of heroin users. In several users there were also reduced amplitudes and temporal dispersion of the evoked muscle response.

Lysergic Acid Diethylamide (LSD)

DiBenedetto (56) recently found evidence of axonal degeneration in LSD users. Sensory amplitudes were approximately one-half normal, but other parameters were within normal limits.

3. Organic Compounds

N-hexane

N-hexane is an organic solvent widely used in printing and in commercial glues. There have been recent reports of polyneuropathy in persons exposed to this compound in industrial adhesives and in "glue sniffers" (57–59). Clinically, an insidious, symmetric stocking-glove sensory-motor disturbance develops several months after exposure to the substance and requires many months to recover. Recovery is relatively complete in mild cases and partial in severe cases.

In the cases which have been reported, motor nerve conduction velocities and distal motor latencies in the upper extremities average about two-thirds normal (59). Lower extremity motor nerve conduction velocities are reduced about the same degree. Sensory conduction velocities are either unobtainable or in the same range as motor velocities. EMG shows denervation potentials of an acute neuropathic process.

Acrylamide

Motor nerve conduction velocities are either normal or just below normal limits, but terminal latencies are very prolonged. Sensory nerve action potentials are either reduced in amplitude or absent (60). There appears to be selective destruction of the large myelinated fibers, which may account for the slight reduction in maximal conduction velocity (51).

Tri-ortho-cresyl Phosphate (TOCP, Jamaica Ginger Paralysis)

TOCP has probably produced the greatest number of cases of toxic neuropathy in man. In 1929 and 1930, alcoholic extracts of ginger and rum contaminated with TOCP were used as alcoholic drinks, causing many thousands of cases of neuropathy by the end of 1930. Contamination of cooking oil with TOCP has also produced several major episodes of neuropathy, the most recent in Morocco in 1959 affecting about 10,000 people. Although TOCP has affected many thousands of humans, most of the cases occurred before the availability of clinical EMG; therefore, data on humans are not available. However, electrodiagnostic and pathologic information is based on a number of studies in animals.

TOCP causes distal degeneration of axons. In the recovery phase, when distal axonal regeneration has occurred, fairly normal conduction velocities are recorded with prolonged terminal latencies (51). Data from primates indicate that in the acute phase the conduction velocity does not fall; however, the amplitude of the evoked muscle response falls steadily until, at about 40 days, it is approximately 10% of normal. Needle EMG shows denervation in distal muscles (61).

Methyl-butyl-ketone (MBK)

Peripheral neuropathy caused by MBK was first identified in 1973 among the workers of a coated fabric plant. Motor and sensory distal latencies were usually prolonged and nerve conduction velocities either normal or only moderately reduced. Needle EMG showed numerous fibrillations and positive sharp waves in distal muscles (62).

Carbon Disulfide

This industrial solvent can produce peripheral neurotoxicity, but electrodiagnostic findings are minimal and tend to occur predominantly in distal segments of nerve. Nerve conduction slowing is most pronounced in distal sensory fibers (63). Denervation in distal muscles can be seen in more severe cases (60).

Carbon Monoxide

In addition to its effect on the central nervous system in acute poisoning, carbon monoxide can produce symptoms of a peripheral neuropathy. There is a paucity of findings in humans, and no evidence of conduction slowing exists at this time (60).

Dichlorophenoxyacetic Acid

This widely used compound in herbicides has produced several reported cases of peripheral neuropathy. EMG shows partial denervation, but nerve conduction velocity is not slowed (60).

PERIPHERAL NEUROPATHIES ASSOCIATED WITH DISEASES (Table 8.4)

Diabetes Mellitus

Diabetic neuropathy, in all of its varied forms, may be the most common peripheral neuropathy associated with a particular disease. There are at least six different types of diabetic neuropathies: diabetic polyneuropathy (diabetic neuropathy), diabetic mononeuropathy, diabetic amyotrophy, hypoglycemic neuropathy, neuropathy of uncontrolled diabetes and autonomic neuropathy.

Diabetic neuropathy is common. In a classic study, Mulder et al. (64) found that one-third of an unselected group of diabetic patients had polyneuropathy and one-sixth had mononeuropathy, usually at the common sites of nerve entrapment—the median nerve at the wrist, the peroneal nerve at the fibular head, and the ulnar nerve at the elbow. Diabetic polyneuropathy can be present even with good diabetic control. In general, the more severe the clinical signs of neuropathy, the greater the slowing of nerve conduction. Three things tend to adversely affect the electrodiagnostic findings: (a) older age, (b) more severe diabetes and (c) longer duration of diabetes.

Mulder et al. (64) reported that peroneal motor conduction measurement was a more sensitive indicator of diabetic neuropathy than upper extremity motor nerve evaluation. About the same time, Downie and Newell (65) presented data indicating that sensory nerve conduction and evoked poten-

TABLE 8.4. *Peripheral Neuropathies Associated with Diseases*

---

1. Diabetes mellitus
   a. Polyneuropathy
   b. Mononeuropathy
   c. Amyotrophy
   d. Hypoglycemic neuropathy
   e. Uncontrolled diabetic neuropathy
   f. Autonomic neuropathy
2. Alcoholism
3. Chronic renal insufficiency
4. Carcinoma
5. Multiple myeloma
6. Waldenstrom's macroglobulinemia
7. Rheumatoid arthritis
8. Sjogren's syndrome
9. Scleroderma
10. Systemic lupus erythematosus
11. Cranial arteritis
12. Hypothyroidism
13. Polyarteritis nodosa
14. Sarcoidosis
15. Lymphoma
16. Cryoglobulinemia
17. Chronic liver disease
18. Thermal burns
19. Diphteria
20. Leprosy
21. Herpes zoster
22. Thiamine (vitamin B_1) deficiency
23. Riboflavin (vitamin B_2) deficiency
24. Pyridoxine (vitamin B_6) deficiency
25. Pernicious anemia (vitamin B_{12}) deficiency
26. Fasting
27. Postgastrectomy state
28. Tropical (nutritional) ataxia

---

tial amplitude decrements were also very sensitive detectors of diabetic neuropathy. Of electrodiagnostic studies generally available, it is currently felt that sensory nerve studies are more sensitive than motor studies in identifying early diabetic neuropathy (66). Reduction in sensory nerve conduction velocity appears to be greatest in distal segments of peripheral nerves. Buchthal et al. (67) have recently suggested that an increase in temporal dispersion of the sensory potential (prolonged duration and iregular shape) is the earliest sign of diabetic neuropathy and may be observed even when conduction along the fastest fibers and the amplitude of the potential are still within the normal range. Facial nerve latency has also been used as an indicator of diabetic neuropathy (68).

Motor nerve conduction velocity decrements appear to correlate strikingly with diabetic complications. Patients who have normal or only slightly reduced conduction velocities have few diabetic complications, but those who have marked reduction in conduction velocities have multiple and severe complications. We reviewed information on 100 diabetics who had had their conduction velocities determined from 1 to 8 years previously and found that patients who had died since the prior determination (44%) had had conduction velocities which had been considerably lower than the group of diabetics who had survived. The former had had a mean peroneal motor conduction velocity of 27.1 m/sec, whereas the surviving group had had a mean of 35.9 m/sec. Both had shown low normal ulnar motor values (69, 70).

Electrodiagnostic identification of neuropathy in diabetic children under age 5 is negligible. However, over age 5, conduction slows with age, especially in the peroneal nerve; 48% of older children who have had diabetes more than 5 years have abnormal motor nerve conductions (71). Motor nerves in the lower extremity are involved even when sensory nerves in the upper extremities are normal.

There have been histologic reports of both demyelination and axonal degeneration in diabetic neuropathy, and it is unclear whether the demyelination of diabetic neuropathy is primary or secondary (72). Recently a single fiber EMG study by Thiele and Stålberg (73) showed that diabetic fiber density does not differ significantly from normal and that there is a low incidence of jitter, indicating that the main nerve dysfunction in diabetic polyneuropathy is demyelination. We have reviewed our data on patients with diabetic polyneuropathy, including those with markedly reduced conduction velocities, and found that residual latencies in the ulnar nerve were normal and those of the peroneal nerve close to normal. This indicates that the conduction deficit is comparable in middle and distal segments of nerve. We also noted that the residual latency of the median nerve tended to be prolonged, indicating [as did the study of Mulder et al. (64)] that many patients with diabetic polyneuropathy are subject to subclinical carpal tunnel syndrome. F wave studies in diabetics have recently been reported and show significant conduction slowing in the most proximal segments of nerve (74). Thus, the pattern of nerve conduction change in diabetic polyneuropathy is moderate slowing of comparable degree in both proximal and distal segments, with conduction more affected in the lower extremities. Sensory studies appear to be more sensitive than motor for detection of early polyneuropathy.

EMG studies of diabetic polyneuropathy show few, if any, fibrillation potentials. Voluntary motor unit action potentials are of generally normal configuration, amplitude, and duration but may be reduced in number (69, 73). Another electrodiagnostic test which may prove to be of use in diabetic neuropathy is measurement of the refractory period between two stimuli; it has been reported to be prolonged in diabetics prior to development of significant changes in conduction velocity (75).

There is a rapid, clear-cut increase in conduction velocity, which results from adequate treatment of uncontrolled diabetes following either initial diagnosis or an episode of ketoacidosis. Guyton (76) showed an 8 m/sec improvement in peroneal nerve conduction velocity over a 10-hr period following recovery from diabetic coma. Gregersen (77) followed recently diagnosed diabetics treated with insulin for 8–35 days and found conduction velocities in the peroneal nerve to increase as much as 10 m/sec, generally within the first week. These results have been confirmed more recently by others in other motor nerves (78, 79).

Diabetic mononeuropathy generally affects one or two peripheral nerves and can occur either in association with polyneuropathy or in the absence of it. Mulder et al. (64) reported the peroneal nerve to be the most commonly involved. Signs of peroneal conduction deficit were seen in about 12% of diabetics; symptoms and findings are similar to those commonly seen in crossed-leg palsy. Median nerve compression at the wrist and ulnar nerve compression at the elbow were reported to occur with less frequency (64). However, our recent experience indicates that over one-half of diabetic patients may have asymptomatic subclinical "carpal tunnel syndrome" if diagnosed on the basis of prolonged median nerve residual latencies in the presence of normal ulnar residual latencies.

Diabetic amyotrophy is a frequently discussed but poorly understood disorder. It may occur in patients in whom no polyneuropathy is seen. The clinical pattern consists of pain in muscles of the thigh associated with weight loss and an absence of sensory symptoms. The onset of symptoms may be fairly rapid, and clinical improvement, once optimal diabetic management is achieved, can be impressive. Fibrillations and positive sharp waves are commonly encountered in affected muscles, as contrasted to their paucity in diabetic polyneuropathy, and nerve conduction velocities are not usually decreased. In general, the muscles of the thigh and lower paraspinals are most often affected (80).

Hypoglycemic peripheral neuropathy is very rare and associated with various types of hyperinsulinism including insulin-secreting islet cells adenomas of the pancreas. It is a motor-sensory neuropathy with greater involvement of nerves of the upper extremities. Fibrillations can occur in distal hand muscles with little or no motor nerve conduction slowing until late in the disase (81). At times, it may mimic motor neuron disease (82).

Alcoholism

Alcoholic neuropathy is an insidious mixed motor and sensory disorder with symptoms occurring first in the legs. Symptoms are worst in the distal muscles of the extremities. They often start with burning of the feet or painful paresthesias and cramps. Even in severe cases gross slowing of motor conduction velocity is rare; conduction is rarely reduced more than 20%. Sensory conduction may be slightly more reduced than motor. Often the earliest finding will be a decrease in sensory potential amplitude, with distal amplitude reduced more than proximal amplitude (83–85).

Using a variety of electrophysiological techniques to evalute nerve function in alcoholic neuropathy, Blackstock et al. (85) documented only very minimal reduction in maximal motor conduction velocity but much more marked slowing of minimum conduction velocity (smaller nerve fibers). They also noted a prolongation of the H reflex.

Our experience with alcoholic neuropathy and analysis of recent data also indicates that motor nerve conduction velocities in both upper and lower extremities are only minimally reduced and that residual latencies are not prolonged. Unlike diabetic neuropathy, where it appeared that there was a predilection to subclinical carpal tunnel syndrome, no abnormally prolonged distal median latency was observed. Thus, the pattern of involvement of motor nerves in alcoholic neuropathy is one of only very minimal conduction slowing, equally affecting both proximal and distal segments of nerve.

EMG studies show frequent fibrillations, especially in distal muscles. Voluntary action potentials are polyphasic and have a prolonged duration. Single fiber EMG studies show increased fiber density (73). These data, as well as results of histologic studies, indicate that the primary lesion is axonal degeneration.

Chronic Renal Insufficiency

The neuropathy of renal failure has been the subject of considerable study, but its mechanism is still not clear. However, it is clear that dialysis judged to be adequate by blood chemistry standards may not be adequate to arrest peripheral neuropathy. Therefore, since the early reports by Jebsen and coworkers at the University of Washington (86–88) of the value of motor nerve conduction velocity determinations in monitoring uremic neuropathy, nerve conduction velocities have been used as a standard for the evaluation of adequate hemodialysis. These investigators showed that inadequate dialysis resulted in decreased motor nerve conduction velocities, and adequate dialysis resulted in improved conduction velocities.

The neuropathy of chronic renal disease is both motor and sensory; both motor and sensory nerve conduction velocities are slowed equally (89). It is generally believed that patients with chronic renal disease can have subclinical neuropathy detected by slowing of nerve conduction in the absence of signs of clinical neuropathy (88). Although symptoms are more pronounced in the lower extremities, the degree of conduction slowing is approximately equal in nerves of the arms and legs (87). In cases of severe neuropathy, nerve conduction velocities in the range of 20 m/sec may be seen in the peroneal nerve, and nerve conduction velocities in the range of 30 m/sec may be seen in nerves of the upper extremities.

Changes in nerve conduction have been reported to be statistically no different in terminal segments of peripheral nerves than in midextremity segments (90). We have found that residual latencies are not prolonged in most patients we have studied, although in some patients (11% in ulnar nerve, 22% in median nerve), they are prolonged. Codish and Cress (91) reported that distal sensory latencies may be slightly more sensitive indicators of improvement in uremic neuropathy than conventional conduction velocity determinations. H reflex abnormalities parallel changes in conduction in midextremity segments (92).

There appears to be no effect on nerve conduction velocity of a single episode of dialysis (88). In the past, patients occasionally showed an explosive and rapidly progressive peripheral neuropathy during the first weeks of hemodialysis, although this is much more uncommon now with improved dialysis techniques. Increase in conduction velocity with adequate dialysis is slow, and abnormalities may never completely revert to normal. However, with successful renal transplantation, complete recovery can occur (93). Although motor nerve conduction velocity determinations have become a standard means of assessing the effect of long term dialysis on peripheral nerves, some have objected that, in their centers, the error of nerve conduction determinations is so great that data are unreliable (94).

EMG in patients with uremic neuropathy shows fibrillation potentials in the most paretic distal muscles and motor unit potentials which may initially be normal but which become decreased in number and larger in amplitude later in the disease (73, 95).

Thiele and Stålberg found that fiber density and jitter in uremic neuropathy did not differ significantly from normal, indicating that uremic neuropathy has characteristics more in common with a demyelinating than an axonal lesion (73). However, Dyck et al. (95), on the basis of in vitro compound action potential studies, quantitative histologic and teased-fiber studies and electron microscopy on nerves from two patients, felt that there is evidence that the site of primary disease is the neuron, resulting in degeneration of the axis cylinder and secondary demyelination.

Uremic neuropathy is one of the least understood of the common neuropathies. Our data indicate that in most patients there is no predilection for preferential distal conduction slowing; thus, in most patients, neuropathy is compatible with either demyelination or acute axonal dysfunction. However, in approximately one-fifth of our patients, preferential distal slowing, which appears to occur in chronic axonal disease, was prominent. It may be that acute uremic neuropathy has different characteristics from chronic uremic neuropathy, and subclinical carpal tunnel syndrome may occur with some frequency.

Carcinoma

The main symptoms of carcinogenic neuropathies are generally sensory or sensory-motor. When there is motor involvement, distal muscles may show fibrillations and reduction of motor units, with an increased number of polyphasic potentials. Conduction velocities are normal or mildly reduced. Sensory action potentials may be expected to be absent or markedly reduced in patients with sensory neuropathies. Terminal latencies may be slightly prolonged in some patients with normal conduction velocities (96).

Multiple Myeloma

The peripheral neuropathy produced by this disease is probably more common than suspected and is typically a painful sensory-motor neuropathy in a middle-aged male. Nerve conduction velocities in both upper and lower extremities are mildly reduced as are amplitudes of upper and lower extremity sensory action potentials. Midextremity and terminal segments are equally affected (97).

Waldenstrom's Macroglobulinemia

There are only a few published reports of electrodiagnostic studies in this disease and too little data for a complete understanding of the associated neuropathy. The several studies which have been published report motor nerve conduction to vary from normal to minimally slowed. Fibrillations have been reported in clinically affected muscles (98).

Rheumatoid Arthritis

Neuropathy may be seen in as many as 10% of patients with rheumatoid arthritis; it varies in severity from a mild distal sensory neuropathy to acute episodes of mononeuropathy multiplex. The pathogenesis is thought to be due to the vasculitis associated with rheumatoid arthritis. In patients with marked neuropathy, fibrillation potentials may be seen on EMG.

The most commonly encountered peripheral nerve disease in rheumatoid arthritis is considered to be entrapment neuropathy of the median nerve at the wrist (99). However, Herbison et al. (100) have presented data which indicate that, although carpal tunnel syndrome occurs in rheumatoid arthritis, it may not be seen any more frequently than in a matched control population. Furthermore, many patients with rheumatoid arthritis who have symptoms of a carpal tunnel syndrome may have normal nerve latency studies; their symptoms are probably due to rheumatoid synovitis and not carpal tunnel syndrome.

Sjogren's Syndrome

The neuropathy of this disease appears to be identical to that of rheumatoid arthritis and occurs in about 10% of patients with the disease. It is a nonhomogeneous neuropathy, most likely caused by vasculitis. Nerve conduction velocity is low in affected nerves and distal latencies are prolonged. EMG of paretic muscles shows denervation (101).

Scleroderma

Peripheral neuropathy is an extremely rare complication of scleroderma. Histologic sections of affected nerves look similar to nerves from patients with rheumatoid neuropathy, and it might be expected that nerve conduction and EMG changes would be similar (99).

Systemic Lupus Erythematosus

Progressive symmetrical ascending sensory-motor neuropathy is a rare complication of systemic lupus erythematosus. Cases of mononeuropathy multiplex have also been reported. However, sufficient studies have not yet been done to outline the EMG pattern of lupus neuropathy (99, 102).

Cranial Arteritis

Peripheral neuropathy has been described in association with giant cell arteritis and may manifest itself either as a symmetrical polyneuropathy or as mononeuropathy multiplex. Adequate data are not available to determine nerve conduction and EMG changes in this disease (99).

Hypothyroidism

Two types of neuropathy occur in hypothyroidism. The most common type is carpal tunnel syndrome. It is felt that increased amounts of acid mucopolysaccarides, which normally constitute the bulk of the ground substance of extracellular connective tissue, effectively diminish the space available to the median nerve as it passes through the carpal tunnel. Symptoms of the carpal tunnel syndrome of myxedema can, however, usually be successfully treated with hormonal therapy. If a patient can be made to remain euthyroid, abnormally prolonged distal motor latency in the median nerve may return to normal (103).

The second type of neuropathy in hypothyroidism is diffuse peripheral neuropathy. Conduction in motor and sensory fibers of peripheral nerves may be slow, especially in distal segments. These findings may also be reversed with good medical management (103). Fincham and Cape (104) studied motor and sensory nerve conduction in a group of myxedematous patients and found amplitudes of sensory action potentials to be reduced and sensory nerve conduction velocities to be slow; motor nerve conduction was less affected.

Polyarteritis Nodosa

Clinical neuropathy in polyarteritis is common and starts out as a sensory-motor mononeuropathy multiplex which becomes a symmetrical polyneuropathy at a later stage. The pathology of the neuropathy is an acute arteritis, which accounts for the initial segmental symptoms, involving small arteries in segments of nerve. The later polyneuropathy is probably due to the coalescence of multiple segments of nerve lesions. Nerve conduction velocity in affected nerves is decreased, and EMG of affected muscles shows signs of denervation (105).

Sarcoidosis

Peripheral neuropathy is an extremely rare complication of this disease and generally occurs only in the facial nerve. Fluctuating and remitting cranial nerve palsies may occur ("polyneuritis cranialis"). Clinically, this is indistinguishable from idiopathic Bell's Palsy. Needle EMG generally shows fibrillations in affected muscles (106).

Lymphomas (Hodgkin's Disease, Lymphosarcoma, Reticulum Cell Sarcoma, Folicular Lymphoma)

Sensory neuropathies and sensory-motor neuropathies have been described in lymphomas. The neuropathy may be either acute, subacute, or chronic; some are relapsing and remitting. One-third of the patients with lymphomas will show a mild reduction in motor nerve conduction velocities (107). The neuropathy may be due to either a direct infiltration of tumor cells or remote effects of tumor. Histopathologic changes in various stages of disease may show demyelination and axonal degeneration. During acute exacerbations, low conduction velocities can fall even further (108).

Cryoglobulinemia

Peripheral neuropathy is a rare complication of this disorder. EMG may show denervation in affected muscles. Motor conduction velocities are mildly slowed, and it may not be possible to obtain sensory action potentials (98).

Chronic Liver Disease

Peripheral neuropathy can be seen in a variety of disorders producing chronic liver disease: infectious mononucleosis, acute intermittent porphyria, periarteritis nodosa, secondary amyloidosis, celiac disease, and certain intoxications. Although many patients with chronic liver disease have chronic alcoholism, peripheral nerve dysfunction is seen in patients with many other types of liver disease as well.

Electrophysiologic abnormalities have been reported in from 14 to 68% of patients with chronic liver disease. Abnormalities consist of slowing of motor nerve conduction velocities (a slowing which can be quite marked in some patients), denervation in affected muscles, increase in sensory latency, and reduction in the amplitude of the evoked sensory potential (109–111). Careful exclusion of all patients with liver disease who may have other causes for peripheral neuropathy (e.g., alcoholism and diabetes) may reveal very few peripheral neuropathies caused by liver disease alone without other explanations. In addition, there is a distinct disease clinically similar to Guillain-Barré syndrome associated with acute viral hepatitis (111).

Thermal Burns

Henderson et al. (112) reported a 15% incidence of polyneuropathy in a large series of patients on a burn unit. The electrophysiologic abnormality which was reported was a reduction in motor nerve conduction velocity. In general, neuropathy was found to develop approximately 9 weeks after the burn and to be unrelated to the severity of the burn. One-half of the patients recovered spontaneously with discontinuation of antibiotics. The authors considered the neuropathy most likely to be due to antibiotics used in treatment. However, only a few antibiotics have been clearly identified as producing peripheral polyneuropathies; some of the nerve dysfunctions may have been directly related to some unknown toxic effect of the burn.

Diphtheria

Corynebacterium diphtheriae produces an exotoxin which causes segmental demyelination of peripheral nerves. Diphtheritic neuropathy produces mixed sensory and motor symptoms and does not generally occur until 8 weeks after onset of illness. There are only a few case reports in the literature of conduction studies in humans. One indicates that motor conduction velocities at their nadir may be markedly reduced and, with clinical improvement, can return to normal (113). Another case report indicates that in the late stage, even when conduction velocities have returned to normal, distal latencies may still be prolonged (114).

We have had the opportunity to study a patient recovering from diphtheria who, upon discharge from the hospital, developed generalized weakness. Nerve testing showed low normal motor conduction velocities with prolonged distal latencies and decreased amplitude, temporally dispersed muscle action potentials. EMG showed fibrillation potentials and positive sharp waves in affected muscles. Most information on changes in nerve conduction in diphtheria have been done in experimental animals. It may be that in some cases, human diphtheria causes axonal degeneration as well as demyelination.

Leprosy

The neuropathy of leprosy is patchy, affecting different nerves in a spotty manner. In general, conduction slowing occurs through areas where nerves are swollen and palpable, while proximal and distal conduction is normal. Generally, the ulnar nerve is involved earlier and more extensively than other nerves. Distal latencies are often prolonged, and compound muscle action potentials are temporally dispersed and decreased in amplitude. Sensory conduction studies may be difficult to obtain; where they can be obtained, they will generally show a reduction in amplitude of the sensory action potential. EMG may show denervation, and short duration, polyphasic, low amplitude potentials suggestive of myopathy have been reported. Signs of denervation are most frequently seen in the orbicularis oris muscle (115).

Herpes Zoster

Five percent of the patients with clinical herpes zoster will have zoster-induced motor nerve involvement at the same root level as their sensory lesion. It always follows cutaneous zoster. Fibrillation potentials are universally present in affected muscles, including those innervated by the posterior primary division of the spinal nerve. Voluntary motor unit potentials are compatible with a neuropathic disease. Motor and sensory conduction values are generally normal (116).

Thiamine (Vitamin B₁) Deficiency

Thiamine deficiency causes a distal sensory-motor neuropathy, more pronounced in the lower extremities. In animals, thiamine deficiency causes degenerative changes of nerves of the feet commonly seen in "dying back" polyneuropathies (117). The largest and longest nerve fibers are the first to degenerate; if the deficiency is prolonged, smaller nerve fibers degenerate as well (118). Nerve conduction and EMG studies have been carried out in thiamine deficient rats. It has been found that motor nerve velocities decrease to nearly half the normal value and that this decrease is associated with a decrease in amplitude of the evoked muscle response. Experimental studies have shown that electrical stimulation of peripheral nerves causes release of thiamine and that a thiamine antagonist impairs the conductivity of peripheral nerves. Therefore, nerve conduction might be appreciably slowed in thiamine deficiency without having significant histologic changes in peripheral nerve (118). Consequently, such marked conduction slowing as has been seen does not necessarily imply structural changes. EMG shows fibrillations in affected muscles (119).

It is difficult to study thiamine deficiency in man because of the rarity of the deficiency without a deficiency of other vitamins as well. Consequently, there is a paucity of pathologic and electrical information on changes in peripheral nerves in man. However, a recent pathologic study by Takahashi and Nakamura (120) in nine patients showed axonal degeneration of large myelinated fibers to be the major change. EMG observations in man might be expected to be similar to those in experimental animals.

Riboflavin (Vitamin B₂) Deficiency

A deficiency of riboflavin is possibly related to the etiology of Strachan's syndrome: painful neuropathy, amblyopia, and oro-genital dermatitis. Adequate pathologic or electrodiagnostic data are not available in this disease, but it is postulated to be a dying back neuropathy and might be expected to show the EMG and nerve conduction velocity changes associated with such a condition (118). Painful paresthesias or burning feet can occur in the absence of the other components of Strachan's syndrome and may respond favorably to riboflavin injections. Lai and Ransome (121) reported such a case. Burning feet may also occur with alcoholic neuropathy, beri-beri, or pellagra.

Pyridoxine (Vitamin B₆) Deficiency

It is thought that deficiency of pyridoxine is responsible for the neurologic aspects of pellagra; whereas the other manifestations of this deficiency state, dermal lesions and gastrointestinal symptoms, are probably due to lack of niacin. The distribution of the neuropathy is a stocking-glove motor sensory loss. Pathologic sections of peripheral nerve show degeneration of myelin sheaths in early cases, although in advanced pellagra, Wallerian degeneration is evident (118). EMG might be expected to show a picture of axonal degeneration in advanced deficiency states.

Pernicious Anemia (Vitamin B_{12} Deficiency)

Because of the posterior column lesion of pernicious anemia, the clinical identification of polyneuropathy is often difficult. The most complete conduction study of this disorder was by Mayer (122), who evaluated 53 patients with vitamin B_{12} deficiency. He found that nerve conduction abnormalities were present only when patients had neurologic signs; they consisted mainly of conduction slowing in distal sensory fibers and prolongation of the H reflex. The amplitude of the sensory action potential, motor nerve conduction in the lower and upper extremities and proximal sensory conduction were normal. Needle EMG was not done. His conclusion was that the number of nerve fibers conducting was normal and that the primary pathology was a distal dysfunction of myelin.

Fasting

Nerve conduction velocities were determined in a group of patients who fasted from 14 to 28 days and received no vitamin supplements. Motor conduction velocities in the upper and lower extremities and sensory latencies in the upper extremities were found to be statistically unchanged during the period of fasting (123). In spite of the absence of electrodiagnostic changes, approximately one-fourth of the patients developed paresthesias.

Postgastrectomy State

Symptoms of peripheral neuropathy are common in patients following gastrectomy, but a recent electrodiagnostic study of postgastrectomy patients with symptoms of peripheral neuropathy failed to reveal any nerve conduction or EMG abnormalities (124).

Tropic (Nutritional) Ataxia

This disease is endemic in certain parts of Africa and thought to be due to a vitamin deficiency. Others have speculated that it may be due to chronic cyanide intoxication from diets of cassava plants prepared in a particular way. Histologically, peripheral nerves show segmental demyelination with relative sparing of axons. Motor nerve conduction velocities are markedly decreased in the lower extremities and normal or mildly decreased in the upper extremities. Only occasionally are fibrillation potentials noted in paretic muscles (125).

TABLE 8.5. *Idiopathic Neuropathies*

1. Guillain-Barré syndrome
2. Chronic polyradiculoneuropathy
3. Fisher's syndrome
4. Shoulder girdle neuropathy

IDIOPATHIC NEUROPATHIES (Table 8.5)

Guillain-Barré Syndrome (Idiopathic Polyradiculoneuritis, Landry-Guillain-Barré-Strohl Syndrome)

The Guillain-Barré syndrome is a disorder in which nerve conduction studies and EMG can be of great value in confirming the diagnosis, identifying the segments of diseased nerve and determining prognosis. There are a number of reports of the electrodiagnostic findings in this disease, some showing little change in nerve conduction in the presence of severe weakness, leading to the conclusion by some that there is no correlation between clinical symptoms and nerve conduction studies (126).

The explanation for this lack of correlation is most likely that pathologic changes do not occur equally in all parts of a peripheral nerve at the same time. The first area of dysfunction may be the nerve root, shortly followed by dysfunction of the terminal portion of the nerve (127). Radiculitis is generally associated with the most profound clinical weakness, but nerve conduction velocities in conventional segments may be normal. Later, as clinical strength improves, a centrifugal pattern of demyelination may develop and successively more distal nerve segments may show slowing of conduction velocity. Most of the conduction studies in the Guillain-Barré syndrome have not been serial evaluations but have been single determinations in patients with a variety of stages of disease. This has led to a lack of appreciation of the pattern of nerve conduction changes in Guillain-Barré polyneuritis.

The pathologic changes in peripheral nerve consist of mononuclear cellular infiltration and segmental demyelination in the motor and sensory roots, eventually involving the entire length of the neuraxis. Probably because lesions are spotty, there is a greater probability of dysfunction and a greater preponderance of clinical signs in distal muscles, reflecting the greater probability that the longer the individual axon at risk the more likely it is to be affected at one or more points along its course. Axonal degeneration can occur in severe cases and has traditionally been considered to be secondary to the inflammatory process associated with demyelination. The mononuclear inflammatory process in the peripheral nervous system may persist in low grade fashion for months and years after clinical recovery (128).

Early studies by Cerra and Johnson (129) showed that motor nerve conduction velocity determinations were helpful in the diagnosis of Guillain-

Barré syndrome by showing slowing of conduction in midextremity segments of peripheral nerves. Lambert and Mulder (130) showed that during the first 3 weeks of illness, 61% of patients diagnosed as having the Guillain-Barré syndrome had slowing of motor nerve conduction in one or more peripheral nerves, and an additional 25% had temporal dispersion of the muscle action potential. But what of the 14% of patients showing no abnormalities of conduction velocity or terminal latency? If the demyelinating process starts in the nerve roots, radicular nerve conduction velocity should be reduced in the early stages of the disease before conduction slowing occurs in more distal segments. Kimura et al. (131) measured F wave conduction velocities in 10 patients with Guillain-Barré syndrome during the first 4 weeks after onset of symptoms and found them to be slow in 8 out of 10 patients. F wave slowing was approximately 20 m/sec slower than normal, whereas conduction slowing which was observed at that time in more distal segments was much less pronounced. Similarly, Lachman et al. (132) studied patients with Guillain-Barré syndrome within 6 weeks of the onset of symptoms and found the H reflex in the lower extremity and F response to the abductor pollicis brevis muscle to be prolonged in all of seven patients tested. In two of these patients, routine motor and sensory conductions in distal nerve segments were normal. King (133) has also reported F wave latencies to be prolonged in all patients with Guillain-Barré syndrome, even though distal conduction velocity was within the normal range.

In addition to the radicular conduction slowing which occurs during the earliest part of the disease, there is also an early slowing in the small terminal axons, as noted by Lambert and Mulder (130), as well as in the largest terminal fibers, producing a prolongation of the distal latency (131, 134, 135). Conventional nerve conduction velocities may be normal when radicular and terminal latency studies demonstrate slowed conduction (136). We have reviewed our electrodiagnostic data of Guillain-Barré polyneuritis and found many of the distal latency measurements of the median, ulnar, and peroneal nerves to be the longest we have observed in any disease. We have recorded distal motor latencies up to 34 msec in the peroneal nerve, 30 msec in the median nerve, and 18 msec in the ulnar nerve.

Longitudinal studies of changes in nerve conduction in the Guillain-Barré syndrome would be useful to better understand the pattern of development of the nerve lesion and to help the electromyographer interpret his findings. Such data in the literature are limited. In a classic paper, Bannister and Sears (137) reported the serial changes in nerve conduction recorded from one patient starting 12 days after the onset of his illness. At that time, the patient was almost totally paralyzed but had motor nerve conduction velocity in the low-normal range. The distal motor latency which was measured over a relatively short distance (6 cm) was 5.0 msec. On subsequent examinations, the patient was clinically stronger, but the distal motor latency became even more prolonged and motor conduction velocity in the forearm decreased slightly. It was not possible to record any sensory response until the 50th day, at which time the patient had made marked recovery; the distal sensory latency was prolonged (8.0 msec), sensory conduction velocity slow (20 m/sec), and the sensory action potential very low in amplitude. McQuillen and Gorin (138) studied three patients during recovery and found forearm motor conduction velocities to continue to decrease from 2 to 17 weeks after the point of minimum strength had occurred; as conduction velocity fell further, strength returned. Cerra and Johnson (129) also noted that recovery of nerve conduction velocity lags behind the return of clinical strength.

We have studied serial motor nerve conduction velocities over a 17-week period in a 19-year-old male with Guillain-Barré syndrome (Table 8.6). The discrepancy between early clinical improvement and continued deterioration of nerve conduction in mid and distal portions of the extremities can be noted. The pattern is spotty; as conduction in one segment improves, another may worsen. Overall, there is a tendency for a centrifugal movement of dysfunction and repair (Fig. 8.5). What must be stressed is the importance of studying multiple nerves in a patient with Guillain-Barré polyneuritis, since any one segment or any one particular nerve might be normal while other segments might be abnormal (139, 140).

The best indicator of clinical prognosis in the Guillain-Barré syndrome is needle EMG. Patients requiring the longest time to recover demonstrate fibrillation potentials and positive sharp waves in paretic muscles (136). In a study of 50 patients, Ramon and Taori (141) have shown that the presence

TABLE 8.6. *Guillain-Barré Syndrome in a 19-Year-Old Male*

Time After Onset	Motor Nerve	Conduction Velocity (m/sec)	Distal Motor Latency (msec)	Strength
6 weeks	R Ulnar-distal	52.2	4.5	Started to improve
	R Peroneal-distal	31.5	9.0	
11 weeks	R Ulnar-distal	43.1	7.3	Much improved
	R Peroneal-distal	37.1	13.5	
	R Median-distal	40.7	11.2	
	R Median-proximal	32.4		
12 weeks	R Ulnar-distal	40.8	6.4	Continued improve-
	R Ulnar-proximal	38.5		ment
	L Median-distal	43.0	9.5	
	L Median proximal	38.9		
	L Ulnar-distal	43.7	6.5	
	L Ulnar-proximal	38.5		
	L Peroneal-distal	31.1	12.6	
17 weeks	R Ulnar-distal	45.8	4.3	Almost normal
	R Ulnar-proximal	45.7		
	L Median-distal	46.1	6.5	
	L Median-proximal	53.9		
	R Peroneal-distal	52.9	7.7	
	L Ulnar-distal	54.8	11.5	
	L Ulnar-proximal	41.4		

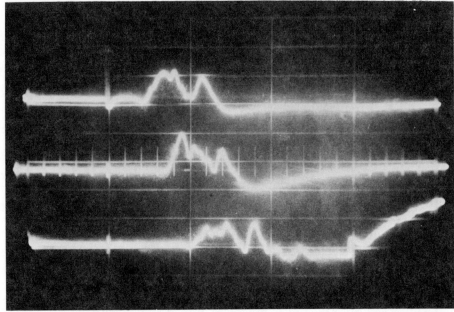

Fig. 8.5. Left median motor studies of a 19-year-old patient with Guillain-Barré polyneuritis 12 weeks after onset of disease. Calibration: each vertical division, 1000 μV; each major horizontal division, 20 msec. All latencies were recorded with surface electrodes. *Top*, distal latency; *middle*, latency at anticubital fossa; *lower*, latency from the supraclavicular point of stimulation. Note the low amplitude temporally dispersed muscle action potential. Proximal nerve conduction velocity, 38.9 m/sec; distal nerve conduction velocity, 43.0 m/sec.

of profuse fibrillation potentials within the first 4 weeks of illness, with or without associated nerve conduction deficits, a condition seen in approximately one-third of their patients, is associated with poor prognosis and pronounced residual deficits.

It is not clear why nerve dysfunction should occur in nerves of Guillain-Barré patients where there is little inflammation. Asbury has noted little inflammatory reaction in terminal segments of peripheral nerves with this disease (131—see Asbury's comments, p. 61). Why, then, is there such striking prolongation of distal motor latency? Is it because radicular inflammation affects the most distant part of the neuraxis, or is it because histologic material has not been taken when terminal latencies were prolonged? Also, why are there classically more motor than sensory symptoms (136)? Arnason (102) has pointed out that there is no preferential histologic involvement of motor over sensory roots.

There are many unanswered questions about idiopathic polyneuritis, but a pattern of nerve conduction and EMG changes can be established. During the 1st month, there is a great likelihood of finding conduction changes in the most proximal segments followed shortly thereafter by changes in the distal latencies. Later, when recovery may be occurring clinically, midextremity conduction velocities may fall even further. An absence of fibrillation potential and positive sharp waves indicates a good prognosis.

Chronic Polyradiculoneuropathy (Chronic Inflammatory Polyradiculoneuropathy)

This term can be applied to an idiopathic polyneuropathy having either a steady (no improvement by 6 months) or progressive course or to a recurring polyneuropathy producing a stepwise progression of symptoms. Dyck et al. (142) have recently reported a series of 53 patients meeting these criteria, with nerve biopsy showing segmental demyelination. Prognosis was poor; complete recovery occurred only occasionally, although patients were followed an average of 7.5 years. Most of the pathologic changes occurred in the spinal roots and proximal portions of nerves.

Chronic polyradiculoneuropathy appears to be characterized by diffusely slow motor conduction velocities and difficulty in obtaining any sensory evoked responses. EMG of severely involved muscles shows denervation. Amplitudes of evoked muscle responses are low, and distal latencies are only minimally prolonged. When sensory conduction velocities can be obtained they are essentially normal. Tasker and Chutorian (143) reported results of electrodiagnostic studies in 16 children with chronic polyneuritis of childhood (persisting longer than 1 year), and they also found decreased nerve conduction velocities and EMG signs of denervation.

Fisher's Syndrome

This rare disease is considered to be a variant of idiopathic polyneuritis in which external ophthalmoplegia and ataxia also occur. However, recent electrodiagnostic studies have shown no conduction abnormalities in peripheral nerves, although areflexia and mild peripheral weakness were present (144).

Shoulder Girdle Neuropathy (Brachial Neuritis)

Symptoms of this disease classically start with an acute, sharp pain in one shoulder, followed several days later by a dull ache. About the same time, the patient notices shoulder weakness, which is followed by atrophy of specific muscles of the shoulder girdle. Sensory loss is very rare. In one-third of the patients, both shoulders are involved, with symptoms developing in the second shoulder at the same time or within hours of the first.

The most commonly affected nerves are the suprascapular nerve to the supraspinatus muscle, the suprascapular nerve to the infraspinatus muscle, and the axillary nerve to the deltoid muscle. The 11th cranial nerve can also be involved. Branches of other peripheral nerves are also occasionally affected, including nerves of the lower extremities (145, 146). Motor nerve conduction velocities from Erb's point to the elbow and from the elbow to the wrist and terminal latencies are normal when recorded to unaffected muscles. However, latencies from Erb's point to paretic shoulder muscles

TABLE 8.7. Nerve Conduction and Electromyographic Findings in Hereditary Neuropathies[a]

Disease	Motor Nerve Conduction Velocity	Site of Maximum Nerve Conduction Velocity Slowing	Amplitude of Muscle Action Potential	Sensory Nerve Conduction Velocity	Amplitude of Sensory Action Potential	Electromyographic Findings	Useful Laboratory Tests
Charcot-Marie Tooth disease	↓↓↓	Distal	↓↓↓	↓↓	↓↓	Fib.	
Hereditary motor sensory neuropathy II	NI	None	NI	NI	↓↓↓		
Dejerine-Sottas disease	↓↓↓	Distal	↓↓↓	Not obtainable	0		
Roussy-Levy syndrome	↓↓↓	Distal	↓↓↓	↓↓	↓↓	Fib.	
Hereditary sensory neuropathy							
Dominant				Not obtainable	0		
Recessive	↓		↓↓	Not obtainable	0		
Hereditary compression neuropathy	↓	At sites of compression				Chronic neuropathic	
Riley-Day syndrome	↓			NI	↓↓↓		
Infantile neural axonal dystrophy	NI					Fib.	
Friedreich's ataxia	↓		↓	Not obtainable	0		
Spinocerebellar degenerations of adulthood	↓			↓		Fib.	
Familial spastic paraplegia	NI		NI	NI	↓	Fib.	

Disease				Distribution	EMG	Special diagnostic test
Pelizaeus-Merzbacher disease	↓↓	↓↓	↓↓			
Refsum's disease	↓↓	↓↓	↓↓		Chronic neuropathic Fib.	↑ Serum phytanic acid
Fabry's disease	NI	NI	NI		NI	↓ Alpha galactosidase
Metachromatic leukodystrophy	↓↓	↓↓	↓↓	General		↑ Sulfatide in urine
Krabbe's leukodystrophy	↓↓	↓↓	↓	General	Fib.	
Tangier disease	↓	↓	↓		Fib.	↓ Plasma high density lipoproteins
Abetalipoproteinemia	↓	↓				↓ Plasma low density lipoproteins
Primary amyloidosis	↓↓			Proximal	Chronic neuropathic	Serum electrophoresis
Myotonic dystrophy	↓ ↓	NI	NI		Myotonia	
Acute intermittent porphyria	↓	↓↓	↓		Fib.	↑ Urine porphyrins

[a] ↓, low normal to slightly reduced; ↓↓, moderately low; and ↓↓↓, extremely low. NI, normal; Fib., fibrillation potentials

Note: When no entries are made in table, adequate electrophysiologic data is not available.

and terminal latencies to paretic distal muscles will be prolonged, have reduced amplitude, and show temporal dispersion (147). The conduction dysfunction parallels the severity of clinical involvement.

An Approach to the Electrodiagnostic Study of Peripheral Neuropathies

More electrodiagnostic information can be obtained from a patient with a peripheral neuropathy than simple determination of conventional motor nerve conduction velocity, although this might be sufficient in many cases. The electromyographer's first step should be to determine the status of peripheral nerve function in different segments of nerve: midextremity, terminal and, sometimes, root. Separate information about conduction velocities and evoked responses in motor and sensory fibers will also be useful. If the neuropathy is evolving, serial conduction studies will provide even more information. Needle EMG will yield valuable data unobtainable from any type of conduction study.

The electromyographer should be familiar with the various electrophysiologic patterns of peripheral nerve dysfunction seen in different peripheral neuropathies and be able to identify conditions compatible with his electrodiagnostic observations. As a starting point, Tables 8.7–8.12 tabulate the motor and sensory nerve conduction velocity, motor and sensory evoked potential amplitude, site of motor nerve conduction velocity slowing, and EMG findings reported from the studies of the 86 diseases discussed in this chapter. By reviewing this chapter and other sources, additional information may be obtained or inferred.

As the sorting-through process continues, certain neuropathies can be excluded because they do not fit the electrophysiologic pattern, while others will be seen to be compatible with electrodiagnostic findings. For example, nerve conduction velocities may be very helpful in separating the Guillain-Barré syndrome from chronic polyradiculoneuropathy. In the former, terminal motor latency prolongation is striking and sensory nerve conduction is slow; whereas, in the latter, motor nerve conduction is equally reduced in midextremity and terminal segments, and sensory nerve conduction may be normal. As another example, Charcot-Marie-Tooth disease can be separated from hereditary motor sensory neuropathy II by the marked slowing of motor nerve conduction in the former and reduction in sensory action potential amplitude in the latter. How many times has an electromyographer been asked to identify the cause of a peripheral neuropathy in an alcoholic patient with diabetes? This may not be possible with a high degree of certainty, but in general, an absence of fibrillation potentials with fairly substantial motor and sensory conduction slowing would identify the latter; and fibrillations, marked reduction in amplitude of sensory action potentials, and only minimal nerve conduction slowing would identify the former.

Acute toxic neuropathies appear to be more likely to cause general axonal failure and diffuse conduction slowing, whereas chronic toxic processes are

TABLE 8.8. *Nerve Conduction and Electromyographic Findings in Heavy Metal Neuropathies*[a]

Heavy Metal	Motor Nerve Conduction Velocity	Site of Maximum Nerve Conduction Velocity Slowing	Amplitude of Muscle Action Potential	Sensory Nerve Conduction Velocity	Amplitude of Sensory Action Potential	Electromyographic Findings	Useful Laboratory Tests
Lead	↓	Distal	↓↓	↓	↓↓	Fib.	↑ Lead in blood, urine
Arsenic	↓↓	General	↓↓↓	↓	↓↓	Fib.	↑ Arsenic in urine
Thallium	↓		↓↓		↓	Fib.	↑ Thallium in urine
Mercury	NI		NI				↑ Mercury in urine
Antimony							
Gold							

[a] Symbols and abbreviations as in Table 8.7.

TABLE 8.9. Nerve Conduction and Electromyographic Findings in Drug Neuropathies[a]

Drugs	Motor Nerve Conduction Velocity	Site of Maximum Nerve Conduction Velocity Slowing	Amplitude of Muscle Action Potential	Sensory Nerve Conduction Velocity	Amplitude of Sensory Action Potential	Electromyographic Findings
Nitrofurantoin	↓↓		↓↓	↓↓	↓↓	Fib.
Diphenylhydantoin	→	Distal		NI		Fib.
Vincristine	→	General	↓↓↓	NI	↓↓↓	
Isoniazide		Distal	→		↓↓	
Dapsone	NI		→	NI	↓↓	Fib.
Corticosteroids	→					
Sodium cyanate		General		↓↑	↓↓	Fib.
Halogenated oxyquinoline deriv.						
Thalidomide	NI			NI	↓↓	
Hydralazine						
Chloramphenical						
Sulfonamides						
Disulfiram	→				↓↓	Fib.
Sulfonamides						
Heroin	NI		→	NI	↓↓	
LSD	NI		NI	NI	↓↓	

[a] Symbols and abbreviations as in Table 8.7.

TABLE 8.10. *Nerve Conduction and Electromyographic Findings in Organic Compound Neuropathies*[a]

Compounds	Motor Nerve Conduction Velocity	Site of Maximum Nerve Conduction Velocity Slowing	Amplitude of Muscle Action Potential	Sensory Nerve Conduction Velocity	Amplitude of Sensory Action Potential	Electromyographic Findings
N-hexane	↓↓	General		↓↓		Fib.
Acrylamide	→	Distal			↓↓↓	Fib.
Tri-ortho-cresyl phosphate	NI	Distal	↓↓			Fib.
Methyl-butyl-ketone	→	Distal		→		Fib.
Carbon disulfide	NI	Disal		→		
Carbon monoxide	NI					
Dichlorophenoxyacetic acid	NI					Fib.

[a] Symbols and abbreviations as in Table 8.7.

TABLE 8.11. *Nerve Conduction and Electromyographic Findings in Diseases Associated with Peripheral Neuropathies*[a]

Disease	Motor Nerve Conduction Velocity	Site of Maximum Nerve Conduction Velocity Slowing	Amplitude of Muscle Action Potential	Sensory Nerve Conduction Velocity	Amplitude of Sensory Action Potential	Electromyographic Findings	Useful Laboratory Tests
Diabetes mellitus							
Polyneuropathy	↓↓	General	→	↓↓	↓↓	NI	↑ Urine and blood glucose
Mononeuropathy	→	Local blocks	↓↓	→	↓↓	Fib.	Same as above
Amyotrophy	NI	Nerves to thigh muscles	↓↓	NI		Fib.	Same as above
Hypoglycemic neuropathy	NI	Nerves of upper extremities				Fib.	↓ Blood glucose
Uncontrolled	→			→			↑ Urine and blood glucose
Autonomic neuropathy							
Alcoholism	→	General		→	↓↓	Fib.	
Renal insufficiency	↓↓	Distal		↓↓		Fib.	↑ Blood urea and creatinine
Carcinoma	NI	Distal			↓↓↓	Fib.	Serum electrophoresis
Multiple myeloma	→	General			↓↓		Serum electrophoresis
Waldenstroms' macroglobulinemia	→					Fib.	Serum electrophoresis
Rheumatoid arthritis	→	Segmental	→			Fib.	↑ Sed rate + rheumatoid factor
Sjogren's syndrome	→	Segmental	→			Fib.	↓ Salivation
Scleroderma							
Systemic lupus erythematosus							+ L.E. prep.

	Location			EMG	Special tests
Cranial arteritis					
Hypothyroidism					
Mononeuropathy	Carpal tunnel	→	→		
Polyneuropathy	Distal	→	↓↓	Fib.	↓ PBI and ↓ T$_4$
Polyarteritis	Segmental			Fib.	+ Kveim reaction
Sarcoidosis	Facial nerve				
Lymphoma					
Polyneuropathy	General			NI	CBC
Mononeuropathy	Local infiltrates			Fib.	
Cryoglobulinemia			↓↓	↓↓	Fib. + Cryoglobulins
Chronic liver disease		↓↓	↓↓	↓↓	Fib. Abnormal liver function tests
Thermal burns					
Diphtheria	Distal	↓↓	↓↓	↓↓↓	Fib.
Leprosy	Segmental; where nerve is enlarged	→	→	↓↓	Fib.
Herpes Zoster	Same root level as cutaneous	NI	NI	Fib.	
Thiamine deficiency		↓↓	↓↓	Fib.	
Riboflavin deficiency					
Pyridoxine deficiency					
Pernicious anemia	Distal	NI	→↓	NI	+ Schilling test
Fasting		NI	NI		
Postgastrectomy		NI			
Tropical ataxia	Lower extremities	↓↓		NI NI	

[a] Symbols and abbreviations as in Table 8.7.

TABLE 8.12. *Nerve Conduction and Electromyographic Findings in Idiopathic Neuropathies*[a]

Disease	Motor Nerve Conduction Velocity	Site of Maximum Nerve Conduction Velocity Slowing	Amplitude of Muscle Action Potential	Sensory Nerve Conduction Velocity	Amplitude of Sensory Action Potential	Electromyographic Findings
Guillain–Barré syndrome	↓↓	Spotty centrifugal	↓↓	↓↓	↓↓	Fib.
Chronic polyradiculoneuropathy	↓↓	General	↓↓	NI	↓↓↓	Fib.
Fisher's syndrome	NI					NI
Shoulder girdle neuropathy	NI	Distal to affected muscles	↓↓			Fib.

[a] Symbols and abbreviations as in Table 8.7.

more likely to produce greater distal axon dysfunction. Similarly, hereditary axonal neuropathies produce the greatest degree of axonal dysfunction distally. The electromyographer should be aware that markedly reduced nerve conduction velocities do not necessarily mean that only demyelination has occurred. Some of the slowest nerve conduction velocities seen are in hereditary neuropathies in which distal axonal failure is severe, resulting in axons with markedly reduced diameter and secondary demyelination. However, the presence of fibrillation potentials is still a reliable sign of axonal disease.

At the conclusion of the sorting-through process, the electromyographer will have compiled those peripheral neuropathies compatible with his electrodiagnostic observations. This list will be shortened further by historical, clinical, and other laboratory data, and final diagnostic impressions can then be made.

In summary, this chapter is not intended to be a comprehensive text, but rather a useful, practical guide to peripheral neuropathies from the electromyographer's viewpoint. Nerve conduction and EMG techniques should become even more useful in the identification and evaluation of peripheral neuropathies as additional techniques (e.g., H and F wave studies, residual latencies, and sensory studies) enter into the electromyographer's armamentarium. Hopefully, this chapter will help the electromyographer identify what studies to do, understand how to interpret them, and learn how maximally to use information obtained to evaluate a patient with a peripheral neuropathy.

REFERENCES

1. LAMBERT, E. H., AND DYCK, P. J.: Compound action potentials of sural nerve in vitro in peripheral neuropathy. In *Peripheral Neuropathy*, vol. 1, pp. 427–441, ed. by P. J. Dyck, P. K. Thomas, and E. H. Lambert, Philadelphia: W. B. Saunders Co., 1975.
2. McDONALD, W.I.: Experimental neuropathy. In *New Developments in Electromyography and Clinical Neurophysiology*, vol. 2, pp. 128–144, ed. by J. E. Desmedt, Basel, Switzerland: Karger, 1973.
3. RASMINSKY, M., AND SEARS, T. A.: Saltatory conduction in demyelinated nerve fibres. In *New Developments in Electromyography and Clinical Neurophysiology*, vol. 2, pp. 158–165, ed. by J. E. Desmedt, Basel, Switzerland: Karger, 1973.
4. KRAFT, G. H.: Serial nerve conduction and electromyographic studies in experimental allergic neuritis. *Arch. Phys. Med. Rehabil.*, 56: 333, 1975.
5. KRAFT, G. H.: Serial motor nerve latency and electromyographic determinations in experimental allergic neuritis. *Electromyography*, 1: 61, 1971.
6. KAPLAN, P. E.: Sensory and motor residual latency measurements in healthy patients and patients with neuropathy. *J. Neurol. Neurosurg. Psychiat.*, 39: 338, 1976.
7. ROBERTSON, W. D., AND LAMBERT, E. H.: Measurement of sensory nerve conduction velocity in children using cerebral evoked potentials. *Arch. Phys. Med. Rehabil.*, 57: 603, 1976.
8. GANS, B. M., AND KRAFT, G. H.: Techniques of quantifying the stimulated M response and their clinical significance. *Arch. Phys. Med. Rehabil.*, 57: 598, 1976.
9. HORNING, M. R., KRAFT, G. H., AND GUY, A.: Latencies recorded by intramuscular needle electrodes in different portions of a muscle: Variation and comparison with surface electrodes. *Arch. Phys. Med. Rehabil.*, 53: 206, 1972.

10. DYCK, P. J., LAIS, A. C., AND OFFORD, K. P.: The nature of myelinated nerve fiber degeneration in dominantly inherited hypertrophic neuropathy. *Mayo Clin. Proc., 49:* 34, 1974.

11. BRIMIJOIN, S., CAPEK, P., AND DYCK, P. J.: Axonal transport of dopamine-β-hydroxylase by human sural nerves in vitro. *Science, 180:* 1295, 1973.

12. DYCK, P. J., AND LAMBERT, E. H.: Lower motor and primary sensory neuron diseases with peroneal muscular atrophy. I. Neurologic, genetic and electrophysiologic findings in hereditary polyneuropathies. *Arch. Neurol, 18:* 603, 1968.

13. HUMBERSTONE, P. M.: Nerve conduction studies in Charcot-Marie-Tooth disease. *Acta Neurol. Scand., 48:* 176, 1972.

14. KIMURA, J.: F-wave velocity in the central segment of the median and ulnar nerves: A study in normal and in patients with Charcot-Marie-Tooth disease. *Neurology, 24:* 539, 1974.

15. DYCK, P. J.: Inherited neuronal degeneration and atrophy affecting peripheral motor sensory and autonomic neurons. In *Peripheral Neuropathy*, vol. 1, pp. 825–867, ed. by P. J. Dyck, P. K. Thomas, and E. H. Lambert, Philadelphia: W. B. Saunders Co., 1975.

16. DYCK, P. J.: Experimental hypertrophic neuropathy. *Arch. Neurol. 21:* 73, 1969.

17. DYCK, P. J., LAMBERT, E. H., SANDERS, K., AND O'BRIEN, P. C.: Severe hypomyelination and marked abnormality of conduction in Dejerine-Sottas hypertrophic neuropathy: Myelin thickness and compound action potential of sural nerve in vitro. *Mayo Clin. Proc., 46:* 432, 1971.

18. KRIEL, R. L., CLIFFER, K. D., BERRY, J., SUNG, J. H., AND BLAND, C. S.: Investigation of a family with hypertrophic neuropathy resembling Roussy-Levy syndrome. *Neurology, 24:* 801, 1974.

19. OHTA, M., ELLEFSON, R. D., LAMBERT, E. H., AND DYCK, P. J.: Hereditary sensory neuropathy, type II: Clinical, electrophysiologic, histologic and biochemical studies of a Quebec kinship. *Arch. Neurol., 29:* 23, 1973.

20. DEWEERDT, C. J., STAAL, A., AND WENT, L. N.: Erfelijke compressie-neuropathie [Hereditary compression neuropathy]: Een classificatieprobleem bij erfelijk neurologische ziekten. *Ned. Tijdschr. Geneeskd., 114:* 1648, 1970.

21. BROWN, J. C., AND JOHNS, R. J.: Nerve conduction in familial dysautonomia (Riley-Day Syndrome). *J. Am. Med. Assoc. 201:* 118, 1967.

22. DUNCAN, C., STRUB, R., McGARRY, P., AND DUNCAN, D.: Peripheral nerve biopsy as an aid to diagnosis in infantile neuroaxonal dystrophy. *Neurology, 20:* 1024, 1970.

23. DYCK, P. J., and OHTA, M.: Neuronal atrophy and degeneration predominantly affecting peripheral sensory neurons. In *Peripheral Neuropathy*, vol. 1, pp. 791–824, ed. by P. J. Dyck, P. K. Thomas, and E. H. Lambert, Philadelphia: W. B. Saunders Co., 1975.

24. ZIEGLER, D. K., SCHIMKE, R. N., KEPES, J. J., ROSE, D. L., AND KLINKERFUSS, G.: Late onset ataxia, rigidity, and peripheral neuropathy. *Arch. Neurol., 27:* 52, 1972.

25. McLEOD, J. G., AND MORGAN, J. A.: Nerve conduction studies in spinocerebellar degenerations. Proc. 5th Int. Congr. EMG Clin. Neurophys., Rochester, Sept. 1975.

26. LOVELACE, R. E., JOHNSON, W. G., AND MARTIN, J.: Peripheral nerve involvement and carrier detection in Pelizaeus-Merzbacher disease. *Arch. Phys. Med. Rehabil., 57:* 600, 1976.

27. REFSUM, S.: Heredopathia atactica polyneuritiformis (Refsum's Disease): Clinical and genetic aspects of Refsum's disease. In *Peripheral Neurophathy*, vol. 1, pp. 868–890, ed. by P. J. Dyck, P. K. Thomas, and E. N. Lambert, Philadelphia: W. B. Saunders Co., 1975.

28. OHNISHI, A., AND DYCK, P. J.: Loss of small peripheral sensory neurons in Fabry disease. *Arch. Neurol., 31:* 120, 1974.

29. BISCHOFF, A.: Neuropathy in leukodystrophies. In *Peripheral Neuropathy*, vol. 1, pp. 891–913, ed. by P. J. Dyck, P. K. Thomas, and E. H. Lambert, Philadelphia: W. B. Saunders Co., 1975.

30. HOGAN, G. R., GUTMANN, L., AND CHOU, S. M.: The peripheral neuropathy of Krabbe's (globoid) leukodystrophy. *Neurology, 19:* 1094, 1969.

31. PLEASURE D. E.: Abetalipoproteinemia and Tangier disease. In *Peripheral Neuropathy*,

vol. 1, pp. 928–941, ed. by P. J. Dyck, P. K. Thomas, and E. H. Lambert, Philadelphia: W. B. Saunders Co., 1975.

32. ARAKI, S., MAWATARI, S., OHTA, M., NAKAJIMA, A., AND KUROIWA, Y.: Polyneuritic amyloidosis in a Japanese family. *Arch. Neurol., 18:* 593, 1968.

33. ROOHI, F., LIST, T., AND LOVELACE, R. E.: Myotonic muscular dystrophy and slow motor nerve conduction velocities. *Arch Phys. Med. Rehabil., 57:* 603, 1976.

34. ALBERS, J. W., ROBERTSON, W. C., AND DAUBE, J. R.: Electromyographic findings in porphyric neuropathy. *Arch. Phys. Med. Rehabil., 57:* 595, 1976.

35. OH, S. J.: Lead neuropathy: Case report. *Arch. Phys. Med. Rehabil., 56:* 312, 1975.

36. FELDMAN, R. G., HADDOW, J., KOPITO, L., AND SCHWACHMAN, H.: Altered peripheral nerve conduction velocity: Chronic lead intoxication in children. *Am. J. Dis. Child., 125:* 39, 1973.

37. FIASCHI, A. F., DEGRANDIS, D., AND FERRARI, F.: Correlations between neurophysiological and histological findings in subclinical lead neuropathy. Proc. 5th Int. Congr. EMG Clin. Neurophys., Rochester, Sept. 1975.

38. FULLERTON, P. M., AND HARRISON, M. J. G.: Subclinical lead neuropathy in man. *Electroencephogr. Clin. Neurophysiol., 27:* 718, 1969.

39. O'SHAUGHNESSY, E., AND KRAFT, G. H.: Arsenic poisoning: Long-term follow-up of a nonfatal case. *Arch. Phys. Med. Rehabil. 57:* 403, 1976.

40. GOLDSTEIN, N. P., McCALL, J. T., AND DYCK, P. J.: Metal neuropathy. In *Peripheral Neuropathy,* vol. 1, pp. 1227–1262, ed. by P. J. Dyck, P. K. Thomas, and E. H. Lambert, Philadelphia: W. B. Saunders Co., 1975.

41. DiBENEDETTO, M.: Evoked sensory potentials in peripheral neuropathy. *Arch. Phys. Med. Rehabil., 53:* 126, 1972.

42. LeQUESNE, P. M.: Neuropathy due to drugs. In *Peripheral Neuropathy,* vol. 1, pp. 1263–1280, ed. by P. J. Dyck, P. K. Thomas, and E. H. Lambert, Philadelphia: W. B. Saunders Co., 1975.

43. McLEOD, J. G., WALSH, J. C., AND LITTLE, J. M.: Sural nerve biopsy. *Med. J. Aust., 2:* 1092, 1969.

44. TOOLE, J. F., GERGEN, J. A., HAYES, D. M., AND FELTS, J. H.: Neural effects of nitrofurantoin. *Arch. Neurol., 18:* 680, 1968.

45. HONET, J. C.: Electrodiagnostic study of a patient with peripheral neuropathy after nitrofurantoin therapy. *Arch. Phys. Med. Rehabil., 48:* 209, 1967.

46. GOODGOLD, J., AND EBERSTEIN, A.: *Electrodiagnosis of Neuromuscular Disease,* pp. 157–205, Baltimore: The Williams & Wilkins Company, 1972.

47. TOOLE, J. F., AND PARRISH, M. L.: Nitrofurantoin polyneuropathy. *Neurology, 23:* 554, 1973.

48. LOVELACE, R. E., AND HORWITZ, S. J.: Peripheral neuropathy in long-term diphenylhydantoin therapy. *Arch. Neurol., 18:* 69, 1968.

49. EISEN, A. A., WOODS, J. F., AND SHERWIN, A. L.: Peripheral nerve function in long-term therapy with diphenylhydantoin. *Neurology, 24:* 411, 1974.

50. SANDLER, S. G., TOBIN, W., AND HENDERSON, E. S.: Vincristine-induced neuropathy: A clinical study of fifty leukemic patients. *Neurology, 19:* 367, 1969.

51. GILLIATT, R. W.: Recent advances in the pathophysiology of nerve conduction. In *New Developments in Electromyography and Clinical Neurophysiology,* vol. 2, pp. 2–18, ed. by J. E. Desmedt, Basel, Switzerland: Karger, 1973.

52. GUTTMAN, L., MARTIN, J. D., AND WELTON, W.: Dapsone motor neuropathy—An axonal disease. Proc. 5th Int. Congr. EMG Clin. Neurophys., Rochester, Sept. 1975.

53. ANSARI, K. A.: Steroids and motor nerve conduction velocity. *Neurology, 20:* 396, 1970.

54. PETERSON, C. M., TSAIRIS, P., OHNISHI, A., LU, Y. S., GRADY, R., CERAMI, A., AND DYCK, P. J.: Sodium cyanate induced polyneuropathy in patients with sickle-cell disease. *Ann. Intern. Med., 81:* 152, 1974.

55. KAESER, H. E., UND WUTHRICH, R.: Zur frage der neurotoxizitat der oxychinoline. *Dtsch. med. Wschr., 95:* 1685, 1970.

56. DiBENEDETTO, M.: Electrodiagnostic evidence of subclinical disease states in drug abu-

sers. *Arch. Phys. Med. Rehabil.*, *57:* 62, 1976.

57. PAULSON, G. W., AND WAYLONIS, G. W.: Polyneuropathy due to n-hexane. *Arch. Intern. Med. 136:* 880, 1976.

58. GONZALEZ, E. G., AND DOWNEY, J. A.: Polyneuropathy in a glue sniffer. *Arch. Phys. Med. Rehabil.*, *53:* 333, 1972.

59. TOWFIGHI, J., GONATAS, N. K., PLEASURE, D., COOPER, H. S., AND McCREE, L.: Glue sniffer's neuropathy. *Neurology, 26:* 238, 1976.

60. HOPKINS, A.: Toxic neuropathy due to industrial agents. In *Peripheral Neuropathy*, vol. 1, pp. 1207–1226, ed. by P. J. Dyck, P. K. Thomas, and E. H. Lambert, Philadelphia: W. B. Saunders Co., 1975.

61. HERN, J. E. C.: Tri-ortho cresyl phosphate neuropathy in the baboon. In *New Developments in Electromography and Clinical Neurophysiology*, vol. 2, pp. 181–187, ed. by J. E. Desmedt, Basel, Switzerland: Karger, 1973.

62. ALLEN, N., MENDELL, J. R., BILLMAIER, D., AND FONTAINE, R. E.: An outbreak of a previously undescribed toxic polyneuropathy due to industrial solvent. *Trans. Am. Neurol. Assoc. 99:* 74, 1974.

63. VASILESCU, C.: Motor and sensory nerve conduction velocity in chronic carbon disulfide poisoning. Proc. 5th Int. Congr. EMG Clin. Neurophys., Rochester, Sept. 1975.

64. MULDER, D. W., LAMBERT, E. H., BASTRON, J. A., AND SPRAGUE, R. G.: The neuropathies associated with diabetes mellitus: A clinical and electromyographic study of 103 unselected diabetic patients. *Neurology, 11:* 275, 1961.

65. DOWNIE, A. W., AND NEWELL, D. J.: Sensory nerve conduction in patients with diabetes mellitus and controls. *Neurology, 11:* 876, 1961.

66. NOEL, P.: Diabetic neuropathy. In *New Developments in Electromyography and Clinical Neurophysiology*, vol. 2, pp. 318–332, ed. by J. E. Desmedt, Basel, Switzerland: Karger, 1973.

67. BUCHTHAL, F., ROSENFALCK, A., AND BEHSE, F.: Sensory potentials of normal and diseased nerves. In *Peripheral Neuropathy*, vol. 1, pp. 442–464, ed. by P. J. Dyck, P. K. Thomas, and E. H. Lambert, Philadelphia: W. B. Saunders Co., 1975.

68. JOHNSON, E. W., AND WAYLONIS, G. W.: Facial nerve conduction delay in patients with diabetes mellitus. *Arch. Phys. Med. Rehabil.*, *45:* 131, 1964.

69. SKILLMAN, T. G., JOHNSON, E. W., HAMWI, G. J., AND DRISKILL, H. J.: Motor nerve conduction velocity in diabetes mellitus. *Diabetes, 10:* 46, 1961.

70. KRAFT, G. H., GUYTON, J. D., AND HUFFMAN, J. D.: Follow-up study of motor nerve conduction velocities in patients with diabetes mellitus. *Arch. Phys. Med. Rehabil.*, *51:* 207, 1970.

71. ENG, G. D., HUNG, W., AUGUST, G. P., AND SMOKVINA, M. D.: Nerve conduction velocity determinations in juvenile diabetes: Continuing study of 190 patients. *Arch. Phys. Med. Rehabil.*, *57:* 1, 1976.

72. THOMAS, P. K., AND ELIASSON, S. G.: Diabetic neuropathy. In *Peripheral Neuropathy*, vol. 1, pp. 956–981, ed. by P. J. Dyck, P. K. Thomas, and E. H. Lambert, Philadelphia: W. B. Saunders Co., 1975.

73. THIELE, B., AND STALBERG, E.: Single fibre EMG findings in polyneuropathies of different aetiology. *J. Neurol. Neurosurg. Psychiat. 38:* 881, 1975.

74. CONRAD, B., AND ASCHOFF, J. C.: The diagnostic value of the F-wave latency. Proc. 5th Int. Cong. EMG Clin. Neurophys., Rochester, Sept. 1975.

75. RAJESWARAMMA, V., PEREZ, S., AND MIGLIETTA, O.: The refractory period of the sensory fibers of the median nerve in normal and diabetic patients. *Arch. Phys. Med. Rehabil.*, *54:* 595, 1973.

76. GUYTON, J. D.: The effects of changes in carbohydrate metabolism on motor nerve conduction velocity. MS thesis, The Ohio State University, 1961.

77. GREGERSEN, G.: Variations in motor conduction velocity produced by acute changes of the metabolic state in diabetic patients. *Diabetologia, 4:* 273, 1968.

78. WARD, J. D., FISHER, D. J., BARNES, C. G., JESSOP, J. D., AND BAKER, R. W. R.:

Improvement in nerve conduction following treatment in newly diagnosed diabetics. *Lancet, 1:* 428, 1971.

79. CAMPBELL, I. W. ET AL.: Peripheral and autonomic nerve function diabetic ketoacidosis. *Lancet, 2:* 167, 1976.

80. DONOVAN, W. H. AND SUMI, S. M.: Diabetic amyotrophy—A more diffuse process than clinically suspected. *Arch. Phys. Med. Rehabil., 57:* 397, 1976.

81. DANTA, G.: Hypoglycemic peripheral neuropathy. *Arch. Neurol., 21:* 121, 1969.

82. MULDER, D. W.: Motor neuron disease. In *Peripheral Neuropathy*, vol. 1, pp. 759–770, ed. by P. J. Dyck, P. K. Thomas, and E. H. Lambert, Philadelphia: W. B. Saunders Co., 1975.

83. CASEY, E. B., AND LeQUESNE, P. M.: Electrophysiological evidence for a distal lesion in alcoholic neuropathy. *J. Neurol. Neurosurg. Psych., 35:* 624, 1972.

84. CASEY, E. B., AND LeQUESNE, P. M.: Alcoholic neuropathy. In *New Developments in Electromyography and Clinical Neurophysiology*, vol. 2, pp. 279–285, ed. by J. E. Desmedt, Basel, Switzerland: Karger, 1973.

85. BLACKSTOCK, E., RUSHWORTH, G., AND GATH, D.: Electrophysiological studies in alcoholism. *J. Neurol. Neurosurg. Psychiat, 35:* 326, 1972.

86. TENCKHOFF, H. A., BOEN, F. S. T., JEBSEN, R. H., AND SPIEGLER, J. H.: Polyneuropathy in chronic renal insufficiency. *J. Am. Med. Assoc., 192:* 91, 1965.

87. HONET, J. C., JEBSEN, R. H., TENCKHOFF, H. A., AND McDONALD, J. R.: Motor nerve conduction velocity in chronic renal insufficiency. *Arch. Phys. Med. Rehabil., 47:* 647, 1966.

88. JEBSEN, R. H., TENCKHOFF, H., AND HONET, J. C.: Natural history of uremic polyneuropathy and effects of dialysis. *N. Engl. J. Med., 277:* 327, 1967.

89. JEBSEN, R. H., AND TENCKHOFF, H.: Comparison of motor and sensory nerve conduction velocity in early uremic polyneuropathy. *Arch. Phys. Med. Rehabil., 50:* 124, 1969.

90. BLAGG, C. R., KEMBLE, F., AND TAVERNER, D.: Nerve conduction velocity in relationship to the severity of renal disease. *Nephron, 5:* 290, 1968.

91. CODISH, S. D., AND CRESS, R. H.: Motor and sensory nerve conduction in uremic patients undergoing repeated dialysis. *Arch. Phys. Med. Rehabil., 52:* 260, 1971.

92. GUIHENEUC, P., AND GINET, J.: The use of the H-reflex in patients with chronic renal failure. In *New Developments in Electromyography and Clinical Neurophysiology*, vol. 2, pp. 400–403, ed. by J. E. Desmedt, Basel, Switzerland: Karger, 1973.

93. TAYLOR, N., HALAR, E. M., TENCKHOFF, H., MARCHIORO, T. L., AND MASOCK, A. J.: Effects of renal transplantation on motor nerve conduction velocity. *Arch. Phys. Med. Rehabil., 53:* 227, 1972.

94. KOMINAMI, N., TYLER, H. R., HAMPERS, C. L., AND MERRILL, J. P.: Variations in motor nerve conduction velocity in normal and uremic patients. *Arch. Intern. Med., 128:* 235, 1971.

95. DYCK, P. J., JOHNSON, W. J., LAMBERT, E. H., AND O'BRIEN, P. C.: Segmental demyelination secondary to axonal degeneration in uremic neuropathy. *Mayo Clin. Proc., 46:* 400, 1971.

96. McLEOD, J. C.: Carcinomatous neuropathy. In *Peripheral Neuropathy*, vol. 1, pp. 1301–1313, ed. by P. J. Dyck, P. K. Thomas, and E. H. Lambert, Philadelphia: W. B. Saunders Co., 1975.

97. WALSH, J. C.: The neuropathy of multiple myeloma: An electrophysiological and histological study. *Arch. Neurol., 25:* 404, 1971.

98. McLEOD, J. G., AND WALSH, J. C.: Neuropathies associated with paraproteinemias and dysproteinemias. In *Peripheral Neuropathy*, vol. 1, pp. 1012–1029, ed. by P. J. Dyck, P. K. Thomas, and E. H. Lambert, Philadelphia: W. B. Saunders Co., 1975.

99. CONN D. L., AND DYCK P. J.: Angiopathic neuropathy in connective tissue diseases. In *Peripheral Neuropathy*, vol. 1, pp. 1149–1165, ed. by P. J. Dyck, P. K. Thomas, and E. H. Lambert, Philadelphia: W. B. Saunders Co., 1975.

100. HERBISON, G. J., TENG C. S., MARTIN, J. H., DITUNNO, J. F., BIRTWELL, W. M., AND TOURTELLOTTE, C. D.: Peripheral neuropathy in rheumatoid arthritis. Paper presented at

American Academy of Physical Medicine and Rehabilitation Annual Meeting, August 23, 1970.

101. KALTREIDER, H. B., AND TALAL, N.: The neuropathy of Sjogren's Syndrome: Trigeminal nerve involvement. *Ann. Intern. Med., 70:* 751, 1969.

102. ARNASON, B. G. W.: Inflammatory polyradiculoneuropathies. In *Peripheral Neuropathy,* vol. 1, pp. 1110–1148, ed. by P. J. Dyck, P. K. Thomas, and E. H. Lambert, Philadelphia: W. B. Saunders Co., 1975.

103. BASTRON, J. A.: Neuropathy in diseases of the thyroid. In *Peripheral Neuropathy,* vol. 1, pp. 999–1011, ed. by P. J. Dyck, P. K. Thomas, and E. H. Lambert, Philadelphia: W. B. Saunders Co., 1975.

104. FINCHAM, R. W., AND CAPE, C. A.: Neuropathy in myxedema: A study of sensory nerve conduction in the upper extremities. *Arch. Neurol., 19:* 464, 1968.

105. LOVELACE, R. E.: Mononeuritis multiplex in polyarteritis nodosa. *Neurology, 14:* 434, 1964.

106. MATTHEWS, W. B.: Sarcoid neuropathy. In *Peripheral Neuropathy,* vol. 1, pp. 1199–1206, ed. by P. J. Dyck, P. K. Thomas, and E. H. Lambert, Philadelphia: W. B. Saunders Co., 1975.

107. McLEOD, J. G., AND WALSH, J. C.: Peripheral neuropathy associated with lymphomas and other reticuloses. In *Peripheral Neuropathy,* vol. 1, pp. 1314–1325, ed. by P. J. Dyck, P. K. Thomas, and E. H. Lambert, Philadelphia: W. B. Saunders Co., 1975.

108. BORIT, A., AND ALTROCCHI, P. H.: Recurrent polyneuropathy and neurolymphomatosis. *Arch. Neurol., 24:* 40, 1971.

109. KNILL-JONES, R. P., GOODWILL, C. J., DAYAN, A. D., AND WILLIAMS, R.: Peripheral neuropathy in chronic liver disease: Clinical, electrodiagnostic and nerve biopsy findings. *J. Neurol. Neurosurg. Psychiat., 35:* 22, 1972.

110. SENEVIRATNE, K. N., AND PEIRIS, O. A.: Peripheral nerve function in chronic liver disease. *J. Neurol. Neurosurg. Psychiat., 33:* 609, 1970.

111. ASBURY, A. K.: Hepatic neuropathy. In *Peripheral Neuropathy,* vol. 1, pp. 993–998, ed. by P. J. Dyck, P. K. Thomas, and E. H. Lambert, Philadelphia: W. B. Saunders Co., 1975.

112. HENDERSON, B., KOEPKE, G. H., AND FELLER, I.: Peripheral polyneuropathy among patients with burns. *Arch. Phys. Med. Rehabil., 52:* 149, 1971.

113. McDONALD, W. I., AND KOCEN, R. S.: Diphtheritic neuropathy. In *Peripheral Neuropathy,* vol. 1, pp. 1281–1300, ed. by P. J. Dyck, P. K. Thomas, and E. H. Lambert, Philadelphia: W. B. Saunders Co., 1975.

114. KOCEN, R. S., McDONALD, W. I., AND FRENGLEY, J. D.: Nerve conduction studies in a patient with diphtheritic neuropathy. Proc. 5th Int. Congr. EMG Clin. Neurophys., Rochester, Sept. 1975.

115. SABIN, T. D., AND SWIFT, T. R.: Leprosy. In *Peripheral Neuropathy,* vol. 1, pp. 1166–1198, ed. by P. J. Dyck, P. K. Thomas, and E. H. Lambert, Philadelphia: W. B. Saunders Co., 1975.

116. THOMAS, J. E., AND HOWARD, F. M.: Segmental zoster paresis—A disease profile. *Neurology, 22:* 459, 1972.

117. PRINEAS, J.: Peripheral nerve changes in thiamine-deficient rats: An electron microscope study. *Arch. Neurol., 23:* 541, 1970.

118. VICTOR, M.: Polyneuropathy due to nutritional deficiency and alcoholism. In *Peripheral Neuropathy,* vol. 1, pp. 1030–1066. ed. by P. J. Dyck, P. K. Thomas, and E. H. Lambert, Philadelphia: W. B. Saunders Co., 1975.

119. KUNZE, K., AND MUSKAT, E.: Thiamine deficiency neuropathy in rats. *Electroencephalogr. Clin. Neurophysiol., 27:* 721, 1969.

120. TAKAHASHI, K., AND NAKAMURA, H.: Axonal degeneration in beriberi neuropathy. *Arch. Neurol., 33:* 836, 1976.

121. LAI, C. S., AND RANSOME, G. A.: Burning-feet syndrome. Case due to malabsorption and to riboflavine responding. *Br. Med. J., 2:* 151, 1970.

122. MAYER, R. F.: Peripheral nerve function in vitamin B12 deficiency. *Arch. Neurol., 13:* 355, 1965.

123. MATTSON, R. H., AND LECOCQ, F. R.: Nerve conduction velocities in fasting patients. *Neurology, 18:* 335, 1968.
124. WILLIAMS, J. A., HALL, G. S. THOMPSON, A. G., AND COOKE, W. T.: Neurological disease after partial gastrectomy. *Br. Med. J., 3:* 210, 1969.
125. WILLIAMS, A. O., AND OSUNTOKUN, B. O.: Peripheral neuropathy in tropical (nutritional) ataxia in Nigeria. *Arch. Neurol., 21:* 475, 1969.
126. DE JESUS, P. V.: Landry-Guillain-Barré-Strohl syndrome: Neuronal disorder and clinico-electrophysiological correlation. *Electromyogr. Clin. Neurophysiol., 14:* 115, 1974.
127. KRAFT, G. H.: Experimental allergic neuritis: A model of idiopathic (Guillain-Barré) polyneuritis. *Arch. Phys. Med. Rehabil., 49:* 490, 1968.
128. ASBURY, A. K., ARNASON, B. G., AND ADAMS, R. D.: The inflammatory lesion in idiopathic polyneuritis: Its role in pathogenesis. *Medicine, 48:* 173, 1969.
129. CERRA, D., AND JOHNSON, E. W.: Motor nerve conduction velocity in "idiopathic" polyneuritis. *Arch. Phys. Med. Rehabil., 42:* 159, 1961.
130. LAMBERT, E. H., AND MULDER, D. W.: Nerve conduction in the Guillain-Barré syndrome. *Am. Assoc. Electromyogr. Electrodiag., 10:* 13, 1963.
131. KIMURA, J., BUTZER, J. F., VAN ALLEN, M. W.: F-wave conduction velocity between axilla and spinal cord in the Guillain-Barré syndrome. *Trans. Am. Neurol. Assoc., 99:* 52, 1974.
132. LACHMAN, T., SHAHANI, B. T., AND YOUNG, R. R.: Late responses as diagnostic aids in Landry-Guillain-Barré syndrome. *Arch. Phys. Med. Rehabil., 57:* 600, 1976.
133. KING, D.: Conduction velocity in the proximal segments of motor nerves in the Guillain-Barré syndrome. *Proc. 5th Int. Congr. EMG Clin. Neurophys.,* Rochester, Sept. 1975.
134. ISCH, F., ISCH-TREUSSARD, C., AND JESEL, M.: Diagnostic and prognostic value of the electromyographic findings in polyradiculoneuritis. *Electroencephalogr. Clin. Neurophysiol., 23:* 387, 1967.
135. SCHNEIDER, C., AND DUMRESE, C.: Le syndrome de Guillain-Barré: Etude clinique et electromyographique de 36 observations. *Schweiz. Med. Wochenschr. 104:* 393, 1974.
136. EISEN, A., AND HUMPHREYS, P.: The Guillain-Barré syndrome: A clinical and electrodiagnostic study of 25 cases. *Arch. Neurol., 30:* 438, 1974.
137. BANNISTER, R. G., AND SEARS, T. A.: The changes in nerve conduction in acute idiopathic polyneuritis. *J. Neurol. Neurosurg. Psychiat., 25:* 321, 1962.
138. McQUILLEN, M. P., AND GORIN, F. J.: Serial ulnar nerve conduction velocity measurements in normal subjects and in patients with idiopathic polyneuritis. *Neurology, 18:* 285, 1968.
139. PLEASURE, D. E., LOVELACE, R. E., AND DUVOISIN, R. C.: The prognosis of acute polyradiculoneuritis. *Neurology, 18:* 1143, 1968.
140. GASSEL, M. M.: Test of nerve conduction to muscles of shoulder girdle as aid in diagnosis of proximal neurogenic and muscular disease. *J. Neurol. Neurosurg Psychiat., 27:* 200, 1964.
141. RAMAN, P. T., AND TAORI, G. M.: Prognostic significance of electrodiagnostic studies in the Guillain-Barré syndrome. *J. Neurol. Neurosurg. Psychiat., 39:* 163, 1976.
142. DYCK, P. J., LAIS, A. C., OHTA, M., BASTRON, J. A., OHAZAKI, H., AND GROOVER, R. V.: Chronic inflammatory polyradiculoneuropathy. *Mayo Clin. Proc., 50:* 621, 1975.
143. TASKER, W. G., AND CHUTORIAN, A. M.: Chronic polyneuritis of childhood. *Neurology, 18:* 302, 1968.
144. SWICK, H. M.: Pseudointernuclear ophthalmoplegia in acute idiopathic polyneuritis (Fisher's syndrome). *Am. J. Ophthalmol. 77:* 725, 1974.
145. KRAFT, G. H.: Multiple distal neuritis of the shoulder girdle: An electromyographic clarification of "paralytic brachial neuritis." *Electroencephalogr. Clin. Neurophysiol., 27:* 722, 1969.
146. MARTIN, W. A., AND KRAFT, G. H.: Shoulder girdle neuritis: A clinical and electrophysiological evaluation. *Mil. Med., 139:* 21, 1974.
147. KRAFT, G. H.: Axillary, musculocutaneous and suprascapular nerve latency studies. *Arch. Phys. Med. Rehabil., 53:* 383, 1972.

9

Entrapment Syndromes

ROBERT J. WEBER, M.D.
DAVID PIERO, M.D.

Peripheral entrapment neuropathies are common and often challenging diagnostic problems for the clinical electromyographer. They represent a specific type of pressure neuropathy in which a nerve is compressed by some other anatomical structure. This usually occurs at a point where the nerve passes through a muscle or a fibro-osseous passageway and is, therefore, more susceptible to compression. Although not technically entrapments, the localized nerve injuries, including those which occur from prolonged pressure or repetitive trauma, frequently produce a similar clinical picture.

Although fibrous bands are frequently reported as the underlying cause of entrapment, numerous other factors favor the development of an entrapment neuropathy. Soft tissue swelling, as may occur with trauma, pregnancy, or myxedema, may lead to nerve compression within an anatomical passageway such as the carpal tunnel. Boney deformity, congenital, post-traumatic, or associated with diseases such as acromegaly, may alter the size or shape of osseous canals, resulting in an increased likelihood of nerve compromise within these passageways. Although nerves whose integrity may have been altered by disease such as diabetes, alcoholism, malnutrition, or Guillain-Barré syndrome are vulnerable to repetitive trauma or pressure, the reason for this vulnerability is not well understood (1–3). Space-occupying lesions such as ganglions, hematomas, vascular anomalies, or tumors may also cause localized pressure on a peripheral nerve. As a nerve courses across a joint, it may be subject to stretching and local irritation.

Pathophysiology of Nerve Compression

Owing to the relatively benign nature of entrapments, there is very little information on the pathological changes which occur with these lesions in human peripheral nerves. Investigators have, however, studied the effects of acute and chronic compression on the nerves of laboratory animals (4). Segmental changes of demyelination and remyelination occur with outer fibers being affected significantly more than centrally located fibers. Experimental models suggest that these outer fibers provide a protective cushioning effect, resulting in relative sparing of the inner fibers. Large diameter myelinated fibers appear to be most sensitive to the effects of compression (5).

Pathological changes may be limited to the specific area of compromise with relatively normal proximal and distal segments. If the area of local compromise is of sufficient severity, distal degeneration occurs. Although less well studied, it appears that once compression is sufficient to produce distal degeneration, pathological changes may be observed in the proximal segments as well. These consist of a reduction in myelinated fiber density and size with myelin debris being present, suggesting retrograde degeneration (6, 7).

The role of ischemia versus direct pressure in the production of the pathological changes observed in experimentally produced entrapment neuropathies is controversial (8). It has been shown that under certain conditions a nerve may be rendered ischemic without significantly affecting conduction velocity. Conduction block which has been produced by pressure appears to have different characteristics from that produced by ischemia. The block appears more slowly with pressure than with ischemia and seems to have a more prolonged recovery (9).

Principles of Electrodiagnosis

EMG and nerve stimulation studies are of established value in the diagnosis of peripheral entrapment neuropathies. Stimulation studies help to localize a site of entrapment by demonstrating an area of partial or complete conduction block. If axonal degeneration has occurred distal to the site of entrapment, the evoked potential may be altered in size and shape. A loss of functioning axons will result in a reduction in the size of the evoked potential, and demyelinated or degenerating fibers that conduct abnormally will produce temporal dispersion of the evoked response.

Although it is well documented that conduction velocity may be reduced proximal to a site of entrapment, the explanation for this slowing is still not clear (10). The previously described evidence of retrograde degeneration with localized nerve lesions may in part explain this. Although reduction in proximal conduction velocity is usually slight, it is important to recognize this phenomenon in order to avoid confusion of a localized lesion with a more generalized neuropathy.

The primary value of needle EMG in the diagnosis of entrapment neuropathies is that of localizing electrical abnormalities to a specific nerve distribution. The relative importance of needle EMG versus nerve stimulation studies will vary depending on the specific entrapment being investigated, but in general the two examinations complement one another.

Interpretation of Nerve Conduction Abnormalities

The functional status of an easily accessible segment of nerve can best be determined by direct nerve conduction studies. Although the conduction velocity across a nerve segment is a valuable index of function, considerable additional information is available to the physician who carefully compares the parameters of the evoked muscle action potentials (EMAP) obtained by stimulating both proximally and distally to the lesion. These parameters include the amplitude, duration, and area of the EMAP.

Individual nerve fibers exhibit two basic types of pathologic responses to injury. The first, demyelination, produces an abnormality or loss of the lipoprotein sheath and may thus result in a marked reduction in conduction velocity along the affected segment of the nerve. This is because rapid (saltatory) conduction is dependent upon normal axonal myelination (Chapter 2). The second category of response involves changes in the axon itself. This ranges from abnormalities of axonoplasmic flow to axonotmesis, in which case no conduction along the axon is possible (11, 12). Peripheral nerves are composed of individual fibers of various diameters and degrees of myelination. In chronic metabolic or toxic neuropathies, relatively pure instances of axonal or myelin disease may be seen; however, in trauma, the nerve presents a mosaic of fibers, each with different degrees of involvement. The electrodiagnostic picture seen depends on the proportion and degree of the various fiber changes present and the time elapsed since the injury. Bauwens (12–15) classified nerve injuries based on the usual electrodiagnostic findings into these categories: neurapraxia, axonostenosis, axonocachexia, and axonotmesis.

Although these categories do not directly represent the pathophysiologic changes, they do provide a conceptual framework for logically analyzing the EMAP.

NEURAPRAXIA

Neurapraxia is the mildest level of nerve injury. It is a temporary segmental block in axonal conduction. Recovery can be rapid and complete if the source of injury is removed; however, with continued injury (swelling, compression, and trauma), axonal damage can progress, leading to the development of a more severe level of nerve injury. Pathologically, the finding is principally that of demyelination of a short segment of the nerve (16). Further, anatomical changes such as telescoping of the myelin sheath and narrowing of the axon diameter may inhibit axon-plasmic flow and axonal membrane function-producing conduction block (8, 12). Thus, a complete neurapraxic lesion is comprised of segmental demyelination and complete axonal conduction block at the injury site: "Incomplete neurapraxia" results when some axons continue to conduct through the injury site.

The EMAP is absent when a neurapraxic axon is stimulated proximally to the lesion (proximal stimulation), but the EMAP is and remains normal with stimulation distally to the lesion (distal stimulation). The conduction velocity of the nerve segment located distally to the lesion (distal segment) will remain normal. Of course, only a certain percentage of the fibers may be neurapraxic, i.e., incomplete conduction block. Thus, some conduction across the lesion may be preserved (but usually slowed) in conjunction with a marked loss of EMAP with proximal stimulation. Thus, in neurapraxic lesions there is a severe decrease in, or absence of, the EMAP with proximal stimulation, but a nearly normal EMAP is obtained with distal stimulation (Fig. 9.1, *a* and *b*). Although normal values are published, a good guide to what is a normal EMAP is comparison to the contralateral side. (Caution: bilateral entrapments may be misleading.)

Acutely damaged nerves remain normally excitable distal to the lesion, regardless of the severity of the injury, until conduction is abruptly terminated by Wallerian degeneration somewhat more than 72 hr following *completion* of the injury (17). Therefore, patients with neurapraxia-like findings when tested early after injury should be restudied 3 or 4 days later to ensure that the EMAP observed was due to neurapraxic axons and not

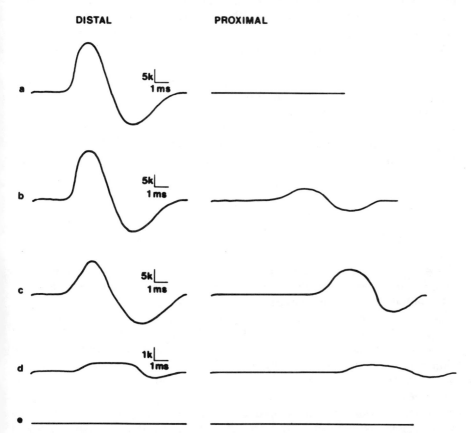

DISTAL   PROXIMAL

Fig. 9.1. Representation of EMAP in various classes of nerve lesions. Illustration represents ulnar nerve lesion at the elbow with stimulation distally at the wrist and proximally above the elbow. (*a*) Complete neurapraxia, (*b*) incomplete neurapraxia, (*c*) axonostenosis, (*d*) axonocachexia, (*e*) axonotmesis.

to axons in which conduction subsequently failed as a result of Wallerian degeneration. An estimate of the degree of neurapraxia versus axonotmesis can be obtained by comparing the area of the EMAP obtained by distal stimulation 4 days after injury with that of the EMAP obtained shortly after symptoms began (or with the contralateral side if no base line studies are available). This is particularly true in idiopathic facial palsy (Bell palsy). (See Estimating Degree of Axonotmesis in this chapter.)

AXONOSTENOSIS

Slowing of conduction along a discreet segment of an axon is termed axonostenosis. While this may not be structural axonal narrowing, it is useful to use this term to indicate chronic localized slowing at an entrapment site. Pathologically, it represents principally demyelination and remyelination along with some axonal degeneration, and, consequently, axons are metabolically stressed, internodal distance are shortened, and smaller diameter axons are present, slowing the conduction velocity. This picture is seen in chronic compression of a nerve segment in problems such as carpal tunnel or ulnar entrapment syndrome. Since noncompressed portions of the axon are little affected, the EMAP obtained by distal stimulation is nearly normal. There is slowing of the conduction velocity across the involved segment. There is a mild amplitude decrease and temporal dispersion (increase in the duration) of EMAP as a result of desynchronization of the arrival of the depolarization signal in the various axons within the entrapped segment, i.e., a spreading out of the nerve action potentials. Again it should be noted that axonostenosis is only a conceptualization and not an actual pathophysiological state (Fig. 9.1c).

AXONOCACHEXIA

In axonocachexia, the entire axonal segment distal to the lesion is affected, so that while conduction is maintained, its velocity is diminished. Both proximal and distal stimulation result in a markedly temporally dispersed EMAP of decreased amplitude. All or most nerve fibers are extensively compromised, and pathologically, axonal degeneration and regeneration, demyelination, and remyelination are seen (Fig. 9.1d).

AXONOTMESIS

Axonotmesis results from injury sufficient to cause Wallerian degeneration with dissolution of the distal segment of the axon. This is death of the axon distal to the lesion. Stimulation at any point along such an axon produces no EMAP (Fig. 9.1e). Muscle membrane instability (positive sharp waves, fibrillations) will develop in from 5 to 28 days after injury. With very short segments of axon distal to the injury, the delay to the onset of abnormalities on needle EMG is often short. Recovery of function (regeneration of nerve) following axonotmesis is slow, being approximately 1 mm/day (18); thus, confusion between potentials due to early reinnervation and those due to preserved function in incomplete injuries is not a problem for some months after injury.

Practical Aspects of Evoked Muscle Action Potential Analysis

The preceding schema is helpful in the logical evaluation of the EMAP; however, as befits a system in which the categories do not directly reflect underlying pathophysiological changes, electrodiagnostic findings intermediate between those described are encountered. In conduction studies of normal nerves (Fig. 9.2), the EMAP obtained by proximal stimulation compared to that obtained by distal stimulation shows a small decrease in the amplitude and a proportionate increase in its duration, such that the area under the negative spike of the EMAP is unchanged. The more separated the two points of stimulation, the quantitatively greater are these changes. This "physiological" change in the EMAP is due to the normal range of fiber conduction velocities within a nerve and the consequent spreading out of the signal as the conduction distance increases (19).

Immediately following a nerve injury in which function is not completely lost (Fig. 9.3a), comparison of the EMAP obtained by proximal with that obtained by distal stimulation demonstrates a more marked change. In this case, the proximal decrease in amplitude is not offset by a proportional duration increase (although duration may increase), so that the area under the negative spike of the EMAP is less than that obtained by distal stimulation. This change reflects the combined effects of demyelination, axonotmesis, and conduction block combined with the physiological dispersion of the EMAP. The EMAP obtained by distal stimulation is normal. The slowing of conduction across the damaged nerve segment is principally due to segmental demyelination with perhaps some portion secondary to loss of the fastest conducting fibers. Neither axonotmetic nor neurapraxic fibers contribute to the EMAP from proximal stimulation. By approximately 4 days after incomplete injury (Fig. 9.3b), Wallerian degeneration causes the abrupt loss of conduction in the axonotmetic fibers (17). (Caution is required in setting the time for this occurrence because the exact time at which Wallerian degeneration occurs is uncertain, particularly when lesions

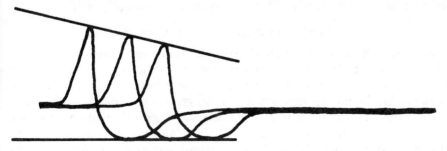

Fig. 9.2. Stimulation along a normal ulnar nerve demonstrating physiological alteration of the EMAP with increasing conduction distances.

DISTAL   PROXIMAL

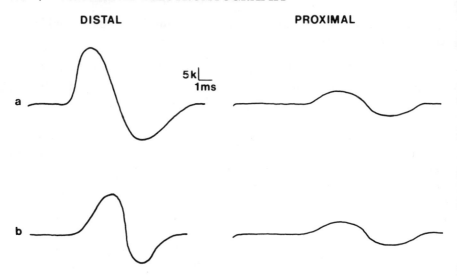

Fig. 9.3. EMAP in ulnar nerve lesion at the elbow in which function is not completely lost, as seen immediately after injury (a) and after Wallerian degeneration (b). In (a), the distal response is composed of all axons, i.e., uninjured, neurapraxic, and those in early stages of Wallerian degeneration, while in (b) only the first two groups of axons are represented.

progress.) After Wallerian degeneration, distal stimulation also results in an EMAP with a decreased amplitude and a decreased area, as axonotmetic fibers are no longer contributing to the distal response, although neurapraxic and undamaged axons continue to respond. Unless the lesion has progressed or conduction block improved, the EMAP from proximal stimulation will have changed little from its immediate post-injury values.

With nerve injuries in which function is completely lost, distal stimulation produces a nearly normal EMAP immediately after injury, and proximal stimulation produces no EMAP. At this stage, complete nerve section cannot be electrophysiologically differentiated from an incomplete lesion with associated complete conduction block (see Neurapraxia). After approximately 4 days, the rapid failure of distal conduction associated with Wallerian degeneration clearly differentiates the two cases (Fig. 9.4).

Estimating Degree of Axonotmesis

A crude estimate of the relative degree of viable versus axonotmetic fibers can be arrived at by determining the area under the negative spike of the evoked potential (20). Approximately 4 days following injury, axons undergoing Wallerian degeneration will no longer conduct; thus, the change in the area of the evoked potential obtained by distal stimulation occurring between the 1st and the 4th day following injury is proportional to the degree of axonotmesis. Those fibers continuing to conduct after sufficient time elapses for Wallerian degeneration to occur may be considered to be viable and, thus, will usually regain normal function. If no EMAP values

DISTAL   PROXIMAL

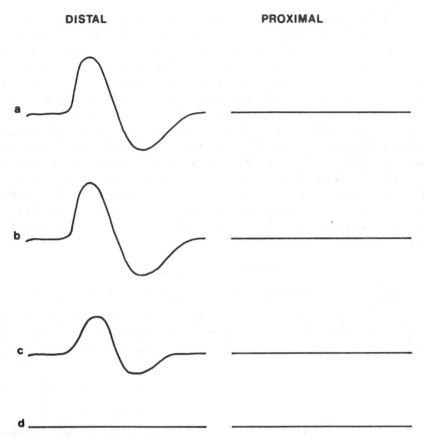

Fig. 9.4. EMAP in ulnar nerve lesion at the elbow in which no volitional function was noted immediately after injury (*a*). After Wallerian degeneration, purely neurapraxic injury (*b*) is clearly separated from purely axonotmetic lesion (*d*). Also after Wallerian degeneration, (*c*) shows an intermediate case in which some fibers are neurapraxic while others are axonotmetic.

from the immediate post-injury period are available for comparison, the evoked potential can be compared with that obtained from identically placed electrodes on the opposite limb. It is the area under the negative spike and not the amplitude of the evoked potential which is important, since this reflects both normal and more slowly conducting axons (Fig. 9.5). Because of the nature of volume conduction, the relationship between area of the EMAP negative spike and the number of axons functioning is not a direct one, i.e., 1:1 or 1:2, etc. The information obtained should be considered qualitative rather than quantitative.

Common Errors

When properly done, EMG and nerve stimulation studies are invaluable diagnostic aids. However, there are many potential sources of error which can mask the value of the electrodiagnostic examination. These include: 1) an inadequate history and physical prior to the electrodiagnostic exam; 2) inadequate knowledge of functional anatomy; 3) failure to recognize cross-over or anomalous innervation; 4) failure to take into account and correct limb temperature; 5) failure to stimulate from a standardized distance when measuring distal latencies; 6) measurement error resulting in false conduction values; 7) failure to measure proximal conduction velocity as well as distal latency; 8) failure to localize the stimulus to the desired nerve; 9) improper placement of recording electrodes; 10) confusion of a volume conducted motor response with a sensory potential; 11) failure to ascertain the correct position of the exploring electrode during needle EMG; 12) failure to examine sufficient number of muscles and/or nerves to establish the presence of a localized lesion; 13) failure to use the same technique as was used to arrive at the standard normal value; and 14) failure to recognize the presence of a generalized neuropathy.

Special Techniques

NEEDLE ELECTRODE USE FOR STIMULATION AND RECORDING

Needle electrode stimulation is not routinely used in conduction studies but does offer a number of advantages over surface stimulation. By bypassing the high impedance of the skin, a monopolar needle electrode can deliver

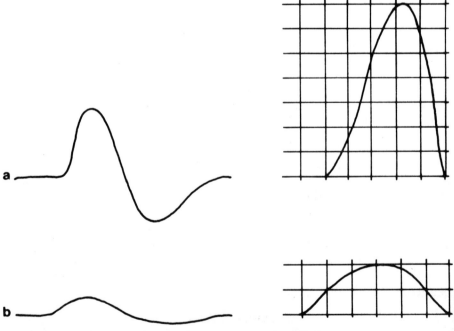

Fig. 9.5. EMAP immediately after injury (a) and following Wallerian degeneration (b). Positive spikes enlarged at right reveal a 64% decrease in EMAP area.

a supramaximal stimulation using much less current. This produces a smaller tissue volume in which the current density is adequate to cause nerve depolarization and thus (coupled with the positioning of the electrode near the nerve trunk) markedly reduces the frequency of stimulation spread to adjacent nerves (Fig. 9.6). Needle stimulation permits access to deep lying nerves, e.g., sciatic nerve and C8 nerve root. It is less painful for the patient, and an extra benefit is that the physician's hands are free to control other aspects of the procedure.

The large, volume-conducted electrical field generated by surface stimulation obscures the actual location along the nerve of initial depolarization and, thus, can seriously affect conduction values when short nerve segments are studied. Needle stimulation by precisely localizing the nerve stimulus has enabled us for the first time to accurately study short nerve segments and to detect narrow areas of entrapment or acute trauma whose slowing effect is lost by dilution when studied as part of longer segments. Needle stimulation above and below the carpal ligament can be particularly helpful in detecting early carpal tunnel syndrome (CTS) or isolated compromise of the recurrent motor branch of the median nerve. In addition to its benefit in short nerve segment studies, we have found its routine use helpful in sciatic, femoral, and lateral cutaneous nerves of the thigh and facial nerves, as well as in H and blink reflex studies. Because of its stimulation localization, it is also helpful in unraveling cases of anomalous innervation.

The reservation concerning needle stimulation most frequently voiced is that it may result in thermal or direct trauma to the nerve. We have had no instance of nerve damage. Direct injury is particularly unlikely if the needle is slowly advanced with the stimulation unit activated as the resultant evoked response signals close approach to the nerve. Studies at Ohio State have indicated that the maximum theoretical temperature increase associ-

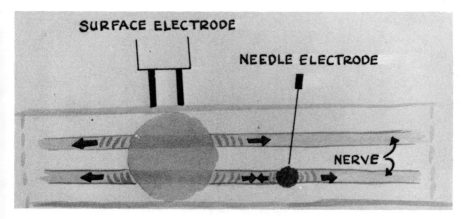

Fig. 9.6. A major advantage of needle electrode stimulation is the ability to isolate the depolarization field to a single nerve trunk. Circles represent relative volumes of tissue in which stimulus is adequate to produce depolarization.

ated with this technique, even assuming that all heat is delivered to a single tissue layer about the needle tip only 1 μ thick and, further, that there is no transport of the heat away from this layer, is less than 3°C (21). In practice, heat transport does occur, thus lowering the actual observed temperature. In any event, a temperature rise of 3°C in this limited tissue volume is not functionally important.

A needle electrode can be used for recording in two ways. When placed subcutaneously, it records a volume conducted response similar to that of the surface electrode. Its use in this way eliminates information about the amplitude and duration of the EMAP available from standard surface recording techniques and is to be condemned for routine studies. When placed intramuscularly, it records the spike potentials of only a few motor units. Such potentials are quite large (many millivolts) and polyphasic. The negative rise time of potentials near the needle tip is very short, and even when recording with settings of 1–2 mV per division, the negative spike of these units is often only a dotted vertical line on the oscilloscope screen (Fig. 9.7). This technique is useful in confirming that a recorded potential

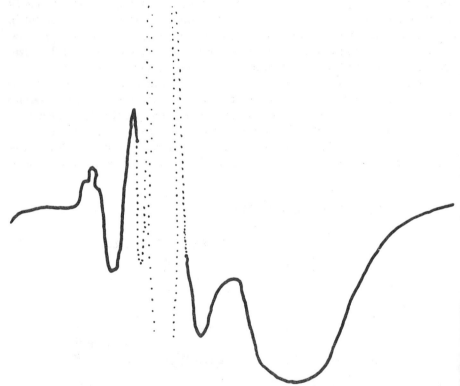

Fig. 9.7. Needle electrode recording of EMAP. Early portion of response is volume-conducted, while spike potential (almost vertical dotted lines) represents discharge of motor fibers near needle tip. It is only these latter deflections which confirm that a response originates in the muscle being investigated by the needle.

actually originated in a specific muscle. This minimizes errors caused by volume conduction from adjacent sources. Because the needle electrode records only from a limited volume of tissue, i.e., several motor units, conduction velocities thus obtained are of limited value. Such a velocity represents only that of a few isolated axons, may not be representative of the entire nerve, and should not be used for comparison to standardized normal values which are for the fastest conducting fibers.

H AND F WAVE USE IN PROXIMAL CONDUCTION STUDIES

The evaluation of a discreet segment of peripheral nerve is routinely accomplished by stimulating the nerve both at the proximal and at the distal end of the segment. With this procedure, a conduction velocity for the segment can be calculated, and changes in the parameters of the evoked response across the segment can be observed. This technique cannot be used when a proximal stimulation point is not readily accessible. This occurs in Guillain-Barré or other diseases in which early conduction changes are found in the area of the nerve roots, in intragluteal sciatic nerve injuries, in the area of the thoracic outlet, and in certain lesions of the brachial or lumbosacral plexes. Here the conduction status of the proximal segment of the nerve can be evaluated by using the H or the F wave.

The F wave is believed to be a recurrent discharge of a small percentage (approximately 5% (22)) of the alpha motor neurons which were antidromically activated during peripheral nerve stimulation (23, 24). Thus, both the afferent and the efferent arcs of this late wave must follow the same alpha motor neuron axons (Fig. 9.8). Which anterior horn cell redischarges varies

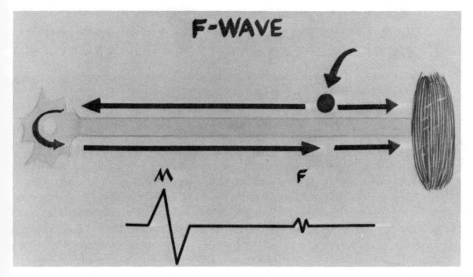

Fig. 9.8. Representation of depolarization course of F wave. Oscilloscope recording is shown below.

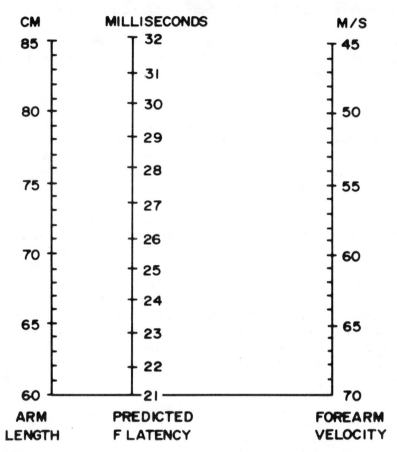

Fig. 9.9. Predicted F wave latency is determined by connecting arm length and forearm velocity by a straight line. Values 2.5 msec greater than predicted are abnormal.

from stimulation to stimulation; thus, the latency and amplitude of the F response varies slightly from stimulation to stimuation. If a number of stimulations are recorded and the shortest latency selected, a consistent value—representing the fastest conducting motor fibers—is obtained.

The F wave occurs in all motor nerves and usually remains present, even in the face of severe disease. Weber (25) has developed the following formula for predicting the F wave in the ulnar nerve: (0.31) times the distance in centimeters from the spine of C7 to the tip of the ulnar styloid) plus (the constant 11.05) minus (0.123 times the forearm velocity of the ulnar nerve). The predicted value may also be obtained from a nomogram (Fig. 9.9). Normal latency should not exceed the predicted value by more than 2.5

msec (2 S.D.). Side to side variation in the ulnar nerve should not exceed 1 msec (2 S.D.), and side to side comparisons in other nerves remain within this general range.

The F wave is not suppressed by a high intensity or frequency of stimulation. Its amplitude is smaller than that of the H wave, being usually less than 500 μV. (26, 27). Care must be taken to ensure that the shortest latency (earliest takeoff) of the wave is used; thus, a recording of multiple potentials is essential for accurate use of this technique. This is accomplished by using a direct paper recorder, memory scope, or polaroid film to record 10 successive stimulations. It is best to slightly displace the vertical axis of the sweep after each three or four superimpositions to facilitate reading the results (Fig. 9.10). For this technique, the ulnar nerve is stimulated at the wrist just as for the usual ulnar motor latency, except that the anode and the cathode positions are reversed (Figs. 9.11 and 9.12). The use of ulnar forearm velocity in the formula avoids the need to stimulate proximally and, thus, the necessity to record an F wave on the up slope of the M wave.

The H wave results from a monosynaptic spinal reflex whose afferent arc is I-a afferent fibers of the muscle spindle and whose efferent arc is the axon

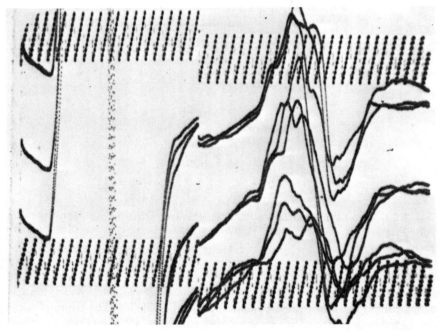

Fig. 9.10. F waves from nine successive ulnar nerve stimulations. Sweep is interrupted at 20 msec to facilitate measurement. Height of time base equals 200 μV. An accurate latency measurement determination results from using a mechanical divider to measure the distance from a straight edge placed between the 20-msec points on the two time bases and the initial F wave deflection. Here the latency is 26.6 msec.

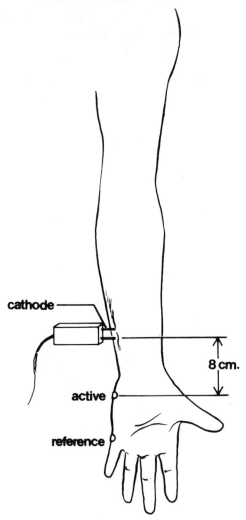

cathode

8 cm.

active

reference

Fig. 9.11. Stimulation procedure for ulnar F wave. The only variation from that used for the ulnar motor latency is that the anode and cathode positions are reversed.

of the alpha motor neuron (26). In infants, the H wave occurs widely; but in normal adults it has a restricted distribution (26, 28–30). The tibial H wave latency for an individual can be predicted from the following formula which was developed by Braddom (31, 32): (0.46 times the length in centimeters from the midpopliteal crease to the tip of the medial malleolus) plus (the patient's age times one-tenth) plus (constant 9.14). This value may also be obtained from a nomogram. The normal variation from the predicted value is rather large (4.8 msec), but it can be reduced in unilateral problems by

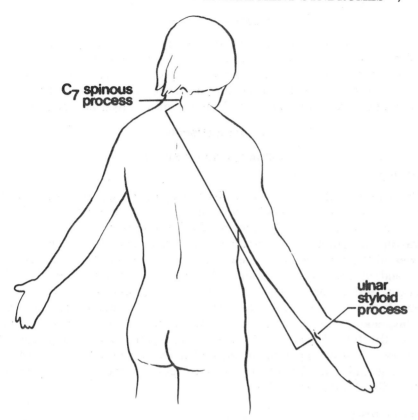

Fig. 9.12. Position for arm measurement when using ulnar F wave technique. Measurement is from the center of the C7 spinous process to the distal tip of the ulnar styloid. The arm is abducted approximately 20° and in the coronal plane of the body.

comparison of the symptomatic to the nonsymptomatic side. In this instance the sides should vary by no more than 1.2 msec (2 S. D.).

The H wave is elicitable by stimulating at an intensity below that which is necessary to evoke the full M response, and it is suppressed by supramaximal stimulation intensities and by stimulation frequencies greater than 0.5/sec; thus, it can be distinguished from the F wave by use of a slowly increasing stimulation intensity (26). Doing this, the H wave will appear before or near the threshold stimulation intensity for eliciting the M response, increase in amplitude to several millivolts, and finally disappear as the intensity of the stimulation increases (see Chapter 2).

Although these techniques offer a method of confirming distal conduction abnormalities (particularly useful in ulnar lesions at the elbow), their routine use in place of direct stimulation studies in readily accessible nerve segments is to be discouraged.

Specific Problems

The following discussion of some of the more common segmental neuro-pathies is organized by specific nerves. Unless otherwise specified, anatom-ical references are from *Gray's Anatomy*. Nerve stimulation techniques, including standardized distances and electrode placements, will be those used at The Ohio State University Department of Physical Medicine.

Upper Extremity

SUPRASCAPULAR NERVE

Anatomy

The suprascapular nerve (C5,6) diverges from the superior trunk of the brachial plexus in the costoclavicular space. It runs laterally beneath the trapezius muscle, eventually entering the suprascapular fossa through the suprascapular foramen. This foramen is a U-shaped notch at the junction of the root of the coracoid process and the superior border of the scapula. The open end of the notch is bridged by the superior transverse scapular ligament. In the suprascapular fossa the nerve supplies two branches to the supraspinatus muscle and one branch each to the glenohumeral and acro-mioclavicular joints. It then enters the infraclavicular fossa by passing around the lateral margin of the scapular spine. Here it supplies two branches to the infraspinatus muscle, along with a branch to the scapula and the glenohumeral joint. The suprascapular nerve has no cutaneous sensory distribution (Fig. 9.13).

Pathogenesis

Nerve compromise may be due to an isolated "neuritis"; compression by the transverse scapular ligament; relatively minor, repeated trauma to a metabolically compromised nerve; or stretching of the nerve during an extreme motion of the scapula (forced scapular protraction).

Symptoms

Weakness or paralysis of the supraspinatus and infraspinatus muscles disrupts normal glenohumeral motion by decreasing stabilization of the humeral head during shoulder abduction. Often, paralysis of the supra-spinatus prevents initiation of shoulder abduction. This can be overcome by dipping the shoulder and flexing the trunk toward the side of the injury, using the resultant pendular motion of the arm to initiate abduction.

Deep pain may be referred to the glenohumeral joint as a result of suprascapular nerve entrapment. This pain may be a cause of acute shoulder pain and of subsequent restricted shoulder motion (frozen shoulder) (33).

Electrodiagnosis

Entrapment produces a prolonged motor latency to the supraspinatus and infraspinatus muscles. When the nerve is stimulated in the supraclavic-

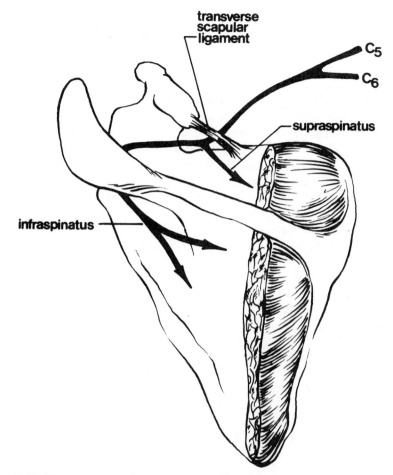

Fig. 9.13. The suprascapular nerve may suffer entrapment or trauma as it passes through the suprascapular foramen under the transverse scapular ligament. Such injury produces no cutaneous sensory changes but can result in shoulder pain.

ular fossa, normal latency should not exceed 3.7 msec (34, 35). Recording with a concentric needle electrode in the supraspinatus muscle may be necessary to avoid confusion by volume conducted potentials when dealing with small EMAPs (Fig. 9.14). The presence of EMG abnormalities confined to the supra- and infraspinatus muscles coupled with a normal paraspinal muscle EMG examination confirms the diagnosis. (*Editor's Note*: EMG abnormalities or membrane irritabilities means positive waves and/or fibrillation potentials.)

RADIAL NERVE

Three particular problems relating to the radial nerve may occur: sleep palsy, midarm trauma, and posterior interosseous syndrome.

Anatomy

The radial nerve (C5 through T1) is a direct continuation of the posterior cord of the brachial plexus. It enters the arm anteromedially to the long head of the triceps. As it passes distally along the middle third of the humerus, it swings dorsolaterally, following the spiral groove (Fig. 9.15). Here it is covered by the long and lateral heads of the triceps, and in turn, it lies upon the more proximal fibers of the medial triceps head. It next pierces the lateral intermuscular septum and continues into the anterior compartment of the arm running along the lateral aspect of the brachialis muscle, deep to and between the brachioradialis and the extensor carpi radialis longus musles.

The radial nerve gives off branches sequentially in its course (Fig. 9.16). The first muscle innervated is the triceps: its most proximal supply originates in the axilla and its most distal (along with the supply for the anconeus), while the nerve is still in the spiral groove. A sensory branch (posterior cutaneous nerve of the forearm) also originates as the nerve follows the spiral groove. As the nerve emerges from the intermuscular septum, it supplies branches to the brachioradialis, extensor carpi radialis longus, and (variable) the brachialis muscles.

Anterior to the lateral epicondyle, the nerve divides into superficial (sensory) and deep (posterior interosseous) branches. The deep branch winds around the lateral aspect of the radius to the posterior forearm where it enters the supinator muscle. As the nerve emerges from the supinator, it gives off its terminal muscular branches.

Two frequent sites of radial nerve entrapment are the lateral aspect of the arm, where compromise may occur during sleep, and in the upper forearm, where compromise is associated with repetitive pronation-supination.

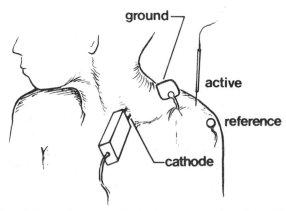

Fig. 9.14. Stimulation in the supraclavicular space (Erb point) with recording from the supraspinatus muscle. Particularly with a small amplitude response, a needle recording electrode may be necessary to detect or isolate the response. Angling the needle toward the base of the scapular spine ensures proper placement.

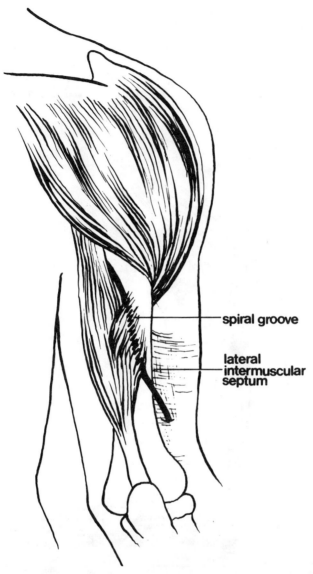

spiral groove

lateral
intermuscular
septum

Fig. 9.15. Posterior view of the arm showing the course of the radial nerve and its penetration of the intermuscular septum. This is the area of nerve compromise from fractures, injections, and crutch pressure. Sleep palsies compromise the nerve just distal to the septum.

The Sleep Palsies

Mechanism. The radial nerve is vulnerable to compression near its emergence from the intermuscular septum. When this occurs in a patient who is in an alcoholic stupor, it is referred to as a "Saturday night palsy." "Honeymoon palsy" (an often misleading term) is a sleep palsy in which compression results from the pressure of a second person's head resting in the crooked arm of the patient (Fig. 9.17).

Symptoms. Radial nerve palsy produces weakness or paralysis of wrist extension and metacarpo-phalangeal joint finger extension. Triceps function is not compromised in the sleep palsies (36); thus, triceps involvement should trigger a search for a more proximally located cause of neurological

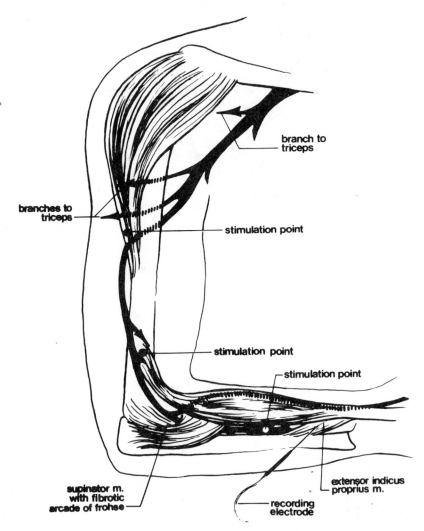

Fig. 9.16. Segmental stimulation points for the radial nerve shown in relation to the nerve, its branches, and muscular landmarks. Proximal stimulation point is along the deltoid insertion, and the middle point is deep between the brachialis and the brachiorachialis. The distal point (4 cm proximal to the recording electrode) requires needle electrode stimulation. Note that the triceps muscle receives innervation from a very proximal branch.

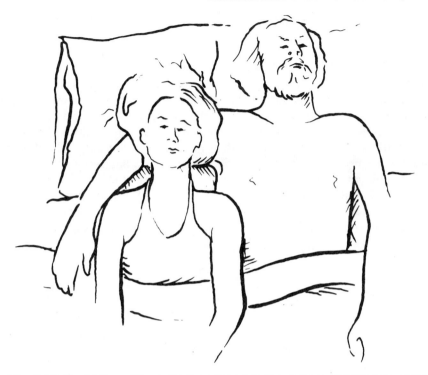

Fig. 9.17. Illustration of the patient position which results in radial nerve compromise from compression as it emerges from the intermuscular septum in "honeymoon palsy." In "Saturday night palsy" compression occurs in the same anatomical location when the arm is draped over the back of a bench or chair (see text).

compromise. The brachioradialis and, less often, the extensor carpi radialis longus muscles may be spared in this syndrome.

Sensory changes (hypesthesia and hypalgesia) are not prominent features, perhaps, because few areas have an exclusive radial sensory supply. When changes are present, they are usually confined to the dorsum of the hand, frequently involving only the dorsum of the thumb (36).

Electrodiagnosis. In motor conduction studies, the nerve is stimulated proximally to the lesion in the supraclavicular space or lateral to the deltoid at its entrance to the spinal groove and stimulated again distally to the lesion 5–6 cm proximal to the lateral epicondyle in the groove between the brachialis and brachioradialis muscles. Recording can be from any wrist extensor, but use of the extensor indicis proprius enables the investigator to determine a conduction velocity for the forearm segment of the radial nerve by using a third stimulation site 3–4 cm proximal to the recording electrode (37) (needle stimulation) (Figs. 9.16 and 9.18).

In normal individuals the radial nerve motor conduction velocity in the forearm is faster than 60 m/sec, and the arm segment velocity is approximately 10% faster than that of the forearm segment (38, 39). A reversal of this velocity relationship suggests nerve compromise.

Immediately after the onset of a sleep palsy, conduction across the lesion may be altered or completely blocked. Conduction velocity in the forearm usually remains normal. Difficulty can arise because of spread by volume conduction of stimulation to adjoining nerves and subsequent recording of volume conducted responses. This can be alleviated by using needle electrodes (see section on use of needle electrodes). The significance of changes in the evoked muscle action potential is discussed earlier in the chapter and should be reviewed for the clinical significance in radial nerve palsy.

EMG following a sleep palsy often shows a marked amount of abnormal membrane irritability in the wrist extensors. Despite this finding, prognosis for recovery (generally within 2 months) is excellent if stimulation distal to the injury remains possible after 4 or 5 days or if volitional motor units are preserved (40).

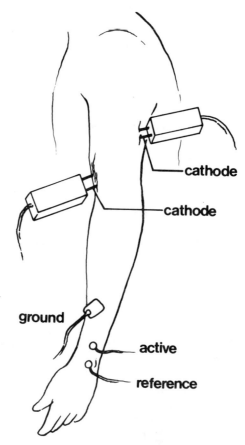

Fig. 9.18. Electrode placement for radial nerve conduction study. Note that the stimulator is pressed deeply between the muscles.

Midarm Trauma

The radial nerve can also be damaged by pressure from axillary crutches, errant intermuscular injection, fractures of the humerus, or an intra-axillary mass. In these instances, the clinical course varies from that of the sleep palsies in that residual functional impairment is more common. Here, the most important use of electrodiagnosis is to determine if the nerve remains in functional continuity. Immediately after injury, the ability to conduct across the lesion or the preservation of volitional motor units on EMG confirm function. After 4 or 5 days, the presence of an EMAP on distal stimulation is also a favorable prognostic sign.

Posterior Interosseous Nerve Syndrome

Anatomy. The posterior interosseous nerve described earlier (see Anatomy of the Radial Nerve) gives motor branches to the brachioradialis, the extensor carpi radialis longus, the extensor carpi radialis brevis, and the supinator prior to passing through the supinator mass. It is a pure motor nerve.

Pathogenesis. Posterior interosseous nerve palsy has been described in cases of direct trauma, compression by a ganglion or vascular anomaly, and rheumatoid synovitis (41–45). However, the nerve is most vulnerable to repeated trauma or entrapment as it passes through the supinator muscle at the tendonous arcade of Frohse (Fig. 9.19). In addition, full pronation of the forearm may exert pressure on the nerve at the sharp tendonous edge of the extensor carpi radialis brevis (46–48).

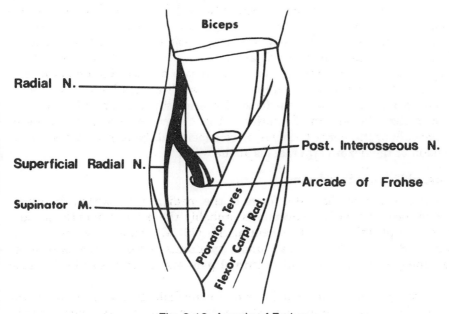

Fig. 9.19. Arcade of Frohse.

Clinical Findings. The patient complains of difficulty extending the fingers and the thumb, frequently associated with dull, aching pain on the posterior aspect of the forearm. The radial wrist extensors are intact, as their innervation is proximal to the usual site of compromise. Sensory loss is not present.

Electrodiagnosis. Needle EMG may show abnormalities in the extensor digitorum, the extensor digiti minimi, the extensor carpi ulnaris, the abductor pollicis longus, the extensor pollicis longus, the extensor pollicis brevis, and the extensor indicis proprius. (*Editor's Note:* EMG abnormalities mean positive waves and fibrillation potentials and reduced number of MVP.) The absence of abnormalities in the brachioradialis, the extensor carpi radialis longus, the extensor carpi radialis brevis, and the supinator establishes the site of the lesion. Stimulation of the radial nerve above and below the site of entrapment is also a useful diagnostic procedure. The nerve can be easily stimulated at the posterior fold of the deltoid, 5–6 cm proximal to the lateral epicondyle and over the dorsolateral aspect of the radius at about the junction of the middle and distal third. Using a monopolar pin as the stimulating electrode may facilitate this procedure. Conduction values are described under The Sleep Palsies. By using a surface recording electrode placed over the extensor indicis proprius and comparing the M response obtained with proximal and distal stimulation, the examiner can estimate the degree of neurapraxia present (see Estimating Degree of Axonotmesis).

MEDIAN NERVE

The median nerve is formed by the union of the medial and lateral cords of the brachial plexus. It descends into the arm lying lateral to the brachial artery and crossing in front of it at about the insertion of the coracobrachialis. At the level of the elbow, the nerve lies medial to the brachial artery behind the bicipital aponeurosis and in front of the brachialis. As it enters the forearm, the nerve passes between the two heads of the pronator teres giving rise to the anterior interosseous branch at this level. The median nerve then passes between the flexor digitorum superficialis and the profundus, being adherent to the former. About 5 cm proximal to the flexor retinaculum, the nerve becomes more superficial, lying just medial to the tendon of the flexor carpi radialis at the wrist.

Carpal Tunnel Syndrome

Compression of the distal fibers of the median nerve within the carpal tunnel (carpal tunnel syndrome) is probably the most frequently encountered peripheral entrapment neuropathy (49). Originally described by Sir James Paget in 1863, carpal tunnel syndrome is now recognized as an extremely common cause of nocturnal pain and paresthesias in the hand (1).

Anatomy. The carpal tunnel is bordered medially by the pisiform and the hook of the hammate and laterally by the crest of the trapezium and the tuberosity of the scaphoid. The floor of the canal comprises the lunate and the capitate bones, and the transverse carpal ligament forms the roof. The median nerve, along with the flexor tendons to the fingers and the thumb and the tendon of the flexor carpi radialis, lies within this anatomical tunnel (Fig. 9.20). After passing through the carpal tunnel, the median nerve gives rise to its motor branch to the thenar muscles (abductor pollicis brevis, opponens, and generally the superficial head of the flexor pollicis brevis). Distally, the nerve supplies the lateral two lumbricales.

Pathogenesis. Any condition which alters the size or shape of the carpal tunnel or its contents can render the median nerve more vulnerable to compromise at this point. Examples are post-Colles' fracture deformity, acromegaly, myxedema, amyloidosis, ganglion cysts, gouty tophi, local tumors, and the edema of pregnancy (50–53). Phalen (54) maintains that thickening or fibrosis of the synovia of the flexor tendons within the carpal tunnel is the most frequent cause of the syndrome.

Clinical Findings. The carpal tunnel syndrome is diagnosed most frequently in middle-aged females (3:1 over males). This syndrome appears to be more common in individuals who do repetitive manual tasks such as typing, knitting, etc. Typically, the patient complains of burning pain and tingling, worse at night, and frequently disturbing sleep. Shaking and rubbing the hands or hanging the hands in a dependent position generally gives some temporary relief of symptoms. This syndrome is frequently bilateral but typically affects the dominant hand first and most severely (1).

Physical examination reveals weakness of opposition of the thumb as an early sign, while atrophy of the thenar muscles is a later finding. Careful examination may show some loss of sensation, especially 2 point discrimination, in that portion of the hand supplied by the median nerve. Lightly tapping over the median nerve at the wrist often produces an electric shock-like sensation in the hand (Tinel sign). Acutely flexing the wrist may produce a tingling sensation in the hand (Phalen sign). These physical findings are not present in every case, which sometimes leads to difficulty in diagnosis.

Electrodiagnosis. The carpal tunnel syndrome is undoubtedly the most well studied, from an electrodiagnostic standpoint, of all the entrapment neuropathies. Various authors have emphasized the importance of many different electrical parameters in establishing the diagnosis of carpal tunnel syndrome (10, 55–61). Of these, the measurement of the distal sensory latency appears to be of most value, with the distal motor latency being a slightly less sensitive diagnostic indicator (58). Prolongation of the median sensory latency characteristically precedes that of the distal motor latency and remains prolonged longer than does the motor latency after appropriate surgical treatment. While of interest, the amplitudes of the thenar motor action potential or the sensory evoked potential are variable enough in normal individuals so to be confusing in most cases of carpal tunnel syndrome when used as the sole diagnostic indicator (58).

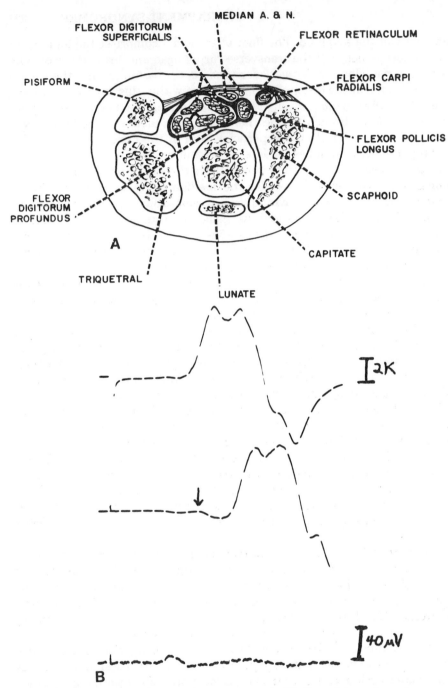

Fig. 9.20. (*A*) Contents of the carpal tunnel. (*B*) Carpal tunnel syndrome and Martin-Gruber syndrome. *Top trace*, wrist latency—6.4 msec; *middle trace*, proximal latency—8.2 msec, distance 20 cm, C.V. 110 m/sec; *bottom trace*, sensory latency. Sweep interrupted at 1 msec intervals. Arrow indicates positive deflection on proximal stimulation (Martin-Gruber syndrome).

When recorded over a standard distance of 14 cm, the distal median sensory latency should not exceed 3.2 ± 0.2 mec (antidromic or orthodromic) with the normal motor latency value being 3.7 ± 0.3 msec. In addition, the hands, if cool, should be warmed to avoid the physiologic prolongation of distal latency which occurs with cold. Generally the amplitude of the sensory action potential will be normal when the latency is prolonged due to cooling of the nerve. Thus, the finding of a prolonged sensory latency with a normal amplitude sensory action potential should signal caution to the examiner.

Measurement of the proximal median conduction velocity, as well as the ipsilateral ulnar latency, aids in establishing the diagnosis of localized entrapment as opposed to a more generalized peripheral neuropathy. Since retrograde slowing of median motor conduction velocity may be occasionally present in carpal tunnel syndrome (7), it is frequently necessary to examine several other nerves for comparison.

While needle EMG alone is a relatively insensitive diagnostic indicator of carpal tunnel syndrome (10, 49), this procedure serves to further localize the lesion to the distal median distribution and occasionally will confirm the presence of a coexisting cervical radiculopathy or other unsuspected lesion.

Carpal tunnel syndrome, when present along with median-ulnar crossover in the forearm (Martin-Gruber anastomosis), may lead to a confusing electrodiagnostic picture (62). In this instance, the distal median motor latency will be prolonged as expected. However, with proximal stimulation at the elbow, the impulse is conducted initially through the median nerve but crosses over to the ulnar nerve in the forearm, producing a motor action potential in the ulnar innervated thenar muscles. Since this impulse by-passes the area of median compromise within the carpal canal, it is not slowed and gives a normal proximal latency. Thus, when a conduction velocity is calculated using the prolonged median motor latency and the normal proximal latency, which is, in reality, the result of crossed ulnar conduction, an artificially fast conduction velocity frequently in the range of 100–150 m/sec results. In addition to the finding of an extremely fast conduction velocity in the presence of carpal tunnel syndrome, the finding of an initially positive deflection of the motor action potential when stimulating at the elbow should alert the examiner to the possibility of the median-ulnar crossover in the forearm.

Although electrodiagnostic studies cannot directly predict the outcome of surgical treatment of carpal tunnel syndrome (63), comparison of the amplitude of the evoked muscle action potential when stimulating the median nerve proximally and distally to the carpal ligament can help one to estimate the approximate degree of neurapraxia present. It should be noted that conduction studies may remain abnormal while showing a return toward a normal values, despite excellent postsurgical subjective relief of symptoms (64).

Anterior Interosseous Syndrome

Anatomy. The anterior interosseous nerve arises from the posterior aspect of the median nerve as it passes between the two heads of the pronator teres. It runs with the anterior interosseous artery along the anterior aspect of the interosseous membrane deep to the flexor pollicis longus and the flexor digitorum profundus giving branches to these muscles. The nerve then runs deep to the pronator quadratus, supplying this muscle as well. In general, only the lateral two heads of the profundus are innervated by this nerve, with the medial two heads being supplied by the ulnar nerve.

Pathogenesis. Although often attributed to "isolated neuritis" (65), the anterior interosseous syndrome may in some cases be a true entrapment neuropathy. In those cases explored surgically, a fibrous constricting band has frequently been found (66, 67). This syndrome is occasionally described with sudden onset following alcoholic stupor, suggesting that local pressure may be a factor in some cases. It also has been described after prolonged or repetitive actions requiring pronation of the forearm.

Clinical Findings. Typically, the patient seeks medical attention because of vague aching pain in the forearm which may be sudden or gradual in onset. The patient frequently is not aware of weakness, but physical examination will reveal weakness of the flexor pollicis longus, the flexor digitorum profundus (lateral two heads), and pronator quadratus. The sensory examination is normal.

Electrodiagnosis. Needle EMG typically reveals abnormal membrane irritability, with a loss of motor units in any or all of the muscles supplied by the anterior interosseous nerve. The characteristic pattern of abnormalities combined with the normal sensory examination confirms the diagnosis (68). However, a complete EMG examination of the involved muscles, including cervical paraspinals, should be done to ascertain the peripheral nature of the lesion. Stimulation studies using needle recording electrodes may also be of benefit in confirming the diagnosis (69).

ULNAR NERVE

General Anatomy

The ulnar nerve arises from the medical cord of the brachial plexus. It lies medial to the brachial artery until the middle of the arm. At this point it pierces the intermuscular septum and follows the medial head of the triceps to the groove between the olecranon and the medial epicondyle of the humerus. The ulnar nerve enters the forearm between the two heads of the flexor carpi ulnaris and subsequently lies between this muscle and the flexor digitorum profundus. In the distal half of the forearm, the nerve lies just medial to the ulnar artery being covered by the tendon of the flexor carpi ulnaris at the wrist. The nerve gains access to the hand anterior to the transverse carpal ligament through the canal of Guyon.

Ulnar Compromise at the Elbow

Anatomy. While in the ulnar groove at the elbow, the ulnar nerve is covered only by skin and fascia which affords it little protection against external trauma. The nerve is fixed proximally as it passes through the intermuscular septum and distally as it runs between the two heads of the flexor carpi ulnaris. The motor branch to the flexor carpi ulnaris may arise proximal to, within, or distal to the ulnar groove.

Pathogenesis. Compromise of the ulnar nerve at the elbow can occur in a variety of ways. Acute compromise can occur following direct trauma to the elbow, as is frequently seen in athletic injuries. Direct pressure on the nerve may occur during surgery, sleep, or coma and is frequently the result of the left elbow being positioned on the arm rest of an automobile during driving. Minor repetitive trauma may result in chronic compromise of the ulnar nerve at the elbow, a situation often seen in diabetic individuals. Hypermobility or complete subluxation of the ulnar nerve on elbow flexion may be observed in normal individuals (70), a circumstance which also renders the ulnar nerve more vulnerable to repetitive external trauma. The term "tardy ulnar palsy" properly refers to ulnar nerve dysfunction following a remote supracondylar humeral fracture.

Clinical Findings. The patient typically relates numbness and tingling in the ring and little fingers, with pain in the forearm being a frequent complaint as well. In the case of acute ulnar compromise, the Tinel sign is usually present with mild percussion of the nerve at the elbow. Passive elbow flexion may reveal hypermobility or complete subluxation of the ulnar nerve. The little finger assumes a slightly abducted posture as an early sign of ulnar intrinsic weakness. Dorsal interosseous atrophy may be present if the lesion has been present for a sufficient length of time. As the examiner attempts to pull a piece of paper from between the patient's thumb and forefinger, substitution of the median innervated long thumb flexor for a weak adductor pollicis (Froment sign) is automatic. (Fig. 9.21) The sensory examination shows a deficit in the ulnar distribution, especially two point discrimination.

Electrodiagnosis. Comparison of the ulnar conduction velocity of the forearm segment to the segment across the elbow is of established value in making the diagnosis of ulnar compromise at the elbow. It has been shown that varying the position of the elbow has a considerable effect on the calculated conduction velocity of the across elbow segment of the ulnar nerve. Cadaver studies have shown that a true length of the across elbow segment is most accurately measured with the elbow flexed, and we routinely place the elbow at about 90° of flexion when determining ulnar conduction velocities across the elbow (Fig. 9.22). Conduction velocity in the across elbow segment will usually be equal to or faster than the forearm velocity in normal individuals. However, due to the problems associated with measurement of nerve length, there may be a normal variation in the calculated conduction velocity of the across elbow segment. This can result in the

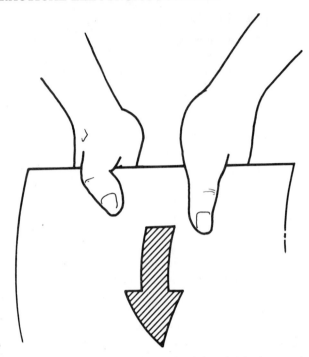

Fig. 9.21. The Froment sign, demonstrating ulnar intrinsic muscle weakness.

calculated conduction velocity in the across elbow segment being up to 7% slower than that of the forearm velocity in normal individuals (71). However, equally as important as the conduction velocity is the character of the M response when the ulnar nerve is stimulated above and below the elbow. Thus, even if the conduction velocity of the across elbow segment of the ulnar nerve is in the normal range, a significant decrease in amplitude or an increase in duration of the negative spike of the M response when stimulating above the elbow should arouse suspicion.

In addition to motor conduction velocity studies, sensory conduction velocity determined by either orthodromic or antidromic methods is also helpful in the diagnosis of ulnar compromise at the elbow. Balmaseda and Checkles (72) reported that the variation normally present in ulnar sensory conduction velocity across the elbow makes the use of absolute conduction velocities more reliable. They reported that 95% of normal individuals tested had an ulnar sensory conduction velocity in the across elbow segment of not less than 50 m/sec.

Needle EMG may show abnormal irritability (positive waves and fibrillation potentials) with a loss of motor units in any of the muscles supplied by the ulnar nerve. Since the flexor carpi ulnaris may receive its innervation above, within, or below the ulnar groove, involvement of this muscle, or the lack thereof, does not reliably localize the site of ulnar compromise.

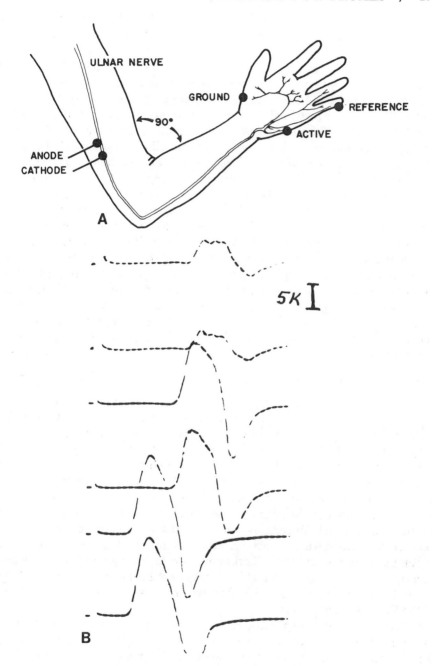

Fig. 9.22. (A) Position for above elbow stimulation of the ulnar nerve. (B) Ulnar nerve entrapment. *Top two traces*, stimulation above elbow; *middle two traces*, stimulation below elbow; *bottom two traces*, stimulation at wrist. Sweep interrupted at 1 msec intervals.

In the case of acute ulnar compromise at the elbow, early electrical abnormalities include a reduction in number of voluntary motor unit action potentials in muscles supplied by the ulnar nerve and a reduction in the amplitude of the M response when stimulating above the elbow. If the lesion is of sufficient severity to cause axonal degeneration, positive waves may be observed in 14 days and fibrillation potentials as early as 18 days. Generally, the more proximal muscles will demonstrate abnormal membrane irritability earlier. The effects of local demyelinization are manifested as slowing in conduction velocity in the across elbow segment of the ulnar nerve, with conduction velocity in the forearm segment being relatively well maintained. With the chronic compromise of repetitive trauma, abnormal membrane irritability may be minimal. The number of voluntary motor units in the ulnar distribution will be reduced, and the existing motor units may be increased in amplitude and duration, reflecting the effects of reinnervation. A slowing of conduction velocity in the across elbow segment, with a marked reduction in the amplitude of the M response, as well as temporal dispersion, is typically present. In the specific case of tardy ulnar compromise, abnormal membrane irritability is often absent, with surviving motor units being greatly increased in amplitude and duration. A profound decrease in conduction velocity in the across elbow segment of the ulnar nerve is present, with a loss of amplitude and a temporal dispersion of the M response.

Ulnar Compromise at the Wrist

Anatomy. Approximately 6 cm proximal to the wrist, the ulnar nerve gives off the dorsal cutaneous branch to the hand. The main nerve, along with the ulnar artery, then enters the hand through the canal of Guyon. Originally described in 1861 by Felix Guyon, a French urologist, the canal is bordered laterally by the pisiform and medially by the hook of the hammate and is covered by the volar carpal ligament. While in the canal, the ulnar nerve divides into a superficial and a deep branch. The superficial branch gives a twig to the palmaris brevis and continues as a sensory branch to the ring and little fingers, as well as to the hypothenar eminence. The deep branch, along with the artery, winds around the hook of the hammate to run between the abductor digiti quinti and flexor digiti quinti brevis and subsequently supplies the dorsal interossei, the third and fourth lumbricals, the adductor pollicis, the first dorsal interosseous, and usually the deep head of the flexor pollicis brevis.

Pathogenesis. Although many causes of ulnar nerve lesions at or distal to the wrist have been reported, compression by a ganglion, occupational trauma, and traumatic laceration appears to be most frequent. Other less common causes include fracture of the hammate or other wrist bones, disease of the ulnar artery, and contracted scar tissue.

Clinical Findings. Distal ulnar nerve lesions fall into three distinct groups, depending on the site of compromise (73, 74):

1. Ulnar intrinsic muscle weakness with sensory deficit due to compression proximal to or within Guyon's canal—if the lesion is distal to the dorsal cutaneous sensory nerve, sensation will be normal on the dorsum of the medial aspect of the hand but decreased on the palmar surface of the hypothenar eminence and the ring and little fingers.
2. Normal sensation with ulnar intrinsic muscle weakness as a result of compression of the deep branch of the ulnar nerve as it exits Guyon's canal or at any point distal as it courses through the hand—the muscles involved will depend on the exact site of the lesion.
3. Normal muscle strength with sensory deficit involving the volar surface of the hypothenar eminence and the ring and little fingers due to compression of the superficial sensory branch of the ulnar nerve— the site of the lesion may be within the canal of Guyon sparing the deep motor branch or anywhere along the superficial course of the sensory branch.

Electrodiagnosis. If only the superficial branch is involved, needle EMG and motor conduction studies will be normal. The distal ulnar sensory potentials, however, may be absent or the latency prolonged. Normal for the distal ulnar sensory latency (orthodromic or antidromic) is 3.2 ± 0.25 msec or less, stimulating at 14 cm from the active electrode. A lesion proximal to the canal of Guyon may prolong the distal ulnar motor latency to the abductor digiti quinti (normal being $3.7 \pm .3$ msec or less, stimulating 8 cm from the active electrode). In this case, needle EMG of the ulnar intrinsic muscles may be abnormal as well. A lesion of the deep branch of the ulnar nerve distal to the hypothenar muscles may produce EMG abnormalities in any of the muscles in its terminal distribution. The terminal motor latency measured to abductor digiti quinti will be normal but may be prolonged when measured to the adductor pollicis or the first dorsal interosseous (75, 76). Although reports of normal latencies to these muscles vary, our experience, in general, agrees with that of Carpendale (77), who states that the difference between the latency to the abductor digiti quinti and to the adductor pollicis should be less than 1 msec in normal individuals.

THORACIC OUTLET SYNDROME

Anatomy

The anterior rami of spinal roots C5 through T1 pass downward from their respective neural foramen, intermingle as the brachial plexus, and form the peripheral nerves, which accompany the axillary vessels into the arm. In this course, the neurovascular bundle passes through the scalene triangle, the costoclavicular space, and the axilla.

Pathogenesis

As the neurovascular bundle passes from the neck into the arm, it can be compressed at various sites. Each of these compression points represents a separate clinical entity. Collectively, they constitute the thoracic outlet syndrome. Contributing etiologic factors include congenital structural anomalies, muscular hypertrophy, muscular weakness, structural alteration due to trauma (particularly fractured clavicle), and atherosclerosis (78). Compression may be constant or may occur only with certain positions of the shoulder, e.g., hyperadduction or depression with retraction (exaggerated military posture). Entrapment is felt to occur through one of the following mechanisms: compression between the first rib and the clavicle, a cervical rib or large transverse process producing elevation and stretching of the neurovascular bundle, compression between the pectoralis minor tendon and the ribs, and scalene muscles tightness (78–80).

Symptoms

Symptoms result from compression of either the neural or the vascular components of the bundle or by compression of both. In our experience, it is most often a vascular phenomena. The most frequent symptoms are paresthesia and numbness on the ulnar aspect of the hand. Objective sensory abnormalities are much less frequent than are subjective complaints. Pain, weakness, swelling, discoloration, ulceration, gangrene, and the Raynaud phenomenon are also encountered.

Electrodiagnosis

Determination of conduction velocity values for a transaxillary ulnar nerve segment following stimulation in the supraclavicular fossa is a traditional method of evaluation in this syndrome (79, 80); however, the value of this technique has been challenged (25, 81). One major problem is that the point of stimulation is located distally to some points of entrapment. Other disadvantages of this method include its susceptibility to errors in segment measurement, volume-conducted spread of the stimulation to adjacent nerves due to the deep location of the posterior cord and patient discomfort. These problems may explain why reported normal values for this study vary widely (25).

Ulnar F wave latency or C8 root stimulation circumvent many of these problems. In C8 root stimulation, a monopolar needle stimulating electrode is inserted to the C7 transverse process, and an evoked potential is obtained at the hypothenar eminence (Fig. 9.23). The latency of this response is recorded, and from it is subtracted the value for the distal wrist (8 cm) stimulation. The mean value for conduction over this segment (elbow straight, shoulder abducted 90°) is 54 ± 2 m/sec and a side-to-side variation in latency of less than 1 msec (82).

F wave latency studies provide a simple method of evaluating the proximal segment. Predicted values for the latency can be easily calculated (see H and F Wave Use In Proximal Conduction Studies).

Needle EMG is unrewarding in most cases of thoracic outlet syndrome. However, since the clinical findings in many upper extremity pain syndromes

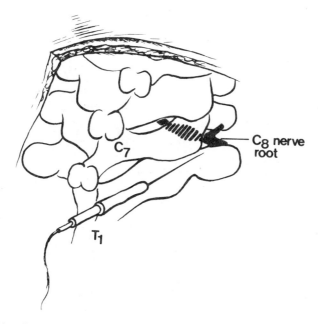

Fig. 9.23. Needle stimulation of the C8 nerve root. Note the limited area of nerve root exposure. Needle is lateral to C7 spinous process.

are strikingly similar, a complete evaluation, including EMG and conduction studies, should be performed to exclude the coexistence of radiculopathy, carpal tunnel syndrome, or other entrapments.

Lower Extremity

THE LATERAL CUTANEOUS NERVE OF THE THIGH

Anatomy

The lateral cutaneous nerve of the thigh, a purely sensory nerve, supplies the lateral one-third of the thigh through the dorsal branches, ventral rami of lumbar roots 2 and 3. The nerve emerges from the lateral margin of the iliopsoas muscle and passes around the pelvis to emerge into the thigh beneath or through the inguinal ligament approximately 1 cm medial to the anterior superior iliac spine. Just distal to the inguinal ligament, the nerve divides into anterior and posterior branches. The posterior branch passes several centimeters distally and posteriorly before penetrating the fascia lata and becoming subcutaneous. It supplies sensation to the posterolateral aspect of the thigh. The anterior branch runs directly distally for approximately 10 cm, at which point it pierces the fascia lata and continues its distal course subcutaneously. It supplies the anterolateral aspect of the thigh (Fig. 9.24).

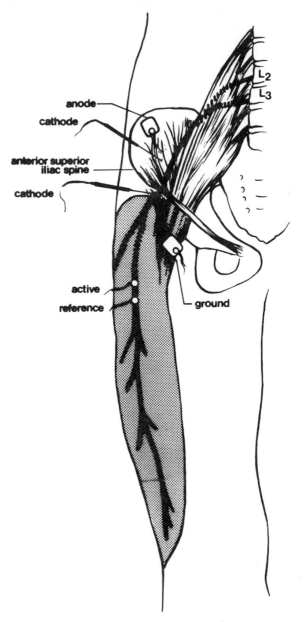

Fig. 9.24. Lateral cutaneous nerve of the thigh. Hash-marked area of nerve indicates portion covered by dense fascia lata; stippled area represents the usual cutaneous innervation. The recording point (12 cm distal to the inguinal ligament) is distal to the nerve's emergence from beneath the fascia but proximal to its terminal arborization. Stimulation points are approximately 1 cm medial to the anterior superior iliac spine.

Pathogenesis

The nerve is susceptible to compression by intrapelvic masses such as tumor or abdominal aortic aneurysm (83). Its close anatomic relationship to the cecum and to the lower descending colon makes it vulnerable to compromise by processes involving these organs. The usual point of entrapment, however, is during its passage through the inguinal ligament. Obesity, underlying metabolic or toxic neuropathies, direct trauma, and indirect trauma by corsets or braces have been implicated in this process. Another potential site of entrapment is the point of penetration of the distal branches through the fascia lata.

Symptoms

Patients complain of burning pain and numbness over the lateral aspect of the thigh, worse during sitting; however, anesthesia in this area rarely occurs. Symptoms are the same for both proximal and distal points of entrapment. Since this nerve is purely sensory, the presence of weakness in the thigh muscles indicates a different etiology for the patient's symptoms.

Electrodiagnosis

The evaluation of nerve function is by means of antidromic sensory conduction along the anterior branch. Stimulation is by means of a pin electrode both proximally and distally to the inguinal ligament. Recording is at a point along the anterior branch, 12 cm distal to the ligament (Fig. 9.24). Normal latency is less than 3.1 msec, and there is little change in the latency across the ligament (84).

In mild, chronic entrapments there is a prolongation of the latency of the evoked potential. In an acute neurapraxic injury, the only abnormality may be a decrease in the size of the evoked potential obtained by stimulation above the ligament as compared to stimulation below the ligament. In severe cases, no evoked potential will be recordable. Because there is anatomic variation in nerve location, the asymptomatic extremity should always be examined when the potential is absent on the symptomatic side.

FEMORAL NERVE

Anatomy

The femoral nerve is the largest branch of the lumbar plexus. It arises from the dorsal branches of the ventral rami of the second, third, and fourth lumbar nerves. It passes through the psoas major and subsequently lies between this muscle and the iliacus. While in the abdomen, the femoral nerve supplies the iliacus and the pectineus. The nerve subsequently passes deep to the inguinal ligament and divides into anterior and posterior branches. The anterior branch supplies the sartorius and gives off the intermediate and medial cutaneous branches to the thigh as well. The posterior branch gives off the saphenous nerve (the largest cutaneous branch of the femoral nerve) and gives motor branches to the quadriceps femorus and articular branches to the knee joint.

Pathogenesis

Femoral neuropathy has been ascribed to many causes, including alcoholism, diabetes, polyarteritis nodosa, trauma from hip fracture, pressure during the birth process and hemorrhage into the psoas muscle secondary to anti-coagulant therapy (85, 86). Self-retaining retractor blades used in an abdominal hysterectomy can injure the femoral nerve high in the abdomen, and femoral nerve palsy has been reported as a complication of prolonged dorsal lithotomy position (87). Presumably, the latter is due to compression of the femoral nerve beneath the inguinal ligament.

Clinical Findings

The patient presents with knee instability, and weakness of the quadriceps muscle is easily demonstrable. Decreased sensation is present on the medial aspect of the thigh and leg. The patellar reflex may be decreased or absent.

Electrodiagnosis

Needle EMG shows positive waves and fibrillation potentials with a loss of motor units in the various portions of the quadriceps femorus and in the sartorius muscle. Since multiple lumbar radiculopathy, common in diabetes mellitus, can simulate femoral neuropathy, EMG examination of the paraspinal muscles is essential. Femoral nerve conduction studies can be helpful in the diagnosis of femoral nerve entrapment or compression beneath the inguinal ligament (89). The femoral nerve is easily stimulated above and below the inguinal ligament. Above the inguinal ligament, the nerve lies lateral to the pulsation of the femoral artery and may be easily stimulated with a needle electrode if surface stimulation proves inadequate. The active electrode is placed on the skin over the center of the vastus medialis with the reference electrode being placed over the quadriceps tendon just proximal to the patella.

Johnson et al. (87) showed the mean delay across the inguinal ligament to be 1.1 ± 0.4 msec. In the case of femoral entrapment at the inguinal ligament, stimulation of the femoral nerve above the inguinal ligament results in a prolonged motor latency. There is usually a decrease in amplitude of the M response as well. Conduction studies distal to the inguinal ligament are normal.

SCIATIC NERVE—INJECTION PALSY

Anatomy

The sciatic nerve is formed within the sacral plexus from portions of the ventral rami of L4 through S2. The nerve exits the pelvis through the sciatic notch, enters the buttock beneath the lower margin of the piriformis muscle, and passes into the posterior thigh between the ischial tuberosity and the greater trochanter. While in the buttock, it is located beneath the gluteus maximus muscle and lies upon the quadratus femorus muscle. In the thigh, it follows the adductor magnus muscle. At the apex of the popliteal fossa, it divides to become the common peroneal and the tibial nerve (Fig. 9.25).

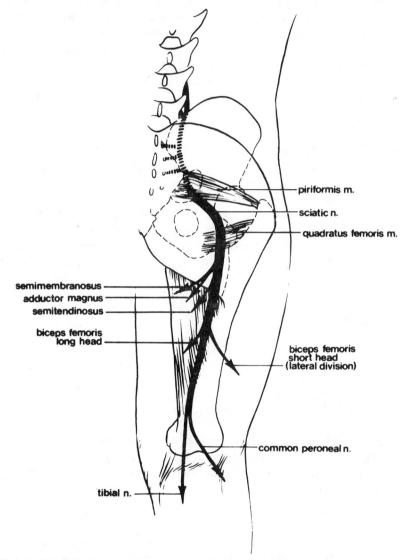

Fig. 9.25. Sciatic nerve course and distribution. The separation between the medial and lateral divisions is complete and is responsible for the frequent limitation of sicatic injuries to a single division of the nerve. Note that the short head of the biceps femoris is the only thigh muscle supplied by the lateral division.

Throughout its course, the sciatic nerve is well differentiated into its constituent parts: medial division (tibial), lateral division (peroneal), and branches to the hamstring muscles. In the thigh, the peroneal portion of the nerve is located laterally and supplies the short head of the biceps femoris. The remainder of the hamstring muscles are supplied by the medially located tibial portion of the nerve: the adductor magnus and semimembranosus innervation arise from a single trunk and the semitendinosus and long head of the biceps femoris are each supplied by separate twigs. Although the two major components of the sciatic nerve normally course together until reaching the apex of the popliteal fossa, they may diverge at any point along the course of the nerve. In up to 15% of individuals, the peroneal component of the nerve passes through the substance of the piriformis muscle rather than (with the medial division) along its lower border.

Pathogenesis

Injection palsy appears to be more frequent in infants and may result from either direct, intraneural injection, or from delayed effects of perineural injection with subsequent tissue reaction (88–90). In the first instance, the needle penetrates the neural sheath and the injected substance damages the nerve through pressure or direct toxic effect. The lateral division is positioned such that it is more likely to receive a direct injection. In the second instance, late sciatic palsy, medication and/or blood envelope the sciatic nerve as a result of either perineural injection or dissection along fascial planes. Compromise is due to constriction of the nerve by the maturing of scar tissue associated with inflammatory tissue reaction.

Symptoms

Direct injection of the nerve usually produces intense pain which radiates along the posterior thigh and calf into the lateral aspect of the foot (91). The onset of numbness and weakness in the sciatic distribution is immediate. For unknown reasons, direct injection may be unaccompanied by pain, exhibiting only the immediate onset of weakness and numbness in the sciatic distribution.

In instances of late sciatic palsy, onset of symptoms (weakness, numbness, and paresthesia in the sciatic distribution) is delayed for up to several months following the injection. Occasionally, patients will have noted pain at the time of the injection.

Electrodiagnosis

EMG immediately following direct injection of the nerve may reveal a reduced number of volitionally activated motor units. Positive waves and, later, fibrillation potentials will appear in the sciatic distribution in approximately 10–21 days following the injection. Months later, motor unit changes consisting of increased amplitude, duration, and polyphasicity may be noted. In late sciatic palsy, abnormal membrane irritability will be minimal or absent. The major EMG finding will involve reduction of motor unit numbers and chronic motor unit changes of increased amplitude and duration.

Conduction studies 72 hr following direct injection may reveal a decrease in amplitude and area of the EMAP in muscles of the involved side compared to those of the uninvolved side. Later some slowing of conduction along the thigh segment of the sciatic nerve plus temporal dispersion of the EMAP may be seen in both direct and late sciatic palsy (Fig. 9.26).

Because it is not practical to stimulate the sciatic nerve above the level of injury, the most effective means of evaluating the function of the proximal nerve segment is the use of late waves. In this regard, H and F wave changes can be present early in direct injection palsy and develop along with the symptoms in late palsy. Both the tibial (H or F wave) and the peroneal (F wave) branches should be tested, since compromise of a single division of the nerve is possible (see H and F Wave Use In Proximal Conduction Studies).

When sciatic nerve compromise occurs in the thigh, it can be evaluated using direct conduction studies. The nerve is located proximally between the ischial tuberosity and the femoral trochanter approximately one-third the distance from the ischium, and a needle electrode must be used for stimulation at that point. The distal stimulation point is in the popliteal fossa (needle or surface stimulation) and recording is from the abductor minimi. Normal conduction velocity for the thigh segment is 51.3 ± 4.4 m/sec (92).

PERONEAL NERVE

Anatomy

The peroneal nerve diverges from the tibial nerve at the apex of the popliteal space and passes through the popliteal fossa along the medial border of the lateral hamstring muscles. From a position directly posterior to the fibular head, it spirals around the caudolateral margin of the fibular head and divides into its two terminal branches: the deep and the superficial peroneal nerves (Figs. 9.27 and 9.28).

Two sensory branches originate from the common peroneal nerve in the popliteal fossa. The lateral cutaneous nerve of the leg supplies sensation to the lateral portion of the upper one-half of the leg, while the second branch joins in the midcalf with its tibial counterpart to form the sural nerve. Neither of these branches are affected by compression at the fibular head; thus, sensation in the upper leg is unaffected by peroneal nerve entrapment at the fibular head.

The deep peroneal nerve provides motor innervation to the anterior tibialis, the extensor digitorum longus, the peroneus tertius, the extensor hallucis longus, the extensor digitorum brevis, and, occasionally, the first dorsal interosseous muscles. It provides cutaneous sensation for the first web space.

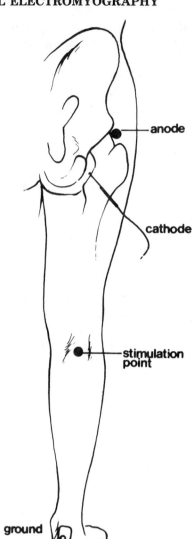

Fig. 9.26. Sciatic conduction studies can utilize either the medial division (shown) or the lateral division. Needle stimulation is necessary proximally with the point of stimulation lateral to the ischium one-third the distance to the greater trochanter. This technique will not be effective in injection palsy since the proximal point of stimulation is distal to the point of compromise.

The superficial peroneal nerve provides motor innervation to the peroneus longus and peroneus brevis muscles. Its sensory field is the lateral aspect of the distal one-third of the leg and the dorsum of the foot, with the exceptions of a variable number of lateral toes and the first web space.

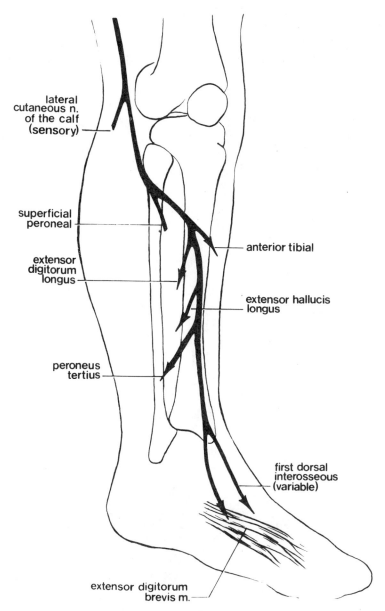

Fig. 9.27. Deep branch peroneal nerve. Peroneal nerve studies should include investigation of both branches, as either can receive isolated compromise. When the EMAP from distal stimulation is absent or smaller than the proximal response, an accessory peroneal nerve should be suspected (see Fig. 9.28).

Pathogenesis

There are several major mechanisms for compromise of the peroneal nerve. The first, "crossed leg palsy," results from compression of the peroneal nerve between the ipsilateral fibular head and the contralateral patella and contralateral femoral condyle (93). This often occurs in people with a

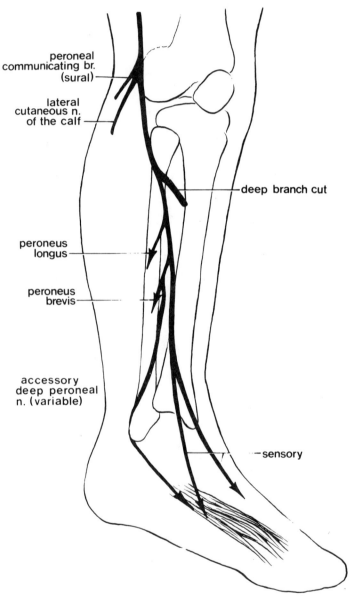

peroneal communicating br. (sural)

lateral cutaneous n. of the calf

deep branch cut

peroneus longus

peroneus brevis

accessory deep peroneal n. (variable)

sensory

Fig. 9.28. Superficial branch peroneal nerve. Note the accessory peroneal nerve which, when present, supplies a variable portion of the extensor digitorum brevis.

recent, large weight loss. A second cause is prolonged, unaccustomed squatting or kneeling, often appearing after weekend projects such as laying a patio or painting a floor. Persons with diabetes or other metabolic diseases or those who are receiving neurotoxic drugs are more susceptible to these injuries (1). Damage to the knee and leg can result in peroneal palsy by direct trauma or, secondarily, as a result of cast pressure or during surgical procedures. Inversion ankle sprains can produce stretch injuries to the peroneal nerve, resulting in susceptibility to recurrent sprains.

Symptoms

The major finding in peroneal palsy is painless foot drop or dorsiflexion weakness. This may be accompanied by a decrease in sensation on the dorsum of the foot. Compression by a ganglion cyst may produce pain on the lateral aspect of the foot (94).

Electrodiagnosis

Conduction studies are most helpful in diagnosing a peroneal palsy. The common peroneal nerve is stimulated in the popliteal fossa and at the lower limit of the fibular head. Distal stimulation of the deep branch of the common peroneal nerve is at the border of the anterior tibialis tendon or, occasionally, at the posterior border of the lateral malleolus (Fig. 9.29) when an accessory peroneal nerve is present (95). This provides conduction values for segments of the nerve both across the fibular head and distal to the fibular head (Fig. 9.29).

Peroneal palsy from compression or entrapment at the fibular head results in slowing of the conduction velocity in the segment of the nerve across the fibular head. The normal peroneal conduction velocity is 49.9 ± 5.9 m/sec (96); that of the proximal segment should be equal to or greater than that of the leg segment. In addition to conduction slowing, there should be changes in the EMAP as described earlier in the chapter.

Before reporting complete axonotmesis, it is important to investigate both the deep and the superficial branch distribution of the nerve. When no clear response is detected using surface recording electrodes, stimulation studies using a concentric needle electrode for recording should be performed, as should routine EMG, in order to fully assess the situation.

EMG changes should be confined to the peroneal nerve distribution. However, the concomitant occurrence of a chronic peripheral neuropathy is possible; thus, the presence of abnormalities in the distal tibially innervated muscles does not necessarily exclude this diagnosis. Stretch injuries associated with ankle sprains may produce only mild distal segment conduction slowing. Here, needle electrode EMG is helpful. Trauma can be confined to a single nerve branch; thus, conduction and needle electrode EMG should routinely be performed in the distribution of both branches.

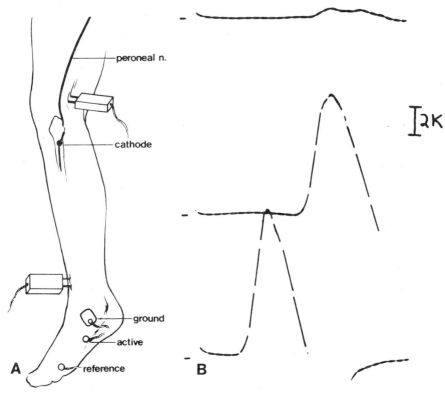

Fig. 9.29. (*A*) Slightly rotated view of the leg showing standard stimulation points along the course of the peroneal nerve. Note how deeply the stimulator depresses the surrounding tissue. (*B*) Crossed leg palsy. *Top trace*, stimulation above knee; *middle trace*, stimulation below fibular head; *bottom trace*, stimulation at ankle. Sweep interrupted at 1 msec intervals.

TIBIAL NERVE—TARSAL TUNNEL SYNDROME

Anatomy

The tibial nerve, the medial and larger terminal branch of the sciatic nerve, receives contributions from the ventral branches of the ventral rami of the fourth and fifth lumbar and first, second, and third sacral nerves. It runs in the posterior aspect of the thigh and is superficial in the middle of the popliteal fossa where it lies lateral to the popliteal vessels. In the lower aspect of the popliteal fossa, the nerve is covered by the heads of the gastrocnemius. In the leg, the nerve runs deep to the soleus until the distal one-third, where it is covered only by skin and fascia.

The nerve subsequently enters the tarsal tunnel, which is posterior and inferior to the medial malleolus and covered by the flexor retinaculum (lancinate ligament) (Fig. 9.30). The contents of the tarsal tunnel include the tibial nerve and vessels, as well as the tendons of the posterior tibialis, flexor digitorum longus, and flexor hallucis longus muscles. At the distal border of the flexor retinaculum, the nerve gives off the medial and lateral plantar nerves and the calcaneal branch, which gives cutaneous and deep sensation to the heel (Fig. 9.31). The medial plantar nerve supplies the abductor hallucis, the flexor digitorum brevis, the flexor hallucis brevis, and the first lumbrical. The lateral plantar nerve has both a superficial and deep branch. The superficial branch may give muscular branches to the third plantar and fourth dorsal interosseous muscles. The deep branch supplies the two or three lateral lumbricals and the remaining interossei, as well as both heads of the adductor hallucis. The motor and sensory distribution of the medial and lateral plantar nerves is roughly analogous to the median and ulnar nerves in the hand.

Pathogenesis

The flexor retinaculum, unlike the transverse carpal ligament, is composed of multiple deep fibrous septa which blend with the periosteum on the medial aspect of the calcaneus (97, 98). The neurovascular bundle in the tarsal tunnel may be attached to the septum, making it susceptible to traction or compression. Specific etiological factors include post-traumatic fibrosis due to ankle fracture, compression by a ganglion or varix of the posterior tibial vein, tendon sheath cysts, valgus deformity of the ankle, and compression by an accessory or hypertrophied abductor hallucis muscle

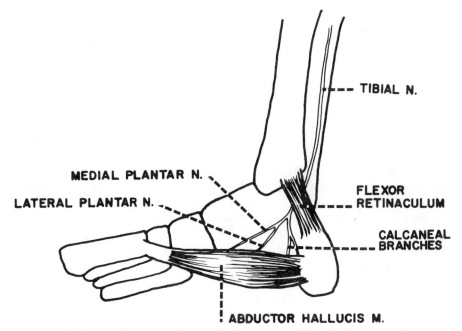

Fig. 9.30. Anatomic relationship of the branches of the tibial nerve in the tarsal tunnel.

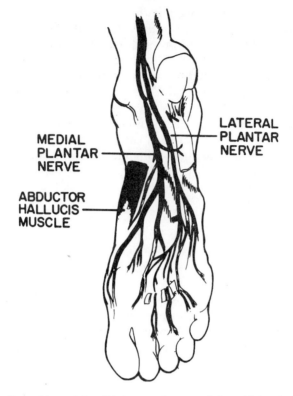

Fig. 9.31. Branching of the tibial nerve into medial and lateral plantar nerves.

(98–100). This syndrome has also been described with sudden weight gain or fluid retention. In the majority of surgically explored cases, however, no underlying cause has been identified.

Clinical Findings

In contrast to the carpal tunnel syndrome, females seem to be affected only slightly more often than males. The patient typically complains of intermittent burning pain and tingling in the foot, usually worse with prolonged standing. Symptoms are usually most prominent at night and seem to be proportional to the amount of standing or walking done during the day. The distribution of sensory impairment depends on the site of compromise and may involve either or both the medial and lateral plantar nerves. Sensation on the dorsum of the foot should be normal with the exception of the distal phalanges of the toes. Tapping over the nerve may produce tingling in the foot, and tenderness proximal and distal to the site of compression (the Valleix phenomenon) may be present. In addition, holding the ankle in forced inversion or application of a venous tourniquet on the calf may reproduce symptoms (98).

Electrodiagnosis

EMG and tibial nerve stimulation studies are of value in establishing the diagnosis of tarsal tunnel syndrome (101). The tibial nerve should be stimulated at the level of the superior border of the medial malleolus to ensure its being proximal to the flexor retinaculum. Motor latencies to the abductor hallucis and abductor digiti quinti pedis muscles may be easily recorded with surface electrodes. Assuming a normal conduction velocity in the proximal segment of the tibial nerve, the latency should not exceed 6.1 msec for the medial plantar and 6.7 msec for the lateral plantar branch. More than a 1.0 msec difference between the latency to the abductor hallucis and the abductor digiti quinti pedis is indicative of lateral plantar nerve compromise. Since the feet are more susceptible to temperature changes than are hands, special emphasis should be given to measurement of skin temperature prior to determining tibial nerve latencies. The distribution of abnormalities on needle EMG will depend on the specific site of compromise and may involve the medial or lateral plantar distribution either separately or in combination.

REFERENCES

1. AGUAYO, A.: Neuropathy due to compression and entrapment. In *Peripheral Neuropathy*, pp. 691–692, ed. by P. Dyck, P. Thomas and E. Lambert, Philadelphia: W. B. Saunders Co., 1975.
2. HOPKINS, A., AND MORGAN-HUGHES, J.: The effect of local pressure in diphtheritic neuropathy. *J. Neurol. Neurosurg. Psychiat., 32:* 614, 1969.
3. SKILLMAN, T. G., JOHNSON, E. W., HAMWI, G. J., AND DRISKILL, H. J.: Motor nerve conduction velocity in diabetes mellitus. *Diabetes, 10:* 46, 1961.
4. FULLERTON, P., AND GILLIATT, R.: Pressure neuropathy in the hind foot of the guinea pig. *J. Neurol. Neurosurg. Psychiat., 30:* 18, 1967.
5. AGUAYO, A., NAIR, C., AND MIDGLEY, R.: Experimental progressive compression neuropathy in the rabbit. *Arch. Neurol., 24:* 358, 1971.
6. AITKEN, J., AND THOMAS, P.: Retrograde changes in fiber size following nerve section. *J. Anat., 96:* 121, 1962.
7. ANDERSON, M., FULLERTON, P., GILLIATT, R., AND HERN, J.: Changes in the forearm associated with median nerve compression at the wrist in the guinea pig. *J. Neurol. Neurosurg. Psychiat., 33:* 70, 1970.
8. OCHOA, J., DANTA, G., FOWLER, T., AND GILLIATT, R.: Nature of the nerve lesion caused by a pneumatic tourniquet. *Nature, 233:* 265, 1971.
9. BENTLEY, F., AND SCHLAPP, W.: The effects of pressure on conduction in peripheral nerve. *J. Physiol., 102:* 72, 1943.
10. THOMAS, P.: Motor nerve conduction in the carpal tunnel syndrome. *Neurology, 10:* 1045, 1960.
11. SPENCER, P.: Reappraisal of the model for "bulk axoplasmic flow." *Nature [New Biol.], 240:* 283, 1972.
12. WEISS, P.: The life history of the neuron. *J. Chronic Dis., 4:* 340, 1955.
13. BAUWENS, P.: Electrodiagnostic definition of the site and nature of peripheral nerve lesions. *Ann. Phys. Med., 5:* 149, 1960.
14. BAUWENS, P.: Electrodiagnosis revisited. *Arch. Phys. Med. Rehabil., 42:* 6, 1961.
15. SEDDON, H. J.: Three types of nerve injury. *Brain, 66:* 237, 1943.
16. LEHMAN, H.: Segmental demyelination and changes in nerve conduction in experimental circumscribed neuropathy. In *New Developments in Electromyography and Clinical Neurophysiology*, ed. by J. Desmedt, Basel, Switzerland: Karger, 1973.

17. GILLIATT, R.: Recent advances in the pathophysiology of nerve conduction. In *New Developments in Electromyography and Clinical Neurophysiology*, ed. by J. Desmedt, Basel, Switzerland: Karger, 1973.

18. JACOBSON, S., AND GUTH, L.: An electrophysiological study of the early stages of peripheral nerve regeneration. *Exp. Neurol., 11:* 48, 1965.

19. GASSER, H., AND ERLANDER, J.: *Electrical Signs of Nervous Action.* Philadelphia: University of Pennsylvania Press, 1937.

20. DeJONG, R. H.: Relation between electromyogram and isometric twitch tension in human muscle. *Arch. Phys. Med. Rehabil., 48:* 539, 1967.

21. STOW, R.: Tissue heating in nerve stimulation by needle electrode (unpublished data).

22. FULLERTON, P., AND GILLIATT, R.: Axon reflexes in human motor nerve fibers. *J. Neurol. Neurosurg, Psychiat., 28:* 1, 1965.

23. DAWSON, G., AND MERTON, P.: "Recurrent" discharges from motoneúrones. XX Congr. Int. Physiol. Bruxelles, Abstract Comm., Bruges, Belgioú, St. Catherine Pr. 221, 1956.

24. TRONTELJ, J. V.: A study of the F response by single fiber electromyography. In *New Developments in Electromyography and Clinical Neurophysiology*, ed. by J. Desmedt, Basel, Switzerland: Karger, 1973.

25. WEBER, R. J., AND PIERO, D. L.: F wave evaluation of thoracic outlet syndrome: A multiple regression derived F wave latency predicting technique. *Arch. Phys. Med. Rehabil., 59:* 464, 1978.

26. MAGLADERY, J. W., AND McDOUGAL, D. B.: Electrophysiological studies of nerve and reflex activity in normal man. *Bull. Johns Hopkins Hosp., 86:* 265, 1950.

27. MAYER, R. F., AND FELDMAN, R. G.: Observation on the nature of the F wave in man. *Neurology, 17:* 147, 1967.

28. HOHMANN, T., GOODGOLD J.: Study of abnormal reflex patterns in spasticity. *Am. J. Phys. Med., 40:* 52, 1967.

29. MAGLADERY, J., PORTER, W., PARK, A., AND TEASDALL, R.: Electrophysiological studies of nerve and reflex activity in normal man. IV. Two-neurone reflex and identification of certain action potentials from spinal roots and cord. *Bull. Johns Hopkins Hosp., 88:* 499, 1951.

30. MAGLADERY, J., TEASDALL, R., PARK, A., AND LANGUTH, H.: Electrophysiological studies of reflex activity in patients with lesions of nervous system. I. Comparison of spinal motoneurone excilatrility following afferent nerve volleys in normal persons and patients with upper motor neurone lesions. *Bull. Johns Hopkins Hosp., 91:* 219, 1952.

31. BRADDOM, R. I., JOHNSON, E. W.: H reflex: Review and classification with suggested clinical uses. *Arch. Phys. Med. Rehabil. 55:* 412, 1974.

32. BRADDOM, R. I., AND JOHNSON, E. W.: Standardization of H reflex and diagnostic use in S_1 radiculopathy. *Arch. Phys. Med. Rehabil., 55:* 161, 1974.

33. KOPELL, H. P., AND THOMPSON, W. A. L.: *Peripheral Entrapment Neuropathies*, 2nd ed., p. 152, Huntington, N.Y.: Kruger 1976.

34. GASSEL, M. M.: A test of nerve conduction to muscles of the shoulder girdle as an aid in the diagnosis of proximal neurogenic and muscular disease. *J. Neurol. Neurosurg. Psychiat., 27:* 200, 1964.

35. KRAFT, G. H.: Axillary, musculocutaneous and suprascapular nerve latency studies. *Arch. Phys. Med. Rehabil., 53:* 383, 1972.

36. TROJABORG, W.: Rate of recovery in motor and sensory fibers of the radial nerve: Clinical and electrophysiological aspects. *J. Neurol. Neurosurg. Psychiat., 33:* 625, 1970.

37. JEBSEN, R. H.: Motor conduction velocity of distal radial nerve. *Arch. Phys. Med. Rehabil., 47:* 12, 1966.

38. JEBSEN, R. H.: Motor conduction velocity in proximal and distal segments of the radial nerve. *Arch. Phys. Med. Rehabil., 47:* 597, 1966.

38. TROJABORG, W., AND SINDRUP, E. H.: Motor and sensory conduction in different segments of the radial nerve in normal subjects. *J. Neurol. Neurosurg. Psychiat., 32:* 354, 1969.

40. GASSEL, M. M., AND DIAMANTOPOULOS, E.: Pattern of conduction times in the distribution of the radial nerve. *Neurology, 14:* 222, 1964.

41. BOWEN, T., AND STONE, K.: Posterior interosseous nerve paralysis caused by a ganglion at the elbow. *J. Bone Joint Surg., 48B:* 774, 1966.
42. CAPENER, N.: The vulnerability of the posterior interosseous nerve of the forearm. *J. Bone Joint Surg., 48B:* 770, 1966.
43. MILLANDER, L., NALEBUFF, E., AND HOLDSWORTH, D.: Posterior interosseus-nerve syndrome secondary to rehumatoid synovitis. *J. Bone Joint Surg., 55A:* 753, 1973.
44. MULHOLLAND, R.: Non-traumatic progressive paralysis of the posterior interosseous nerve. *J. Bone Joint Surg., 48B:* 781, 1966.
45. SHERRARD, W.: Posterior interosseous neuritis. *J. Bone Joint Surg., 48B:* 777, 1966.
46. BRYAN, F., MILLER, L., AND PANIJAYANOND, P.: Spontaneous paralysis of the posterior interosseous nerve. *Clin. Orthop. Related Res., 80:* 9, 1971.
47. GOLDMAN, S., HONET, J., SOBEL, R., AND GOLDSTEIN, A.: Posterior interosseous nerve palsy in the absence of trauma. *Arch. Neurol., 21:* 435, 1969.
48. SPINNER, M.: The arcarde of Froshe and its relationship to posterior interosseous nerve paralysis. *J. Bone Joint Surg. 50B:* 809, 1968.
49. KOPELL, H., AND GOODGOLD, J.: Clinical and electrodiagnostic features of carpal tunnel syndrome. *Arch. Phys. Med. Rehabil., 49:* 371, 1968.
50. JOHNSON, E. W., WELLS, R., AND DURAN, R.: Diagnosis of carpal tunnel syndrome. *Arch. Phys. Med. Rehabil., 49:* 414, 1962.
51. LYNCH, A., AND LIPSCOMB, P.: The carpal tunnel syndrome and Colles fracture. *J. Am. Med. Assoc. 185:* 363, 1963.
52. MELVIN, J., BURNETT, C., AND JOHNSON, E.: Median nerve conduction in pregnancy. *Arch. Phys. Med. Rehabil., 50:* 75, 1969.
53. TOMPKINS, D.: Median neuropathy in the carpal tunnel caused by tumor-like conditions. *J. Bone Joint Surg., 49A:* 737, 1967.
54. PHALEN, G.: Reflections on 21 years' experience with the carpal tunnel syndrome. *J. Am. Med. Assoc. 212:* 1365, 1970.
55. BUCHTHAL, F., AND ROSENFALCK, A.: Sensory conduction from digit to palm and from palm to wrist in the carpal tunnel syndrome. *J. Neurol. Neurosurg. Psychiat., 34:* 243, 1971.
56. DAUBE, J. R.: Percutaneous palmar median nerve stimulation for carpal tunnel syndrome. Presented at 38th AAEE Meeting, San Diego, Nov. 1976.
57. MELVIN, J., HARRIS, D., AND JOHNSON, E.: Sensory and motor conduction velocities in the ulnar and median nerves. *Arch. Phys. Med. Rehabil., 47:* 511, 1966.
58. MELVIN, J., SCHUCHMANN, J., AND LANESE, R.: Diagnostic specificity of motor and sensory nerve conduction variables in the carpal tunnel syndrome. *Arch. Phys. Med. Rehabil., 54:* 69, 1973.
59. WIEDERHOLT, W.: Median nerve conduction velocity in sensory fibers through carpal tunnel. *Arch. Phys. Med. Rehabil., 51:* 328, 1970.
60. JOHNSON, E. W., AND MELVIN, J.: Sensory conduction studies of median and ulnar nerves. *Arch. Phys. Med. Rehabil., 48:* 25, 1967.
61. THOMAS, J., LAMBERT, E., AND CSEUZ, K.: Electrodiagnostic aspects of the carpal tunnel syndrome. *Arch. Neurol., 16:* 635, 1967.
62. GUTMANN, L.: Carpal tunnel syndrome and median-ulnar communications. Presented at 38th AAEE Meeting, San Diego, Nov. 1976.
63. CSEUZ, K., THOMAS, J., AND LAMBERT, E., ET AL.: Long-term results of operation for carpal tunnel syndrome. *Mayo Clin. Proc., 41:* 232, 1966.
64. MELVIN, J., JOHNSON, E., AND DURAN, R.: Electrodiagnosis after surgery for the carpal tunnel syndrome. *Arch. Phys. Med. Rehabil. 49:* 502, 1968.
65. FEARN, C., AND GOODFELLOW, J.: Anterior interosseous nerve palsy. *J. Bone Joint Surg., 47B:* 91, 1965.
66. FARBER, J., AND BRYAN, R.: The anterior interosseous nerve syndrome. *J. Bone Joint Surg., 50A:* 521, 1968.
67. STERN, M., ROSNER, L., AND BLINDERMAN, E.: Kiloh-Nevin syndrome. *Clin. Orthop. Related Res. 53:* 95, 1967.

68. O'BRIEN, M., AND UPTON, A.: Anterior interosseous nerve syndrome. *J. Neurol. Neurosurg. Psychiat., 35:* 531, 1972.

69. NAKANO, K.: Anterior interosseous nerve (AIN) syndrome: Diagnosis by EMG and nerve conduction studies and alternative treatments. Presented at 38th AAEE Meeting, San Diego, Nov. 1976.

70. ASHENHURST, E.: Anatomical factors in the etiology of ulnar neuropathy. *Le Journal De L'Association Medicale Canadienne, 87:* 159, 1962.

71. CHECKLES, N., RUSSAKOV, A., AND PIERO, D.: Ulnar nerve conduction velocity—Effect of elbow position on measurement. *Arch. Phys. Med. Rehabil., 52:* 362, 1971.

72. BALMASEDA, M., AND CHECKLES, N.: Standardization of ulnar sensory fiber conduction velocity. Presented at 38th AAEE Meeting, San Diego, Nov. 1976.

73. EBELING, P., GILLIATT, R., AND THOMAS, P.: A clinical and electrical study of ulnar nerve lesions in the hand. *J. Neurol. Neurosurg. Psychiat., 23:* 1, 1960.

74. SHEA, J., AND MCCLAIN, E.: Ulnar nerve compression syndromes at and below the wrist. *J. Bone Joint Surg., 51A:* 1095, 1969.

75. BHALA, R., AND GOODGOLD, J.: Motor conduction in the deep palmar branch of the ulnar nerve. *Arch. Phys. Med. Rehabil., 49:* 460, 1968.

76. PAYAN, J.: Electrophysiological localization of ulnar nerve lesions. *J. Neurol. Neurosurg. Psychiat., 32:* 208, 1969.

77. CARPENDALE, M.: The localization of ulnar nerve compression in the hand and arm: An improved method of electroneuromyography. *Arch. Phys. Med. Rehabil., 47:* 323, 1966.

78. LORD, J. W., JR., AND ROSATI, L. M.: Thoracic outlet syndromes. *Clin. Symp., 23:* 2, 1971.

79. CALDWELL, J. W., CRANE, C. R., AND KRUSEN, E. M.: Nerve conduction studies: An aid in the diagnosis of the thoracic outlet syndrome. *S. Med. J., 64:* 210, 1971.

80. URSCHEL, H. C., RAZZUK, M. A., WOOD, R. E., MANAHARLAL, P., AND PAULSON, D. L.: Objective diagnosis (ulnar nerve conduction velocity) and current therapy of the thoracic outlet syndrome. *Ann. Thorac. Surg., 12:* 608, 1971.

81. DAUBE, J. R.: Nerve conduction studies in the thoracic outlet syndrome. *Neurology, 25:* 347, 1975.

82. JOHNSON, E. W., AND TAYLOR, R.: Personal communication.

83. GHENT, W.: Further studies on meralgia paresthetic. *Can. Med. Assoc. J., 85:* 871, 1961.

84. BUTLER, E. T., JOHNSON, E. W., AND KAYE, Z. A.: Normal conduction velocity in the lateral femoral cutaneous nerve. *Arch. Phys. Med. Rehabil., 55:* 31, 1974.

85. ROSENBLUM, J., SCHWARZ, G., AND BENDLER, E.: Femoral neuropathy—A neurological complication of hysterectomy. *J. Am. Med. Assoc. 195:* 115, 1966.

86. GASSEL, M. M.: A study of femoral nerve conduction time. *Arch. Neurol. 9:* 607, 1963.

87. JOHNSON, E. W., WOOD, P., AND POWERS, J.: Femoral nerve conduction studies. *Arch. Phys. Med. Rehabil., 49:* 528, 1968.

88. COMBES, M. W., AND CLARK, W. K.: Sciatic nerve injury following intragluteal injection: Pathogenesis and prevention. Speech before the Society for Pediatric Research Program and Abstracts 30th Annual Meeting, Levampscott, Mass., 1960.

89. JOHNSON, E. W., AND RAPTOU, A. D.: A study of intragluteal injection. *Arch. Phys. Med. Rehabil. 46:* 167, 1965.

90. LACHMAN, E.: Applied anatomy of intragluteal injections. *Am. Surg. 29:* 236, 1963.

91. TARLOV, I. M., PERLMUTTER, I., AND BERMAN, A.J.: Paralysis caused by penicillin injection: Mechanism of complication—A warning. *J. Neuropathol. Exp. Neurol. 10:* 158–176, 1951.

92. YAP, C., AND HIROTA, T.: Sciatic nerve motor conduction velocity study. *J. Neurol. Neurosurg. Psychiat., 30:* 233, 1967.

93. WOLTMAN, H.: Grossing the legs as a factor in the production of peroneal palsy. *J. Am. Med. Assoc. 93:* 670, 1929.

94. STACK, R. E., BIANCO, A. J., AND MACCARTY, C.S.: Compression of the common peroneal nerve by ganglion cysts. *J. Bone Joint Surg., 47A:* 773, 1965.

95. LAMBERT, E. H.: The accessory deep peroneal nerve—A common variation in innervation of extensory digitorum brevis. *Neurology, 19:* 1169, 1969.

96. CHECKLES, N., BAILEY, J., AND JOHNSON, E. W.: Tape and caliper surface measurements in determination of peroneal nerve conduction velocity. *Arch. Phys. Med. Rehabil. 50:* 214, 1969.

97. DISTEFANO, V., SACK, J., WHITTAKER, R., AND NIXON, J.: Tarsal tunnel syndrome. *Clin. Orthop. Related Res. 88:* 76, 1972.

98. LAM, S.: Tarsal tunnel syndrome. *J. Bone Joint Surg. 49B:* 87, 1967.

99. EDWARDS, W., LINCOLN, R., BASSETT, F., AND GOLDNER, J.: The tarsal tunnel syndrome. *J. Am. Med. Assoc., 207:* 716, 1969.

100. KECK, C.: The tarsal tunnel syndrome. *J. Bone Joint Surg., 44A:* 180, 1962.

101. JOHNSON, E. W., AND ORTIZ, P.: Electrodiagnosis of tarsal tunnel syndrome. *Arch. Phys. Med. Rehabil., 47:* 776, 1966.

10

Pediatric Considerations

MICHAEL A. ALEXANDER, M.D.
MARGARET TURK, M.D.

Any pediatrician can tell you it's folly to treat children as little adults. Any electromyographer who has had some experience with children will agree. If one sets out in the EMG laboratory with the misconception that he can compare values and amplitudes of studies found in children with known adult values, he will be in error. Also, techniques of needle exploration must be modified for infants and small children. Some pathologic conditions affecting children also require special adaptation of the electrodiagnostic examination. The actual approach of the electromyographer to the child similarly must be adjusted to the child's developmental level, cooperation, and parental desires, as well as to the suspected disease or injury.

Ontogeny of the Motor Unit

Many of the neurologic differences between the adult and the child are related to the delay in the developmental sequence of the central nervous system. At the time of birth, the central nervous system is not mature, and there is a lag of several years before the human organism is neurologically mature. One can detect differences in the muscle fibers of the premature newborn and older child. The embryo begins to show a differentiation into muscle fiber types by 8–10 weeks with the type II fibers more predominant (1). At 20 weeks, it can be said that, though there are equal numbers of types I and II fibers, the type II fibers appear to predominate and the type I's are smaller in size (1, 2). By 30 weeks gestation, fiber types I and II are of the same size and number. There is more accelerated growth rate of the type I fibers at that time than occurs later in gestation. It has been speculated that this may account for the selective involvement of type I fibers in many cases of spinal muscular atrophy with onset prenatally (3). With respect to the nerve fibers themselves, there is no myelinization of fibers until the 16th week of gestation (4). It is not until after the first 20 weeks that there is an increase in the conduction velocities of peripheral nerves (5), which corresponds with onset of myelinization.

260

The Pediatric Motor Unit

The gradual increase in conduction velocities has prompted several studies of conduction velocities in the newborn and growing child. The newborn infant full-term has conduction velocities which are 50% of adult values (6–8) (Fig. 10.1). The values approach 100% of the adult by age 4 (6–8). It has been observed that the peroneal velocity in the newborn and infant 1–3 years of age is often faster than the median (7); in fact, the ulnar and median velocities do not approach each other until after age 6 (7). This is probably a measurement artifact, since the surface measurement of the peroneal nerve tends to be longer than the actual length of the nerve. The median

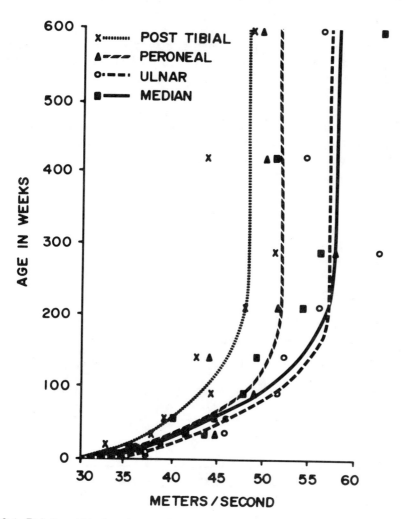

Fig. 10.1. Relationship of motor conduction velocities and age in weeks [after Baer and Johnson (6)].

nerve measures shorter because of the lack of the complete extension of the newborn's elbow.

Nerve conduction velocity studies are consistent and can be used as predictors of length of gestation. When one finds a velocity in the newborn of the elbow to wrist segment of less than 20 m/sec, the probability is greater than 95% that the infant is pre-term (8). Similarly, it has been shown that in the premature there was a rise in velocity over the first few weeks of life (9). In fact, one can look at all infants born with a low birth weight, and on the basis of conduction studies, separate them into two distinct populations. One group will fall within the full-term infant velocities, and the other group will fall in the pre-term ranges (10, 11) (Fig. 10.2). A closer look at the group with the low weight but higher velocities, suggestive of a full-term infant, will show these infants are postmature category or have some serious medical problem contributing to small size (dysmature). At the time the pre-term infant is equivalent in age to its full-term counterpart, it will have velocities which are in the full-term infant's ranges (12). The amplitudes of the evoked muscle action potentials have been shown to increase with age (13). It has also been shown that the duration of the residual latency increases with the age (13). Residual latency is that portion of the distal latency remaining after the calculated velocity has been subtracted.

Low threshold afferent fibers of the ulnar nerve in the newborn can be

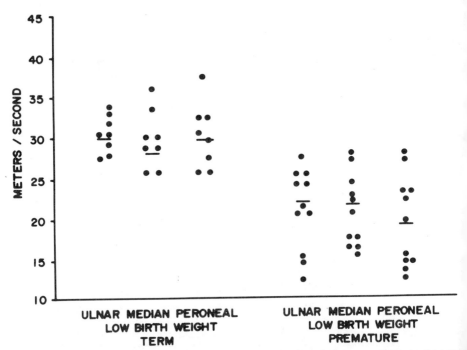

Fig. 10.2. Comparison of motor conduction velocity of ulnar, median, and peroneal nerves in premature and dysmature newborns [after Ruppert and Johnson (11)]

stimulated with a current to elicit the H reflex response; this is usually not present in this nerve in the adult or in children over a year of age (7, 13, 14). The latency of the H reflex is longer in the newborn and approaches normal as the velocities do (14), by the 4th year of life.

Amplitude and duration of motor unit potentials vary with the age of the child as well as maturation of the central nervous system. The mean amplitude of the motor unit potential has been shown to increase from 3 months to 20 years of age and the duration of the motor unit potential increase by 20% in that same period of time (15). The electromyographer studying infants and small children must be familiar with these differences in order to interpret the electrodiagnostic results properly.

Equipment and Technique

One should preferably begin with a warm, quiet setting away from any distractions if possible. Temperature is critical in the newborn and premature infant. The infant's surface area to mass ratio and immaturity of temperature control mechanism will lead to a low temperature in the extremities and the resultant decreased velocities (16). The studies can be done easily with the infant still in the incubator. However, the open crib with the overhead warmer facilitates the examination.

While the parents may be present for studies in the newborn, it is best to have the parents wait outside the examining room for all children. It is amazing how much better the child will behave when he is alone with the electromyographer than when mother or dad is present for soliciting sympathy. In children under 4, plan on needing an assistant and using restraints. The young child can be most heroic in his attempts to thwart the EMG assault. The child over 4 may be able to help with the steps of the examination. Explaining that he will see his muscles on television and will see how they work may gain the needed cooperation for detecting and measuring the first recruited potentials.

The EMG in an adult may be planned as a sequence of five steps (muscle at rest, insertional activity, minimal contractions, maximal contractions, and distribution of abnormalities). In the child, it is expedient to consider these five steps from two aspects: first, the need for electrical silence and second, the requirement for recruitment of motor units.

As the most discomfort may be felt on electrode insertion through the skin, avoid multiple skin reinsertions. It may be difficult at times to get electrical silence in the young infant; therefore, begin the EMG by exploring muscles which are inactive at the developmental stage, such as the extensor digitorum brevis, abductor digiti quinti pedis, opponens pollicis, hypothenar muscles, and first dorsal interosseus (17). The intrinsic muscles are generally not active in early infancy.

As a rule, to minimize motor unit recruitment, a muscle should be put into its shortest length from origin to insertion (17). For example, to test the anterior tibialis, dorsiflex the foot maximally (Fig. 10.3). Two-joint muscles

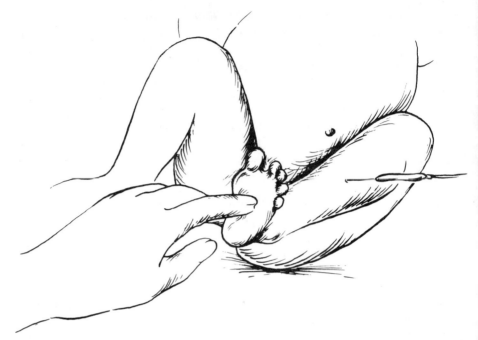

Fig. 10.3. For steps 1 and 2 of EMG, the muscle should be at its shortest length to ensure electrical silence.

such as the gastrocnemius require control of both joints; in this case, bend the knee as the foot is forcefully plantarflexed. Conversely the long head of the triceps is usually not active with the elbow flexed to more than 120° (17).

In the older child, do not use the word needle, since this conjures visions of hypodermics and previous painful injections. Even phrases such as "pin sticks" and "mosquito bite" may end cooperation. Do *not* show the child the electrode. Its length may be equated with pain anticipated by the child. Select the finest and shortest needle electrode and proceed with the examination. Also, the Teflon-coated monopolar electrodes are the least painful (18). Coincident with insertion of the electrode, a pinch or light slap will often distract the child and mask the discomfort of the monopolar needle.

Conduction studies require meticulous technique to avoid error in measurements. Extremities are quite short, so nerve segments studied may be 6–8 cm in the newborn. Errors of 1 cm could introduce an error of 15%. The baby fat layer, in effect, leads to a longer measurement than the true length of the nerve.

Surface electrodes are satisfactory for recording because of ease of securing and because of the added information of amplitude and duration of the evoked muscle action potential at the proximal and distal sites of stimulation. Bipolar stimulation electrodes do not need the separation of 4 cm used in adult studies. This permits study of a longer segment. One may also use a needle electrode as the stimulating cathode with a large surface anode on the opposite surface of the limb. Avoid excessive electrode paste since current leakage may occur between electrodes. Also, excessive perspiration may result in surface current shunts. These technique problems are obviated by using needle electrodes for stimulation. Securing recording electrodes is critical, and, as a rule, the younger the child, the more the adhesive tape is needed. Sedation is not necessary for carefully planned electrodiagnostic examinations.

A detailed history and careful physical examination are essential prior to planning the electrodiagnostic study. Especially in the infant, the EMG must be considered an extension of the history and physical.

Physical Examination

A proper pre-EMG screening physical examination is essential. Anticipated reflexes of the newborn will bring out recruitment in the desired muscle. The moro responses elicit activity in shoulder abduction, elbow, and finger extensors (Fig. 10.4). Note that the infant completely opens the hand in the normal moro response. The asymmetric tonic reflex allows screening of flexion and extension of both elbows. The positive supporting and placement responses (Fig. 10.5) activate all muscle groups in the lower

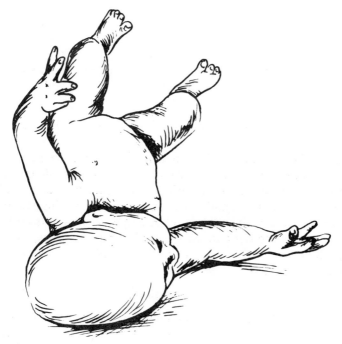

Fig. 10.4. Moro response to activate motor unit potentials in steps 3 and 4 of EMG.

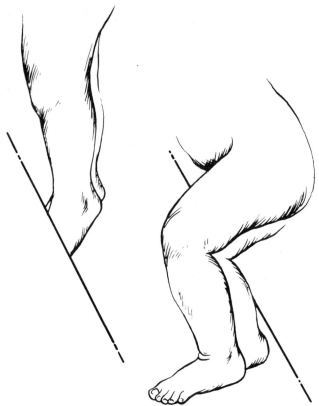

Fig. 10.5. Placement response is elicited by sensation on dorsum of foot, to activate motor unit potentials in foot dorsiflexor, e.g., steps 3 and 4.

extremities. Finally, the grasp and Babinski reflexes elicit distal extremity function.

The older child who walks, if taken away from his mother and placed on the floor, will, in sequence, get up from the floor, run to his mother, reach up and stand on his toes in anticipation of being picked up (17) (Fig. 10.6). Observing the child dress and undress can be an evaluation of muscle function. Finally, even when the child attempts to escape from the physician's examination, activity in various muscle groups may be observed. Planning EMG exploration on the younger child, the weakest muscles should be examined first.

Hypotonia

The problem of the limp or immobile infant has long been of concern to the clinician. A variety of medical writers have discussed the definition and causes of hypotonia and have classified the etiologies in a number of ways (19–21).

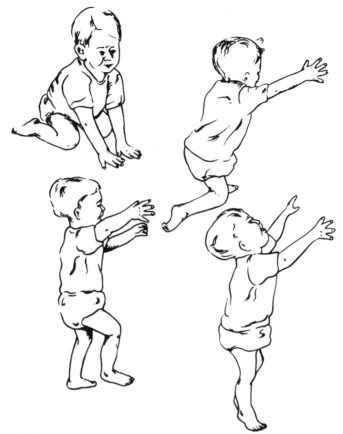

Fig. 10.6. Getting up from floor to run to mother to observe functional activity in various muscle groups.

Hypotonia, however, must first be defined. There are three clinical features associated with hypotonia: lack of spontaneous movement, poor adjustment to postural demands, and little resistance of the joints to passive movement (19). Increase in the range of movement of the joints is often included as a sign (21). In the newborn period, there may be unusual posturing or a lack of muscle activity; delay in developmental milestones usually presents at about 6 months or older (21, 23).

Commonly, hypotonia is a symptom of an underlying disease. Age of onset can be of critical importance in determining the cause. Muscular hypotonia may be associated with neuromuscular syndromes, cerebral palsy, metabolic disorders, or simply prematurity. The diagnosis becomes more complex because of confusion with multiple classifications and nomenclature.

A system of classifying hypotonia initially on clinical criteria and then progressing with a detailed laboratory investigation has been proposed by

Dubowitz (21). His classification is based on the presence or absence of significant weakness. Weakness is present if the infant is unable to move the limbs spontaneously or after stimulus or if he is unable to maintain his limb in an elevated posture. Therefore, the two subdivisions are: (a) a paralyzed child with evidence of hypotonia and (b) a hypotonic child with weakness.

The paralytic group is composed primarily of children with neurogenic muscular atrophy (Werdnig-Hoffmann disease). Other causes include congenital myopathies and various neuromuscular disorders.

Hypotonia is also the predominant symptom in the nonparalytic group. The main disorders which are likely to present in this way are central nervous system, connective tissue, and metabolic disorders. There appears to be an association of hypotonia with mental deficiency, often with no apparent underlying disease; it is often difficult to assess the degree of motor delay from intellectual or developmental causes. However, until the pathogenesis of hypotonia is clarified, this confusion is likely to remain.

Also included in the nonparalytic group is a subdivision of children with hypotonia as an isolated feature with no apparent underlying muscle weakness of associated disease. This group has been termed "benign congenital hypotonia" or "essential hypotonia." As originally described by Walton (23), these infants were generally hypotonic with some weakness at birth, with a gradual improvement or disappearance of symptoms in time. Those children with residual weakness would now probably be defined as a congenital myopathy.

The logical sequence of various diagnostic procedures in evaluation of the floppy infant is determined by the original clinical assessment. In the paralytic group, the goal is identifying the neuromuscular disorder. The possibilities in the nonparalytic group are much broader. Important studies include muscle biopsy, serum enzymes, and, of course, EMG and nerve stimulation studies.

Neurogenic Muscular Atrophy

The classification of neurogenic muscular atrophy has been a debated issue since the first clinical descriptions of the entity in 1891 (21). Werdnig and Hoffmann both described healthy children with the onset of hypotonia, weakness, and atrophy during the first 6 months of life (24). Soon, cases were reported beginning during the fetal or neonatal periods. The disease entity became confused with the advent of Oppenheim's description of children with severe muscular hypotonia in the neonatal period who later improved. However, his long term follow-up of these patients diagnosed as amyotonia congenita have not been published (24). Review by Walton (23) and Brandt (25) of patients previously classified as amyotonia congenita revealed new diagnoses of Werdnig-Hoffmann disease or other neuromuscular disorders. Brandt concluded Oppenheim's diagnosis was one of a symptom complex, not a specific entity. Wohlfart and Kugelberg and Welander described another variant of spinal muscular atrophy in a group of patients who began to show weakness, atrophy, and fasciculations in late childhood (24). Since that time, a number of cases have been reported which seem to represent transitional forms between Werdnig-Hoffmann disease and Kugelberg-Welander disease.

Presently, there continues to be confusion in terms of classification, and the confusion will, no doubt, remain until there is clarification of the pathogenesis in terms of enzyme or metabolic defects and of etiology in regard to heredity (26).

There appear to be some generalities that can be made about this disease entity, despite its wide range (27). The distribution of muscle weakness is symmetrical, affecting the proximal limb most often, but may involve the distal limb, the bulbar, scapuloperoneal, or fascioscapulohumeral muscle groups. The weakness may be generalized with gradual progression upwards. There can be sensory involvement more severe in the longer surviving cases (28). The muscular involvement can be noted at any time from embryonic to late middle age life. The disease process is progressive, usually more severe in the earlier onset. An exception to this is found in arthrogryposis multiplex congenita, in which the disorder seems to have arrested in utero.

All of these diseases have a genetic pattern. The forms that are fatal in early childhood show an autosomal recessive inheritance (26). In the more benign forms with longer survival there may be autosomal dominant as well as recessive inheritance.

EMG is useful in the diagnosis of neurogenic muscular atrophy. The EMG feature unique to infantile spinal muscular atrophy is spontaneous activity in relaxed muscles (29). The activity is irregularly discharged, 5–15/sec, and occurs in functioning motor units. Positive waves and fibrillation potentials are infrequent in the earliest stages of the disease. However, this membrane irritability can be seen on insertional activity in later stages. Also present may be increased amplitude and duration with reduced number of motor unit potentials as compared to strength of contraction (30). This increased amplitude and duration of motor unit potentials has been attributed to reinnervation of denervated muscle fibers (31). Bizarre high frequency discharges can also be observed.

There have been reports of low amplitude and short duration motor units associated with neuropathic changes or even found as the only EMG feature (32).

Fasciculations can be found clinically in older patients (29). However, fasciculations were reported electromyographically on a child 25 months old, about 1½ years before they were observed clinically (33). Clinically observed fasciculations can be seen in 20% of cases (34).

In all cases, nerve conduction studies are normal (30).

Myopathy

EMG can be useful in evaluation of childhood neuromuscular disorders, particularly in differentiating neuropathic and myopathic changes.

Myopathies can be divided into four groups: the congenital nonprogressive myopathies, a few rare congenital progressive myopathies, the noncongenital progressive muscular dystrophies, and the myotonic syndromes (26). An EMG can identify abnormalities which are quite helpful diagnostically in evaluation of the muscular dystrophies and the myotonic syndromes. In Duchenne muscular dystrophy and some of the myotonias in infancy, the most consistent EMG abnormalities found in the myopathies are increased polyplasicity and short duration motor unit potentials, particularly those first recruited (35).

There are two types of benign myotonia disorders. The first is Thomson disease, autosomal dominantly inherited, with symptoms appearing at birth or sometimes delayed into the first or second decade of life (26). The myotonia is widespread. Myotonic bursts can be found on an EMG. The second variety of myotonia was described by Becker (36) and is an autosomal recessive inheritance. This entity is much more common and usually has a later onset. EMG may show a decremental response of muscle-evoked potentials on repetitive stimulation (depolarization block).

Dystrophia myotonica (Steinert disease), inherited as an autosomal dominant trait, may cause symptoms in early infancy. The symptoms may be inconspicuous early with the child presenting as a feeding problem. The disorder is often associated with other congenital disorders, including heart disease, endocrine and gonadal anomalies, and cataracts. The EMG may show evidence of myopathy, besides the typical myotonic "dive bomber" bursts (35).

In paramyotonia congenita, again inherited as an autosomal dominant, there are no myopathic EMG abnormalities seen (35). This myotonia becomes clinically apparent after exercise or exposure to cold and electromyographically presents as trains of positive waves or diphasic spikes varying in frequency and amplitude.

Clinical manifestations of osteo-chondro-muscular dystrophy begin in infancy with slowly progressive boney deformities and a mild muscular dystrophic process. EMG findings in this disorder differ somewhat from that of myotonic dystrophy. There is marked spontaneous activity in muscle that is maintained without relation to mechanical stimulation or to volitional activation (37).

Serum potassium levels may be related to muscle weakness and hypotonia. Hypokalemia may occur in conjunction with gastrointestinal or renal losses, but the familial disorder is rare in young children. During paresis, there is a single unit interference pattern; during paralysis, there is electrical silence (35). Hyperkalemic periodic paralysis may begin in infancy (38). Attacks of weakness are brief and may be confused with myasthenia gravis. Serum potassium levels are variable (26). During paresis, there is increased insertional activity, with a decrease in the number of motor units during voluntary effort (35).

McArdle disease is a hereditary primary myopathy due to a phosphorylase deficiency. Pain is usually the most prominent symptom, associated with easy fatigue and muscle stiffness. EMG changes appear only after fatigue and hypoxia of the muscle. During full effort, there is a progressive decrease in amplitude of the interference pattern until the muscle goes into contracture; there is then electrical silence (39).

Connective tissue disorders can present positive EMG findings. One of the five major criteria used to define polymyositis is the classic EMG triad of short, small, polyphasic motor units, profuse membrane irritability, and bizarre high frequency discharges (40). In both diffuse scleroderma and acroscleroderma, the EMG pattern corresponds to the type recorded in polymyositis. There is a low voltage pattern with an increased number of polyphasic potentials. The most statistically significant finding is a shortened potential duration (41). In circumscribed scleroderma, this is most frequently seen in the muscles underlying the lesions.

Neuropathies

Isolated nerve palsies occur frequently in children. Facial palsy in children is usually idiopathic as in adults (42). Newborns can present with facial paralysis due to direct pressure on the exposed nerve (43); however, unlike adults, otitis media is the second largest cause and hypertension the third (42).

Diabetic neuropathies are present to a greater extent than reported under 6 years of age (44). Conduction velocities of the ulnar and peroneal nerves have been reported to be slower than expected; interestingly, no fibrillation potentials or positive waves were reported but a decrease recruitment pattern has been seen (45). A description of the familial neuropathies will be covered in greater detail in other chapters. An important value of EMG remains in detecting other affected members of Friedreich ataxia (46) and Charcot-Marie-Tooth disease (47, 48). Even isolated nerve lesions warrant a family history as there are families where several members at different times showed isolated nerve involvement (49).

There have been several studies describing children who only manifest a sensory disorder with absence of monosynaptic reflexes, absence of pain, and self-mutilation. Their sensory and H reflex studies are abnormal, yet motor conductions and needle EMG are usually negative (50, 51). Another similar group is associated with spasticity (52) and some populations blend into more traditional neuropathies (53).

Since the almost eradication of polio, the sudden onset of neuropathy in a child is most often diagnosed as Guillain-Barré Syndrome, and often the spinal fluid will show the albuminocytologic dissociation. Often the first EMG changes may be in the proximal segments, and for this, an H or F wave study may be needed (54). A history of toxins or recent immunizations may be relevant. Prophylactic inoculation has been implicated in several rapidly progressing cases of neuropathies (55). As more children with leukemia receive anti-neoplastic agents such as vincristine, methotrexate, and 5-Fluorouracil, one can expect neuropathies (56). Though no longer a medical scourge, in the past, a sudden paralysis heralded the onset of dyphtheria (57). Finally, many chronic ingestions both prescribed, as in diphenylhydantoin (58), and child's gustatory preference, as in lead paint, can produce a neuropathy. Proximity to lead smelters or even families that burn newspapers for heating have children with high enough serum lead levels to correlate with mild neuropathies (59).

In the child with myelomeningocele, there is a correlation between decreased insertional activity and poor prognosis for function in that muscle (60). Often after surgery, fibrillation potentials may be more prominent; this may be due to injury as a result of sac closure (60).

Special Problems

EMG may be of use in evaluating the enuretic child (61). A high number of these children have a neurogenic component manifested by a decreased firing pattern or insertional abnormalities (62). The best firing pattern will be seen just after insertion of the electrode. An assistant on standby is generally necessary.

Torticollis of newborns presents a management problem. When does one use physical therapy and when is surgical intervention warranted? If on EMG there is no electrical activity or electrode movement in the sternocleidomastoid (Fig. 10.7), there is a fibrous band which needs excision. The more electrical activity, the better the prognosis that stretching and positioning will accomplish good results (63).

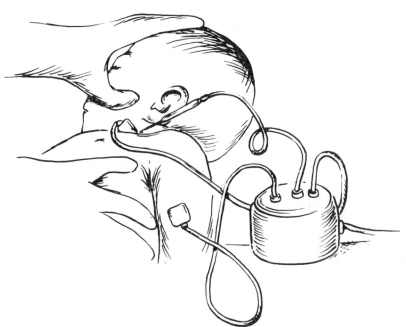

Fig. 10.7. Electrode placement for examination of sternocleidomastoid, e.g., for management of congenital muscular torticollis.

EMG Research in Children

Researchers often imply that the use of EMG lends credibility to their conclusions, and some clinicians are less likely to question such studies if they include EMG. This is probably incorrect.

Orthodontists have set up elaborate studies of the kinesiology of mastication (64). Investigators ran into wide variations in patterns (65). Sequential studies in orthodontically treated groups were done and showed there were phase changes with mandible realignment (66). Inferences were drawn from these studies about treated children. Yet, it was not until years later that studies in the child were performed allowing such comparisons (67).

Kinesiologic studies of phase activity in cerebral palsy show interesting changes in muscles operated on as well as in other muscle groups (68). Studies have implicated medial hamstrings in the production of the internal rotation deformity of the hips (69).

As always, rigid control and previous standardization are mandatory. Studies have been published claiming phase activity of muscles based on surface electrodes which are over muscles which, in fact, are only accessible by needle electrodes. Endplate noise has been confused by investigators and reported as "denervation potentials." There have been a number of papers on EMG findings in idiopathic scoliosis suggesting a neuropathic etiology based on similar misconceptions. Only recently has clarification been made (70). In children, meticulous methods, proper research design, and critical analysis of data are essential in interpreting kinesiologic EMG studies in children.

REFERENCES

1. FENICHEL, G. M.: A histochemical study of developing human skeletal muscle. *Neurology, 16:* 741, 1966.
2. DUBOWITZ, V.: Enzyme histochemistry of skeletal muscle: Part II. Developing human muscle. *J. Neurol. Neurosurg. Psychiat., 28:* 516, 1965.
3. FENICHEL, G. M.: Abnormalities of skeletal muscle maturation in brain damaged children: A histochemical study. *Dev. Med. Child Neurol., 9:* 419, 1967.
4. HAMILTON, W. J., AND MOSMAN, H. W.: *Human Embryology: Prenatal Development of Form and Function,* 4th ed., Cambridge: Heffer, 1972.
5. WYKE, B. D.: *Principles of General Neurology. An Introduction to the Basic Principles of Medical and Surgical Neurology,* Amsterdam and London: Elsevier, 1969.
6. BAER, R. D., AND JOHNSON, E. W.: Motor nerve conduction velocities in normal children. *Arch. Phys. Med. Rehabil., 46:* 698, 1965.
7. GAMSTROP, I.: Normal conduction velocity of ulnar, median, and peroneal nerves in infancy, childhood, and adolescence. *Acta Paediatr., 146:* 68, 1963.
8. WAGNER, A. L., AND BUCHTHAL, F.: Motor and sensory conduction in infancy and childhood: Reappraisal. *Dev. Med. Child Neurol., 14:* 189, 1972.
9. CERRA, D., AND JOHNSON, E. W.: Motor conduction velocity in premature infants. *Arch. Phys. Med. Rehabil., 43:* 160, 1962.
10. SCHULTE, F. J. ET AL.: Motor nerve conduction velocity in term, preterm, small for dates newborn infants. *Pediatrics, 42:* 17, 1968.
11. RUPPERT, E. S., AND JOHNSON, E. W.: Motor nerve conduction velocities in low birth weight infants. *Pediatrics, 42:* 255, 1968.
12. LITTMAN, B.: Peripheral nerve maturation in premature infants. *Neuropaediatrie, 6:* 3, 1975.

13. THOMAS, J. E., AND LAMBERT, E. H.: Ulnar nerve velocity and H reflex in infants and children. *J. Appl. Physiol., 15:* 1, 1960.

14. MAYER, R. F., AND MOSSER, R. S.: Excitability of motor neurons in infants. *Neurology, 19:* 932, 1969.

15. SACCO, G., BUCHTHAL, F., AND ROSENFALK, P.: Motor unit potentials at different ages. *Arch. Neurol., 6:* 44, 1962.

16. HENDRICKSEN, J.: Conduction velocity of motor nerves in normal subjects and patients with neuromuscular disorders. Thesis, University of Minnesota, June 1956.

17. JOHNSON, E. W.: Examination for muscle weakness in infants and children. *J. Am. Med. Assoc., 168:* 1306, 1958.

18. SPENCE, R. W., AND GUYTON, J. D.: Control of pain in electromyography. *Arch. Phys. Med. Rehabil., 47:* 771, 1966.

19. JERSEN, R. H., JOHNSON, E. W., KNOBLACH, H., AND GRANT, D. K.: Differential diagnosis of infantile hypotonia. *Am. J. Dis Child., 101:* 8, 1961.

20. RABE, E. F.: The hypotonic infant. *Pediatrics, 64:* 422, 1964.

21. DUBOWITZ, V.: *The Floppy Infant,* Suffolk: The Lavenham Press Ltd., 1969.

22. WALTON, J. N.: The "Floppy" Infant. *Cerebral Palsy Bulletin, 2:* 10, 1960.

23. WALTON, J. N.: The limp child. *J. Neurol. Neurosurg. Psychiat., 20:* 144, 1957.

24. GAMSTORP, I.: Characteristic clinical findings in some neurogenic myopathies and in some myogenic myopathies causing muscular weakness, hypotonia, and atrophy in infancy and early childhood. *Birth Defects, 7:* 72, 1971.

25. BRANDT, S.: *Werdnig-Hoffmann's Infantile Progressive Muscular Atrophy,* Copenhagen: Munksgaard, 1950.

26. WALTON, J. N. (Ed.): *Disorders of Voluntary Muscle,* Glasgow: Bell and Bain Ltd., 1974.

27. EMERY, A. E. H.: Review: The nosology of the spinal muscular atrophies. *J. Med. Genet., 8:* 481, 1971.

28. MARSHALL, A., AND DUCHEN, L. W.: Sensory system involvement in infantile spinal muscular atrophy. *J. Neurol. Sci., 26:* 349, 1975.

29. BUCHTHAL, F., AND OLSEN, P. Z.: Electromyography and muscle biopsy in infantile spinal muscular atrophy. *Brain, 93:* 15, 1970.

30. MUNSAT, T. L., WOODS, R., FOWLER, W., AND PEARSON, C. M.: Neurogenic muscular atrophy of infancy with prolonged survival. *Brain, 92:* 9, 1969.

31. LAMBERT, E. H.: Neurophysiological techniques useful in the study of neuromuscular disorders. *Res. Publ. Assoc. Res. Nerv. Ment. Dis., 38:* 247, 1960.

32. MASTAGLIA, F. L., AND WALTON, J. N.: Histological and histochemical changes in skeletal muscle from cases of chronic juvenile and early adult spinal muscular atrophy (the Kugelberg-Welander syndrome). *J. Neurol. Sci., 12:* 15, 1971.

33. BYERS, R. K., AND BANKER, B. Q.: Infantile muscular atrophy. *Arch. Neurol., 5:* 38, 1961.

34. VAN WIJINGAARDEN, G. K., AND BETHLEM, J.: Benign infantile spinal muscular atrophy. *Brain, 96:* 163, 1973.

35. GOODGOLD, J., AND ELBERSTEIN, A.: *Electrodiagnosis of Neuromuscular Disease.* Baltimore: The Williams & Wilkins Company, 1972.

36. BERGSMA, D. (Ed.): *The Clinical Delineation of Birth Defects Part VII Muscle.* Baltimore: The Williams & Wilkins Company, 1972.

37. HUTTENLOCHER, P. R., ET AL.: Osteo–chondro–muscular dystrophy. *Pediatrics, 44:* 945, 1969.

38. GAMSTORP, I.: Adymania episoda hereditaria and myotonia. *Acta Neurol. Scand., 39:* 41, 1963.

39. LUBRAN, M. M.: McArdle's disease: A review. *Ann. Clin. Lab. Sci., 5:* 115, 1975.

40. BOHAN, A., AND PETER, J. B.: Polymyositis and dermatomyositis. *N. Engl. J. Med., 292:* 344, 1975.

41. HAUSMANOWA-PETRUSEWICZ, I., AND KOZMINSKA, A.: Electromyographic findings in scleroderma. *Arch. Neurol., 4:* 281, 1961.

42. LLOYD, A. V. D., ET AL.: Facial paralysis in children with hypertension. *Arch. Dis. Child., 41:* 292, 1966.

43. HEPNER, W. R.: Some observations on facial paresis in the newborn infant: Etiology and incidence. *Pediatrics, 8:* 494, 1951.

44. LAWRENCE, D. G., AND LOCKE, S.: Neuropathy in children with diabetes mellitus. *Br. Med. J., 5333:* 784, 1963.

45. EEG-OLOFSSON, O.: Childhood diabetic neuropathy—A clinical neurophysiological study. *Acta Paediatr. Scand., 55:* 163, 1966.

46. DUNN, H. G.: Nerve conduction studies in children with friedreich's ataxia and ataxia-telangectasia. *Dev. Med. Child Neurol., 15:* 324, 1973.

47. EARL, W. C., AND JOHNSON, E. W.: Motor nerve conduction velocity in Charcot-Marie-Tooth disease. *Arch. Phys. Med. Rehabil. 44:* 247, 1963.

48. DYCK, P. J.: Lower motor and primary sensory neuron diseases with peroneal muscular atrophy. *Arch. Neurol., 18:* 619, 1968.

49. ATTAL, C.: Familial nerve trunk paralyses. *Dev. Med. Child Neurol., 17:* 787, 1975.

50. JOHNSON, R. H.: Progressive neuropathy in children. *J. Neurol. Neurosurg. Psychiat., 27:* 125, 1964.

51. OGDEN, T. E.: Some sensory syndromes in children: Indifference to pain and sensory neuropathy. *J. Neurol. Neurosurg. Pychiat., 29:* 267, 1959.

52. KOENIG, R. H.: Hereditary spastic paraparesis with sensory neuropathy. *Dev. Med. Child Neurol., 12:* 576, 1970.

53. FEDRIZZI, E.: Peripheral sensory neuropathy in childhood. *Dev. Med. Child Neurol., 14:* 501, 1972.

54. KIMURA, J.: F wave conduction velocity in Guillain-Barré syndrome. *Arch. Neurol., 32:* 524, 1975.

55. MILLER, H. G.: Neurologic sequellae of prophylactic inoculation. *Q. J. Med., 23:* 1, 1954.

56. WEISS, H. D.: Neurotoxicity of commonly used anti-neoplastic agents. *N. Engl. J. Med., 291:* 75, 1974.

57. KAZEMI, B.: Motor nerve conduction in diphtheria and diphtheric myocarditis. *Arch. Neurol., 29:* 104, 1973.

58. BRUMLIK, J.: The effect of diphenylhydantoin on nerve conduction velocity. *Neurology, 16:* 1217, 1966.

59. LANDRIGAN, P. J.: Increased lead absorption with anemia and slowed nerve conduction in children near a lead smelter. *J. Pediatr., 89:* 904, 1976.

60. INGBERG, H. O., AND JOHNSON, E. W.: Electromyography evaluation of infants with lumbar meningomyelocele. *Arch. Phys. Med. Rehabil., 44:* 86, 1963.

61. BAILEY, J. A., ET AL.: A clinical evaluation of electromyography of the anal sphincter. *Arch. Phys. Med. Rehabil., 51:* 403, 1970.

62. WAYLONIS, G. W., ET AL.: Clinical application of anal sphincter electromyography. *Surg. Clin North Am., 52:* 807, 1972.

63. BAXTER, C. F.: Prognostic significance of electromyography in congenital torticollis. *Pediatrics, 28:* 442, 1961.

64. PRUZANSKY, S.: The application of electromyography to dental research. *J. Am. Dent. Assoc., 44:* 49, 1952.

65. LIEBMAN, F. M., AND COSENZA, F.: An evaluation of electromyography in the study of the etiology of malocclusion. *J. Prosthet. Dent., 10:* 1065, 1960.

66. GROSSMAN, W. J., ET AL.: Electromyography as an aid in diagnosis and treatment analysis. *Am. J. Orthod., 47:* 481, 1961.

67. VITTI, M., AND BASMAJIAN, J. V.: Muscles of mastication in small children: An electromyographic analysis. *Am. J. Orthod., 68:* 412, 1975.

68. PERRY, J., ET AL.: Electromyography before and after surgery for hip deformities in children with cerebral palsy. *J. Bone Joint Surg., 58A:* 201, 1976.

69. SUTHERLAND, D. H., ET AL.: Clinical and electromyographic study of seven spastic children with internal rotation gait. *J. Bone Joint Surg., 51A:* 1070, 1969.

70. ALEXANDER, M. A., AND SEASON, E. H.: EMG studies and idiopathic scoliosis. *Arch. Phys. Med. Rehabil., 59:* 314, 1978.

11

EMG in Upper Motor Neuron Conditions

JOHN PETTY, JR., M.D.
ERNEST W. JOHNSON, M.D.

For the electromyographer, since the basic writing of Denny-Brown and Pennybacker in 1938 (1), the presence of fibrillation and positive sharp wave potentials has been the *sine qua non* of lower motor neuron disease. Conventionally, fibrillation and positive sharp wave potentials have represented the pathognomonic sign of muscle denervation (1–4).

In 1954, Lambert and associates (5) reported finding positive sharp waves and fibrillation potentials in patients with progressive muscular dystrophy and polymyositis. In 1966, Buchthal and Rosenfalck (2) reported fibrillation potentials occurring in 10% of normal subjects (without evidence of denervation or lower motor neuron disease). They also found fibrillation potentials in 29 of 76 patients with progressive muscular dystrophy. More recently, fibrillation potentials have been recorded in cases of muscle trauma, electrolyte disturbance (hyperkalemia and hypokalemia), and upper motor neuron disease (6–10). Thus, fibrillation potentials and positive sharp waves are not synonymous with denervation or lower motor neuron disease.

The positive sharp wave is an artifact produced by mechanical stimulation of the electrode tip, which causes depolarization of the muscle cell membrane or several muscle cell membranes in the zone of injury. It occurs as a result of an abnormal hyperirritable state of the muscle cell membrane, and it is not recorded from normal muscle. The fibrillation potential is the resultant electrical activity of a single muscle cell membrane discharging spontaneously. The spontaneous depolarization takes place because of an abnormal hyperirritable or hypersensitive state of the muscle cell membrane in which there is increased sensitivity to acetylcholine along the entire surface of the muscle fiber instead of the normally localized sensitivity at the motor endplate zone (11, 12). It is thus a conceptual error to assign fibrillation potentials and positive sharp waves as EMG abnormalities occurring only in lower motor neuron disease. Rather, these nonspecific findings should be regarded only as alterations in the excitability of the muscle cell membrane produced by a variety of circumstances.

Due to the lack of specificity of these EMG findings, they must be interpreted in the light of the clinical history, physical examination, and laboratory data. No one EMG finding is pathognomonic of any clinical condition as once was thought. Moreover, diagnostic terms assigned to these EMG abnormalities (for example, denervation potential) need to be discarded, and they should rather be identified as simply neurophysiological abnormalities (for example, fibrillation potential). This terminology is clearly recommended in the Pavia report on EMG terminology (13).

EMG and Spinal Cord Injured Patients

CLINICAL INFORMATION

In patients in whom the case history and clinical picture implicated no other abnormality other than a spinal cord injury secondary to trauma, numerous EMG studies have reported muscle cell membrane hyperirritability (positive sharp waves and fibrillation potentials) (14–20). In general, the findings are distributed bilaterally and diffusely below the level of lesion without confinement to any segmental or peripheral nerve pattern. There has been only an occasional report of paraspinal muscle involvement (Fig. 11.1).

As long as the muscle status allows evoked potentials to be obtained in spinal cord injured patients, nerve conduction studies remain within normal limits (14). Due to early atrophy of the extensor digitorum brevis, more productive results can be acquired by studying the velocity of the posterior

SPINAL CORD INJURY

			PTS	+ %	TIME	ELECTRODE
	1967	O'HARE				
	1968	ISCH				
EMG ABNORMALITIES	1969	NOTERMANS				
	1969	ROSEN	7	86	2–8 mos	monopolar
	1971	NYBOER	10	80	3–10 mos	monopolar
	1972	SPIELHOLTZ	32	47	13 days–21 yr	coaxial
	1974	TAYLOR	22	100	1–40 days	monopolar
	1975	ONKELINX	10	100	4–19 mos	coaxial
	1976	BRANDSTATER	42	100	2–3 mos	

Fig. 11.1. Summary of EMG findings in spinal cord injured patients reported in the literature.

tibial nerve as opposed to that of the peroneal nerve. In the extensor digitorum brevis, the reduction in the amplitude of the M wave response (compound action potential) occurs early and progresses relatively quickly until no response can be obtained. In muscles without voluntary function, it is difficult to evaluate motor unit changes. The quantitative technique of McComas and associates (21) for estimating the number of residual functioning motor units is performed by nerve stimulation and obviates the need for voluntary or reflex muscle activation. The amplitude of the M wave response is measured at threshhold and at subsequent all or none increments as the stimulus voltage is slowly increased. These increments are thought to represent activation of individual motor units, thus giving an estimate of the number of residual functioning motor units. When using this technique to evaluate motor unit changes in spinal cord injured patients, marked reduction in motor unit number is usually found.

Since it is difficult to evaluate motor unit changes in spinal cord injured patients, the EMG abnormality most commonly studied is that of muscle cell membrane hyperirritability (positive sharp waves and fibrillation potentials). Perhaps the most interesting aspect of this alteration is its transient nature. These findings are not found prior to the 15th day postinjury and, in general, develop maximally between the 1st and 4th month postinjury and slowly decrease or vanish between the 5th through the 12th month postinjury, as the patient either regains motor function or develops spasticity. Studies (20, 22) have tried to associate the duration of muscle cell membrane hyperirritability directly with the period of spinal shock following cord trauma. However, as the clinical picture changes from one of flaccid paralysis with absent deep tendon reflexes to one of spasticity, clonus, and hyperreflexia, many have reported the abnormal findings persisting (Fig. 11.2). For the most part, after a spinal cord injured patient develops spasticity or regains some degree of motor function, in time, usually within a year after injury, the abnormal muscle cell membrane irritability will either markedly decrease or vanish.

EXPERIMENTAL INFORMATION

Although many etiologies for the abnormal muscle cell membrane hyperirritability in the spinal cord injured patient have been advanced (23), neurophysiological aberration secondary to interruption of the descending pathways appears to be the most likely cause. In animals with spinal cord hemisection, basic investigations have shown changes in excitability occurring in the anterior horn cell and internuncial pool (24, 25). In 1889, Warrington (26) reported finding marked histiologic changes in the anterior horn cell 30 days after section of the posterior roots. In 1941, Tower and associates (27) found marked chromatolysis (disintegration of Nissel substance—the protein synthesizing machinery of the anterior horn cell) following spinal cord transection in monkeys. Van Alphen and associates (28), in 1962, were the first to report these anterior horn cell histologic changes in

SPINAL CORD INJURY

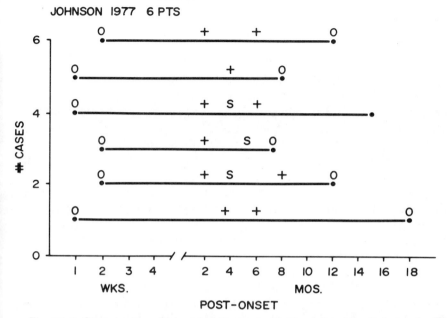

Fig. 11.2. Six spinal cord injured patients studied from time of admission for EMG abnormalities. An "O" indicates there were no positive waves and fibrillation potentials on EMG. A "+" indicates positive waves and fibrillation potentials were found. An "S" means spasticity appeared.

human spinal cords following traumatic injury. In three autopsied patients, each of whom was between the 1st and 2nd month postaccident at the time of death, Van Alphen found marked anterior horn cell chromatolysis.

Spielholz and associates (29), in 1972, adding their own clinical data, hypothesized that the anterior horn cell produces a trophic factor, a protein tentatively labeled "anti-fibrillation factor" which is transported down the axon and is responsible for muscle cell membrane stability in normal muscle. Following spinal cord injury and subsequent anterior horn cell chromatolysis, they propose that there is insufficient production of "anti-fibrillation factor" by the anterior horn cell to stabilize the muscle cell membrane, and, therefore, resultant muscle cell membrane hyperirritability occurs.

From the above, one might postulate that any disorder which disrupts the production, delivery, or reception of "anti-fibrillation factor" from the anterior horn cell down the axon to the muscle cell membrane may cause muscle cell membrane hyperirritability on EMG (positive sharp waves and fibrillation potentials). Since fibrillation potentials have been reported in cases of botulism (8, 10) (inhibited acetylcholine release), acetylcholine may be associated with such an "anti-fibrillation factor." Further support of this postulation rests with the evidence that when acetylcholine has been experimentally eliminated from the muscle cell membrane with an anatomically intact neuromuscular junction, spontaneous EMG activity has been recorded (11, 30).

EMG in Hemiplegia

CLINICAL INFORMATION

In patients in whom the case history and clinical picture pointed to no abnormality other than hemiplegia produced by a cerebral vascular accident, many EMG studies have reported muscle cell membrane hyperirritability (6, 31–35) (Fig. 11.3). The distribution of findings has been confined to the hemiplegic extremities with diffuse involvement, without a segmental or peripheral nerve pattern. There has been no report of muscle cell membrane hyperirritability in the paraspinal musculature.

In general, muscles of the upper extremity show more extensive findings than those of the lower extremity, and distal muscles show more prominent changes than proximal muscles. Nerve conduction studies performed on the hemiplegic side are essentially within normal limits with only one report of significant slowing, that being localized to the proximal segment of the ulnar nerve. Abnormal muscle cell membrane irritability in hemiplegic patients, like that seen in spinal cord patients, is transient in nature. There have been no reports of positive sharp waves or fibrillation potentials occurring prior to 7 days poststroke. The peak incidence of fibrillation potentials is 4.5 weeks post-cerebral accident, and this is preceded by an earlier appearance of positive sharp waves.

In the spastic type hemiplegia, hyperirritability of the muscle cell mem-

HEMIPLEGIA

			PTS	+ %	TIME	ELECTRODE
EMG ABNORMALITIES	1967	GOLDKAMP	116	70	0–13 wks	monopolar
	1968	ISCH				
	1969	BHALA	37	71	0–6 mos	coaxial
	1973	KRUEGER	21	81	$\frac{1}{2}$–10 mos	monopolar
	1975	JOHNSON	20	100	$\frac{1}{4}$–18 mos	monopolar
	1977	NEPOMUCENO	63	61	AVE–45 wks	monopolar
NO EMG ABNORMALITIES	1971	ALPERT	50	0	2 wks–10 yrs	monopolar and coaxial
	1973	ALPERT	15	28	9–22 days	monopolar and coaxial
	1974	HERNESS	4	0	1–3 mos	coaxial

Fig. 11.3. Summary of EMG findings in hemiplegia patients reported in the literature.

brane gradually lessens and finally disappears as volitional activity or spasticity develops. Twitchell (36) has reported a general sequence of development of volitional function or spasticity in hemiplegic patients. Quadriceps spasticity or function is usually the first to appear, followed by the gastrocnemius and the biceps brachii. Interestingly, the disappearance of abnormal muscle cell membrane irritability (positive sharp waves and fibrillation potentials) parallels the appearance of spasticity and volitional activity (35). In general, the abnormal EMG findings disappear centrifugally, starting in the lower extremity and progressing to the upper extremity as spasticity and volitional activity develop. Anti-gravity muscles of the lower extremity (quadriceps and gastrocnemius/soleus) are usually the first to lose spontaneous EMG activity, followed by the anti-gravity muscles of the upper extremity (biceps brachii, wrist, and finger flexors), then the antagonist of these anti-gravity muscles, and lastly, the distal muscles of the hands and feet. It may frequently require more than a year for findings in the hands and feet to return to normal (Fig. 11.4).

Contradictory reports in the literature dispute the presence of EMG abnormalities in hemiplegic patients (31, 37–39). Explanations given for the positive findings range from coincidental brachial plexus injuries to outright

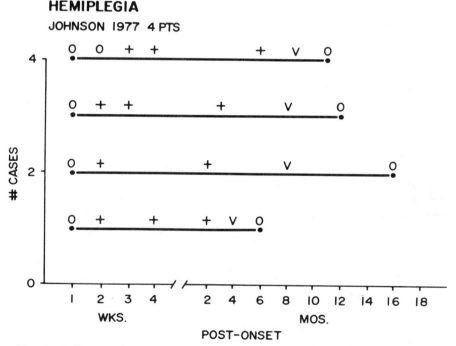

Fig. 11.4. Four stroke patients studied from admission for EMG abnormalities. An "O" indicates there were no positive waves and fibrillation potentials on EMG. A "+" indicates fibrillation potentials and positive waves were found. A "V" means volitional movement appeared.

282 / PRACTICAL ELECTROMYOGRAPHY

denial—apparently to avoid the iconoclastic conclusion that fibrillation potentials and positive waves are not synonymous with lower motor neuron disease. The transient character of the EMG findings in stroke patients is the explanation usually forwarded to explain these investigators' inability to record these findings.

EXPERIMENTAL INFORMATION

The experimental and clinical work of several investigators indicates that the upper motor neuron exerts a definite yet unknown influence on the anatomic and physiologic existence of the lower motor neuron. Baranek and Guttmann (24) observed that physiologic divorce of the lower motor neuron from the upper motor neuron in rabbits reduced the rate of motor fiber regeneration. They referred to this influence of one nerve cell upon the other connected to it as "trans-synaptic trophic influence." Hess (40) demonstrated that neuron maintenance is dependent metabolically on neuronal association and not merely on isolated anatomical integrity. Nyberg-Hansen and Brodal (41), 9 days after cortical lesions in cats, found transneuronal trophic changes in the spinal cords.

In cerebral vascular accidents, the pathway between a motor strip and effector muscle group is compromised, and this circumstance, it has been hypothesized, interferes with CNS influence on the muscle cell membrane. Presumably, this loss of trophic influence (possibly secondary to decreased stimulation of the anterior horn cell's so-called "anti-fibrillation factor" production) introduces instability into the equilibrium of the muscle cell membrane, which can then depolarize spontaneously (fibrillation potentials) or repetitively when disrupted by movement of the needle electrode (positive sharp waves).

Muscle wasting in hemiplegia has been recognized for many years (42–46), but the etiology of the atrophy has remained somewhat obscure. Disuse atrophy has been proposed as an etiology, but EMG of disuse atrophy fails to reveal positive waves and fibrillation potentials. Engel (47), in 1965, reported that muscle fibers affected only by suprasegmental CNS disease may show reduction in diameter and a histologic pattern similar to those encountered typically in lower motor neuron disease. Fenichel (48), in 1964, in biopsies of hemiplegic muscles in stroke patients, reported finding "simple atrophy" characterized by scattered, small, rounded muscle fibers. Thus, the pathogenesis of hemiplegic atrophy may also be due to the loss of a "trophic influence" of the CNS upon a muscle cell via the lower motor neuron. Silverstein (45, 46) has stated that the greatest degree of atrophy most commonly occurs in the small muscles of the hemiplegic hand. One may recall that this is also where the EMG changes have been found to be the most severe and the most persistent. This data suggests a cerebral pattern and possibly a relationship with the portion of the brain supplied by the middle cerebral artery. This cortical pattern is supported in part by the failure of the paraspinal muscles to demonstrate muscle cell membrane hyperirritability, as they have a different area of cortical representation.

Other Applications of EMG in Upper Motor Neuron Disorders

REFLEX STUDIES IN UPPER MOTOR NEURON DISEASE

H Reflex

In 1922, Hoffmann described an evoked response which could be elicited by stimulating a mixed peripheral nerve. This response was later referred to as the H reflex (49). In normal populations without neurological deficit, the H reflex can be commonly recorded from the gastrocnemius or soleus muscle following stimulation of the posterior tibial nerve. An H reflex has been recorded in normal subjects infrequently from the quadriceps muscles after stimulation of the femoral nerve and occasionally from the anterior tibial muscle after stimulation of the common peroneal nerve. Hohmann and Goodgold (50) reported finding positive H waves in the anterior tibial muscle after stimulation of the common peroneal nerve in 75% of cases with upper motor neuron lesions below the level of the midbrain. Similar results were obtained from the extensor indices proprius following stimulation of the radial nerve and from the abductor digiti quinti after stimulation of the ulnar nerve. These studies were performed postspinal shock, as during severe spinal shock associated with upper motor nerve insult, the H reflex, like the tendon jerks, is usually absent. In cases of upper motor neuron damage above the level of the midbrain, the H reflex could not be elicited from the extraposterior tibial innervated muscles, regardless of duration of time after insult.

Before positive sharp waves and fibrillation potentials were found in upper motor neuron disorders, these EMG findings had been used to differentiate lower motor neuron disorders from those of the upper motor neuron. Nepomuceno and associates (23) compared positive sharp waves and fibrillation potentials found in upper motor neuron disorders with those found in lower motor neuron disorders. They found the lower motor neuron positive sharp wave to be of a slightly longer duration than the upper motor neuron positive sharp wave. This finding is of little practical diagnostic value, but a positive H reflex in muscles other than those innervated by the posterior tibial nerve may offer distinguishing diagnostic evidence for upper motor neuron lesion in cases where there is a paucity of clinical findings.

It should be noted that it is very important to have the muscle being tested completely relaxed when trying to elicit an H reflex. With muscle contraction, an H reflex can be facilitated in a nonposterior tibial innervated muscle similar to facilitation of a muscle stretch reflex. Furthermore, the H reflex has been demonstrated in muscles other than those innervated by the posterior tibial nerve in children under the age of 2 years (51). This is due to CNS immaturity and can be related to the presence of a Babinski reflex and other infant neurological reflexes in this age group.

Flexor Reflex

For the past half-century, flexor reflexes of the foot (Babinski counterpart) have been of experimental interest in an effort to gain better understanding of the human spinal cord function and the mechanism of spasticity. A flexor reflex response, consisting of two components, can be obtained by recording from the anterior tibialis muscle and electrically stimulating the sole of the foot (52). The first component is usually of low threshhold and is normally seen isolated well before the second component, which is related to the actual withdrawal of the foot. In Shahani's laboratory (53), the first component is usually seen at a latency of 50–60 msec, with the second component, depending on the strength of the stimulus, usually seen at a latency of 110–400 msec.

In spinal cord injury, the first component is uniformly never seen isolated from the second component. At a prolonged latency of 120–400 msec, a very low threshhold response (due to increased excitability) can be elicited, with the two components appearing merged and difficult to separate. In discrete cerebral lesions, Shahani (52) has recorded finding multiple, varying components quite different from the two normally isolated components and the low threshhold merged components of a prolonged latency seen in spinal cord injury. Thus, using the flexor reflex, one is able to differentiate spasticity secondary to a spinal cord lesion from that secondary to a lesion rostral to the brain stem.

USE OF SOMATOSENSORY POTENTIALS IN UPPER MOTOR NEURON DISEASE

Somatosensory potentials are elicited by repeatedly stimulating a peripheral sensory or mixed nerve with a mild electric shock and recording from one's scalp a summated response (with characteristic latency, wave forms, and amplitude), from which information may be gathered regarding the functional integrity of the anatomical pathways in the spinal cord. Recording somatosensory potentials is performed at the bedside with a mobile cart containing EEG amplifier, averager computer, oscilloscope, and camera (25, 54, 55). Ordinary type EEG electrodes are applied to the scalp over the area of the sensory strip close to where the stimulated afferent nerve is supposed to conduct. Averaging technique is required to extract the small (6–10 μV) repetitively evoked potentials from the intrinsic noise of the electroencephalogram.

Studies of somatosensory evoked potentials have provided some data useful in the early projection of a spinal cord injured patient's prognosis (55). In all cases in which the spinal cord lesion was clinically complete, no evoked potentials were observed when stimulation was performed caudal to a lesion. However, in patients with resulting incomplete lesions, early evoked potentials were recorded in all patients but with an abnormal amplitude and an abnormal W wave form. In some cases it has been noted that as the patient's clinical deficit improved, the characteristic wave form returned to normal.

TRADITIONAL ELECTRODIAGNOSIS IN UPPER MOTOR NEURON DISEASE

Traditional electrodiagnosis, like EMG, has historically been limited to the diagnosis of lower motor neuron lesions (19, 56–58). Upper motor neuron lesions have been characteristically associated with normal strength-duration curves and no significant alterations in rheobase and chronaxie. There have been some reports in spinal cord injured patients in spinal shock of chronaxie elevation caudal to the level of the lesion (59), and this may carry similar significance as EMG changes reported in spinal shock in spinal cord injured patients. With pyramidal tract disease, chronaxies have been found to double, resembling denervation values, with strength-duration curves also resembling those of denervation.

Rheobase elevations found by Panin and Paul (60–62) in paretic muscles in hemiplegic patients have, at present, no explanation. Aserinsky and Shriener's (59) findings of no rheobase changes in altered chronaxie on the affected side of hemisected spinal cords in dogs reveal what might be expected with hypertonicity, although it does contest the "subordination effect" axiom, where any change in chronaxie is supposedly secondary to a change in rheobase.

Clinical Application of EMG in Upper Motor Neuron Disease

It is essential for the electromyographer to realize that EMG findings of muscle membrane hyperirritability (positive sharp waves and fibrillation potentials) do occur in patients with lesions confined solely to the upper motor neuron. Although upper motor neuron and lower motor neuron disease can occur simultaneously, the presence of positive sharp waves and fibrillation potentials in upper motor neuron disease does not always implicate a concomitant axonal neuropathy, radiculopathy, traction brachial plexitis (in hemiplegics), or other abnormality specifically of the lower motor neuron. With their typical distribution and transient existence, these EMG findings quite to the contrary, can be used to rule out the existence of many lower motor neuron disorders, *not* to diagnose them. With knowledge of the general sequence of disappearance of findings in stroke patients, one may find an abnormal distribution of findings helpful in the workup of a suspected concomitant lower motor neuron abnormality. In any event, we emphasize that the interpretation of these nonspecific findings should always be made in the light of the clinical history, physical examination, and laboratory data.

Flaccidity, in itself, is not always a reliable sign of lower motor neuron abnormalities. In these cases, after an EMG is done for degree and distribution of findings, an H reflex performed in muscles other than those innervated by the posterior tibial nerve may be useful in differentiating lesions of the lower motor neuron from those of the upper motor neuron, especially those conditions affecting the corticospinal tract at or below the midbrain.

In cases of spasticity of undetermined origin, flexor reflex studies can be performed and, under proper conditions, may be of benefit in distinguishing spasticity from spinal cord pathology from that of cerebral abnormality.

Information gathered from somatosensory studies can be useful in assessing the "completeness" and prognosis of a spinal cord injury. This knowledge regarding the completeness of a patient's spinal cord lesion is often helpful in management of the patient's neurogenic bowel and bladder, skin, and spasticity problems.

One of us has reported the presence of the H reflex in Huntington disease (Chorea) and also in half of individuals at risk for this disease (63). The presence of an H reflex in the deep peroneal nerve in a relaxed individual may be of help in separating those individuals at risk into those who will and those who will not get the disease.

It should be appreciated that many of the questions regarding the etiology and significance of EMG findings in upper motor neuron disease are currently unanswered. Much of what has been reported in this chapter conflicts with many of the traditional concepts of EMG. However, the clinical electromyographer should be fully informed in order to avoid diagnostic errors. In this relatively new area of EMG diagnosis, the data currently available is at best "sketchy," and a new frontier of EMG investigation lies in the future.

REFERENCES

1. DENNY-BROWN, D., AND PENNYBACKER, J. B.: Fibrillation and fasciculation in voluntary muscle. *Brain, 61*: 331, 1938.
2. BUCHTHAL, F., AND ROSENFALCK, P.: Spontaneous electrical activity of human muscle. *Electroencephalogr. Clin. Neurophysiol, 20*: 321, 1966.
3. GOODGOLD, J., AND EBERSTEIN, A.: *Electrodiagnosis of Neuromuscular Diseases*, Baltimore: The Williams and Wilkins Company, 1972.
4. RODRIGUEZ, A. A., AND OESTER, H. T.: Fundamentals of electromyography. In *Electrodiagnosis and Electromyography*, 2nd ed., pp. 300–306, ed. by S. H. Licht, New Haven: E. Licht, 1961.
5. LAMBERT E. H., SAYRE, G. P., AND EATON, L. M.: Electrical activity of muscle in polymyositis. *Trans. Am. Neurol. Assoc., 79*: 64, 1954.
6. BHALA, R. P.: Electromyographic evidence of lower motor neuron involvement in hemiplegia. *Arch. Phys. Med. Rehabil., 50*: 632, 1969.
7. FUSFELD, R. O.: Electromyographic abnormalities in cases of botulism. *Bull. Los Ang. Neurol. Soc., 35*: 164, 1970.
8. JOSEFSSON, J. D., AND THESLEFF, S.: Electromyographic findings in experimental botulism intoxication. *Acta Physiol. Scand., 51*: 163, 1961.
9. MORRISON, J. B.: Electromyographic changes in hyperkalemia familial periodic paralysis. *Ann. Phys. Med., 5*: 153, 1960.
10. PETERSON, I., AND BROMAN, A. M.: Electromyographic findings in a case of botulism. *Nord. Med., 65*: 259, 1961.
11. BELMAR, J., AND EYZAGUIRRE, C.: Pacemaker site of fibrillation potentials in denervated mammalian muscle. *J. Neurophysiol, 29*: 425, 1966.
12. BROWN, G. C.: Actions of acetylcholine on denervated mammalian and frog muscle. *J. Physiol. (Lond.), 89*: 438, 1937.

13. Report of Committee on Terminology. International Association EEG and Clinical Neurophysiology, Pavia, Italy, 1964.

14. BRANDSTATER, M. E., AND DINSDALE, S. M.: Electrophysiological studies in the assessment of spinal cord lesions. *Arch. Phys. Med. Rehabil.*, *57*: 70, 1976.

15. ISCH, F.: Electromyographie et les lesions du rachis. *Electromyography*, *8*: 215, 1968.

16. NYBOER, V. J., AND JOHNSON, H. E.: Electromyographic findings in lower extremities of patients with traumatic quadriplegia. *Arch. Phys. Med. Rehabil.*, *52*: 256, 1971.

17. O'HARE, J. M., AND ABBOT, G. H.: Electromyographic evidence of lower motor neuron injury in cervical spinal cord injury. *Proc. Ann. Clin. Spinal Cord Inj. Cent.*, *17*: 25, 1967.

18. ONKELINX, A., AND CHANTRAINE, A.: Electromyographic study of paraplegic patients. *Electromyogr. Clin. Neurophysiol.*, *15*: 71, 1975.

19. ROSEN, J. S., LERNER, I. M., AND ROSENTHAL, A. M.: Electromyography in spinal cord injury. *Arch. Phys. Med. Rehabil.*, *50*: 271, 1969.

20. TAYLOR, R. G., KEWALRAMANI, L. S., AND FOWLER, W. M.: Electromyographic findings in lower extremities of patients with high spinal cord injury. *Arch. Phys. Med. Rehabil.*, *55*: 16, 1974.

21. McCOMAS, A. J., FAWCETT, P. R. W., CAMPBELL, M. J., ET. AL.: Electrophysiological estimation of number of motor units within a human muscle. *J. Neurol. Neurosurg. Psychiat.*, *34*: 121, 1971.

22. ANGYAN, A., FEKECS, B., AND HUNDYADI, L.: On changes in peripheral time excitability (chronaxie) accompanying acute shock of central nervous system. *Acta Physiol. Acad. Sci. Hung.*, *5*: 111, 1954.

23. NEPOMUCENO, C., McCUTCHEON, M., MILLER, J. M., GOWENS, H., OH, S., STOVER, S., AND BLACKSTONE, E.: Differential analyses of EMG findings in motor neuron lesions. *Am. J. Phys. Med.*, *56*: 1, 1977.

24. BARANEK, R., AND GUTTMANN, E.: The rate of regeneration of motor and sensory fibers after transection of the spinal cord. *Physiol. Bohemoslov.*, *2*: 41, 1953.

25. McCOUCH, G. P., STEWART, W. B., AND HUGHES, J.: Cord potentials in spinal shock: Crossed effects in monkey, macaca mulatta. *J. Neurophysiol*, *3*: 151, 1940.

26. WARRINGTON, W.: Further observations on structural alterations observed in nerve cells. *J. Physiol.*, *24*: 464, 1889.

27. TOWER, S., HOWE, H., AND BODIAN, D.: Fibrillation in skeletal muscle in relation to denervation and to inactivation without denervation. *J. Neurophysiol.*, *4*: 398, 1941.

28. VAN ALPHEN, H. A. M., LAMMERS, H. J., AND WALDER, H. A. D.: On remarkable reaction of motor neurons of lumbosacral region after traumatic cervical transection in man. *Neurochirurgie*, *8*: 328, 1962.

29. SPIELHOLZ, N. I., SELL, G. H., GOODGOLD, J., RUSH, H. A., AND GREENS, S. K.: Electrophysiological studies in patients with spinal cord lesions. *Arch. Phys. Med. Rehabil.*, *53*: 558, 1972.

30. PURUES, D., AND SAKMANN, B.: Membrane properties underlying spontaneous activity of denervated muscle fibers. *J. Physiol. (Lond.)*, *239*: 125, 1974.

31. ALPERT, S., JARRETT, S., LERNER, I., AND ROSENTHAL, A. M.: Electromyographic findings in early hemiplegia. *Arch. Phys. Med. Rehabil.*, *54*: 464, 1973.

32. HERNESS, D., AND ENDE, J.: Electromyography in hemiplegia. *Bull. Hosp. Joint Dis.*, *35*: 211, 1974.

33. KRUGER, K., AND WAYLONIS, G.: Hemiplegia lower motor neuron electromyographic findings. *Arch. Phys. Med. Rehabil.*, *54*: 360, 1973.

34. GOLDKAMP, O.: Electromyography and nerve conduction studies in 116 patients with hemiplegia. *Arch. Phys. Med. Rehabil.*, *48*: 59, 1967.

35. JOHNSON, E. W., DENNY, S. T., AND KELLEY, J. P.: Sequence of electromyographic abnormalities in stroke syndrome. *Arch. Phys. Med. Rehabil.*, *56*: 468, 1975.

36. TWITCHELL, T. E.: Prognosis of motor recovery in hemiplegia. *Bull. Tufts-N. Engl. Med. Cent.*, *3*: 146, 1957.

37. ALPERT, S., IDARRAGA, S., ORBEGOZO, J., AND ROSENTHAL, A. M.: Absence of electromy-

ographic evidence of lower motor neuron involvement in hemiplegic patients. *Arch. Phys. Med. Rehabil.*, *52*: 179, 1971.

38. MOSKOWITZ, E., AND PORTER, II: Peripheral nerve lesions in the upper extremity in hemiplegic patients. *N. Engl. J. Med.*, *269*: 776, 1963.

39. SUTTON, L. R., COHEN, B. S., AND KRUSEN, U. L.: Nerve conduction studies in hemiplegia, *Arch. Phys. Med.*, *48*: 64, 1967.

40. HESS, A.: Experimental embryology of the fetal nervous system. *Biol. Rev.*, *32*: 231, 1975.

41. NYBERG-HANSEN, R., AND BRODAL, A.: Sites of termination of corticospinal fibers in the cat. An experimental study with silver impregnation methods. *J. Comp. Neurol.*, *120*: 369, 1963.

42. GUTH, L.: "Trophic" influences on nerve and muscle. *Physiol. Rev.*, *48*: 654, 1968.

43. GUTHRIE, L.: Muscular atrophy and other changes in nutrition associated with lesions of the sensory cortex of the brain, with special reference to the possible existence of trophic representation in the post central areas. *Proc. Roy. Soc. Med.*, *11*: 21, 1918.

44. NOTERMANS, S. L. H., AND BLOKZIJL, E. J.: Electromyography in patients with lesions of central motor neuron and so-called parietal muscular atrophy. *Psychiat. Neurol. Neurochir.*, *72*: 557, 1969.

45. SILVERSTEIN, A.: Atrophy of the limbs as a sign of involvement of the parietal lobe. *Arch Neurol. Psychiat.*, *26*: 237, 1931.

46. SILVERSTEIN, A.: Diagnostic localizing value of muscle atrophy in parietal lobe lesions. *Neurology*, *5*: 30, 1955.

47. ENGEL, W. K.: Muscle biopsy. *Clin. Orthop. Related Res.*, *39*: 80, 1965.

48. FENICHEL, G. M., DAROFF, R. B., AND GLASER, G. H.: Hemiplegic atrophy—Histological and etiological considerations. *Neurology*, *14*: 883, 1964.

49. TEASDALE, R. D., PARK, A. M., LANGUTH, H. W., AND MAGLADERY, J. W.: Electrophysiological studies of reflex activity in patients with lesions of the nervous system. *Bull. Johns Hopkins Hosp.*, *91*: 219, 1952.

50. HOHMANN, T. C., AND GOODGOLD, J.: A study of abnormal reflex patterns in spasticity. *Am. J. Phys. Med.*, *40*: 52, 1961.

51. THOMAS, J., AND LAMBERT, E. H.: Ulnar nerve conduction velocity and H reflex in infants and children. *J. Appl. Physiol.*, *15*: 1, 1960.

52. SHAHANI, B.: Flexor reflex afferent nerve fibers in man. *J. Neurol. Neurosurg. Psychiat.*, *33*: 786, 1970.

53. SHAHANI, B. T., AND YOUNG, R. R.: Human flexor reflexes. *J. Neurol. Neurosurg. Psychiat.*, *34*: 616, 1971.

54. CRACCO, R. Q.: Spinal evoked response: Peripheral nerve stimulation in man. *Electroencephalogr. Clin. Neurophysiol.*, *35*: 379, 1973.

55. PEROT, P. L.: The clinical use of somatosensory evoked potentials in spinal cord injury. *Clin. Neurosurg.*, *20*: 367, 1973.

56. DAVIS, H., AND FORBES, A.: Chronaxie. *Physiol. Rev.*, *16*: 407, 1936.

57. HARRIS, R.: Chronaxie. In *Electrodiagnosis and Electromyography*, 2nd ed., pp. 218–298, ed. by S. H. Licht, New Haven: E. Licht, 1961.

58. LAMBERT, E. F., SKINNER, B. F., AND FORBES, A.: Some conditions affecting intensity and duration thresholds in motor nerve, with reference to chroniaxie of subordination. *Am. J. Physiol.*, *106*: 721, 1933.

59. ASERINSKY, E., AND SHRIENER, D. P.: The detection of an upper motor neuron lesions by means of electrical testing of peripheral nerve. I. Immediate and chronic effects of spinal hemisection. *Am. J. Phys. Med.*, *42*: 221, 1963.

60. PANIN, N., PAUL, B. J., AND POLICOFF, L. D.: Nerve conduction velocities in hemiplegia: Preliminary report. *Arch. Phys. Med. Rehabil.*, *46*: 467, 1965.

61. PANIN, N., PAUL, B. J., POLICOFF, L. D., AND ESON, M. E.: Nerve conduction velocities in hemiplegia. *Arch. Phys. Med. Rehabil.*, *48*: 606, 1967.

62. PAUL, B. J., PANIN, N., POLICOFF, L. D., AND ESON, M. E.: Chronaxie and strength duration studies in hemiplegic patients. *Arch. Phys. Med. Rehabil.*, *49*: 96, 1968.

63. JOHNSON, E., RADECKI, P., AND PAULSON, G.: Huntington disease: Early identification by H reflex testing. *Arch. Phys. Med. Rehabil.*, *58*: 162, 1977.
64. SOLANDT, D. Y., AND MAGLADERY, J. W.: Comparison of effects of upper and lower motor neuron lesions on skeletal muscles. *J. Neurophysiol.*, *5*: 373, 1942.
65. WEDDELL, G., FEINSTEIN, B., AND PATTLE, R. E.: Electrical activity of voluntary muscle in man under normal and pathological conditions. *Brain*, *67*: 178, 1944.
66. WIECHERS, D. O., GUYTON, J. D., AND JOHNSON, E. W.: Electromyographic findings in the extensor digitorum brevis in a normal population. *Arch. Phys. Med. Rehabil.*, *57*: 84, 1976.

12

Single Fiber EMG

DAVID O. WIECHERS, M.D.

The basic building block of the neuromuscular system, the motor unit, consists of a motor neuron, its axon, and all the muscle fibers that it innervates. Muscle fibers themselves are of two basic types, determined by ATPase staining. Type I muscle fibers turn on at low frequencies and discharge rhythmically over long sustained periods of time. These muscle fibers are high in oxydative enzymes. Type II muscle fibers turn on in high frequency bursts and are employed in vigorous contractions. Type II motor units fatigue rapidly and are low in oxydative enzymes. The muscle cells belonging to the same motor neuron are all of one histochemical type. Therefore, one can identify type I and type II motor units.

Routine clinical EMG permits examination of the motor unit action potentials produced by the depolarization of type I and type II motor units. The muscle fibers belonging to an individual motor unit are dispersed throughout the muscle. A needle electrode in muscle is recording the summated action potentials from the muscle fibers that belong to the same motor unit and are within the pickup area of the electrode. The spike rangement of the so-called motor unit potential is generated by approximately 5–20 individual muscle fibers. By recording from several motor units throughout different areas of the muscle and noting the size, shape, and firing characteristics of their action potentials, a determination can be made about their physiological functioning as to normalcy or abnormalcy. Certain characteristics of these composite motor unit action potentials recorded from groups of fibers belonging to the same motor unit may give clues as to the underlying pathological process. Fragmentation of the motor unit action potentials, with dropout of individual fibers and overall low amplitude of recorded potentials, is suggestive of a neuropathic process. Motor unit action potentials of increased amplitude and duration or of increased number of fibers available for recording in the pickup area of the standard electrode is suggestive of fiber type grouping or reinnervation.

Single fiber electromyography (SFEMG) allows division of this usually triphasic composite depolarization of a group of muscle fibers belonging to the same motor unit into individual single muscle fiber depolarizations (1) (Fig. 12.1). This technique permits study of the neurophysiology of individual muscle fibers and their functional relationship to individual muscle fibers that belong to the same motor unit. Care must be taken, however, in extrapolating the functioning of an individual fiber to that of the whole motor unit and, subsequently, the entire muscle.

A good analogy is to consider a single muscle being represented as a forest. The forest is made up of many different trees, but they are of two main types, conifers and broadleaf. Routine EMG reveals the characteristics of small groups of trees interacting together. After sampling the characteristics of many of these groups of trees, conclusions may be drawn about the overall condition of the forest. This is routine clinical EMG and there is no substitute for obtaining this vital physiologic information. An adjunct to

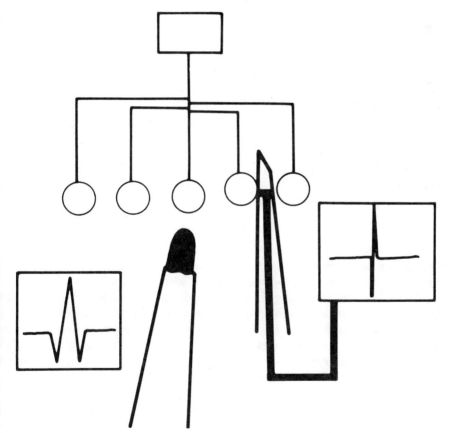

Fig. 12.1. Monopolar electrode (left) records summated depolarization of all five muscle fibers that belong to the motor unit. The SFEMG electrode records from one individual muscle fiber.

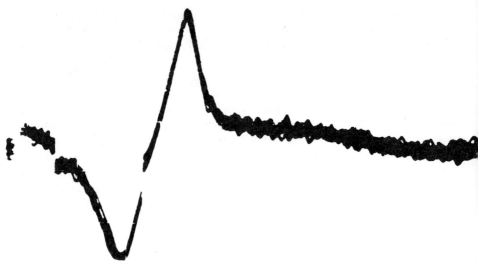

Fig. 12.2. Depolarization of a single muscle fiber.

this testing process, but by no means a replacement for it, is SFEMG (2). SFEMG examines a single tree (muscle fiber) individually and notes its characteristics and those of its closest neighbors and its relationship to them. SFEMG should be performed in conjunction with routine EMG so that one does not miss the forest for the trees.

The single muscle fiber action potential looks like a fibrillation potential (Fig. 12.2). A fibrillation potential is a spontaneous discharge of a single muscle fiber. The parameters of any recording, however, depend highly on the recording techniques and the instrumentation involved.

Instrumentation

The instrumentation and recording techniques employed in order to record from single muscle fibers require marked selectivity. Since muscle fibers normally have a diameter of 60–80 μ, electrode leadoff surface must be quite small. The recording tip of 25 μ in diameter was found to be most satisfactory. The pickup area of the electrode is a hemisphere of approximately 250–350 μ in diameter (3). Therefore, the electrode must be extremely close to the active muscle fiber in order to record it. When studying single fibers, it is very important not to injure the fiber by the electrode itself. Therefore, the leadoff surface is positioned approximately 3 mm along the shaft of the cutting point of the small 28–32-gauge needle. The result is a small high impedance concentric electrode with an exposure tip of 25 μ along the shaft of the cutting edge (Fig. 12.3).

Since these electrodes have a high impedance, the input impedance of the amplifier must be correspondingly high so that the signal is not lost. An input impedance of approximately 100 megohms is, therefore, necessary

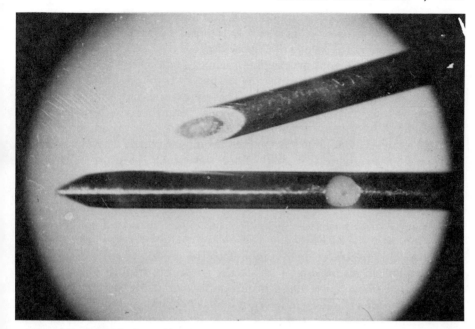

Fig. 12.3. SFEMG electrode with 25-μ exposure leadoff surface in comparison to standard concentric electrode.

when using platinum as the recording metal. The amplifier should have a frequency response of 0.01 Hz to 20 KHz in order to record the characteristics of these potentials. In order to increase the selectivity of the recording low frequency interference from distant fibers, a low frequency filter of about 500 Hz is employed. The band pass then for routine SFEMG is 500 Hz to 20 KHz. These filter settings do not allow any detailed study of the action potential shapes.

Besides the electrodes and the amplifiers, there are several other electronic components which are very helpful for the analysis of SFEMG. Since events occur in the time span of microseconds, it is necessary to have an electronic means of triggering the sweep of the oscilloscope by the presence of the potential to be examined. One triggers on the fastest slope of the positive negative deflection, since this portion of the wave form will be most constant. When triggering on the potential itself, however, the first portion of the potential is lost from the cathode ray tube. An electronic component that will delay the display of the potential once it has triggered the sweep of the oscilloscope displays the entire potential.

Clinical SFEMG concerns the voluntary contractions of individual fibers (4). The frequency of discharge of these fibers can alter the characteristics of subsequent depolarization. It is, therefore, most helpful to have a rate meter which the patient can observe and from which to obtain direct biofeedback as to his frequency of voluntary motor unit discharge. A rate meter can be a modified automobile tachometer or almost any device that can provide a frequency from 0 to 100 Hz. It is desirable to have the rate meter triggered by the sweep of the oscilloscope.

Single fiber motor unit action potentials can be recorded for analysis on direct photosensitive paper, since the frequency response of photosensitive recording is within acceptable limits. These potentials can also be recorded on tape, as long as there is a good carrier system for the tape-recording instrument. A frequency response of 100 Hz to 10 KHz would be adequate for time analysis alone, but a frequency response of up to 20 KHz would be necessary for evaluation of single fiber wave shape. Flutter of the tape should be kept at a minimum and a wow should not exceed 5 msec.

Procedure

After asking the patient to provide a minimal contraction of the muscle to be examined, the SFEMG electrode is inserted perpendicular to the fiber direction. The electrode then is held with the recording surface up and is gently moved in an attempt to slide the recording surface up against an active muscle fiber. Since the recording surface is on the cutting edge of the concentric needle, the fiber to be examined is not damaged by the electrode. The high pitched character of the single fiber potential is noted on the loud speaker as one advances closer to the active fiber.

The single muscle fiber potential is a biphasic wave with an initial positive deflection (Fig. 12.2). Its total duration is usually about 1 msec. The rise time of the potential is in the order of 75–200 msec. The amplitude of the potential is variable due mainly to the distance from the active fiber to the recording surface. It usually is between 1 and 7 mV. The criteria established by Stålberg and Ekstedt (5, 6) for the acceptance of the potential as being truly generated by a single fiber is one with biphasic smooth shape which is constant on repetitive firing when the recording system allows a time resolution of 10 msec.

In approximately 20% of normal SFEMG electrode insertions, a double potential will be recorded (Fig. 12.4). The interval between the two potentials, or the interpotential interval, is usually less than 4 msec. The recording of two action potentials occurs because the active electrode is spaced between two individual muscle fibers that belong to the same motor unit, and both are within the pickup area of the electrode. They occur at different points in time due to variations of terminal axon length, time delay across the myoneural junction of each individual fiber, and the distance down the muscle fiber that the potential must be propagated to arrive at the electrode or the point of recording. One can be sure that these two individual fibers belong to the same motor unit by triggering on one of the potentials and noting that the other potential only occurs when the triggering potential is fired (4).

If one now triggers on the rapid rising slope of the first single fiber potential, there is a variation in time in the appearance of the second

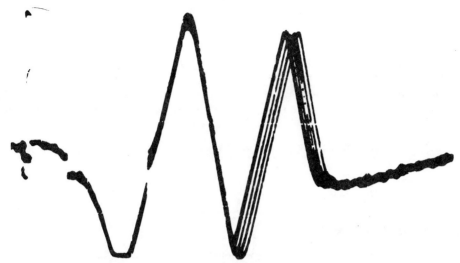

Fig. 12.4. Normal double potential or the depolarization of two individual muscle fibers that belong to the same motor unit.

potential with repetitive voluntary discharge (Fig. 12.4). This is normally in the order of 10–55 msec. This variation in time is called jitter. Jitter is the variability of the interpotential interval with consecutive discharges. This variability of the interpotential interval is dependent upon conduction times through terminal axons, myoneural junctions, and muscle fibers. In normal individuals, nerve fiber transmission is not variable, and if the rate of discharge is kept constant, the muscle fiber conduction velocity will also be constant. This variation in time for the appearance of the second single fiber action potential is mainly due to delays across the myoneural junctions of both fibers (Fig. 12.5).

Since the sweep is triggered by the first potential, a delay of its myoneural junction will result as a shortening of the interpotential interval, where a delay of the myoneural junction of the second fiber will result in a lengthening of the interpotential interval. Thus, the jitter seen in the nontriggering potential (usually the second) is the total jitter in the two motor endplates. At times there is a failure of conduction to one or the other of the individual fibers, and its action potential is not recorded (Fig. 12.6). This is referred to as blocking. Blocking is frequently seen in disorders effecting the myoneural junction when there is failed conduction across the junction. Blocking can also occur at terminal branching sites in distal axons (7). This is seen in pathological situations where there has been extensive reinnervation with axon sprouting. When the blocking occurs at a terminal branching site in the distal axon, it is referred to as neurogenic blocking. With neurogenic blocking, one may see the dropout and return of several individual muscle fibers simultaneously (Fig. 12.7).

The variation in the interpotential interval with consecutive discharges, commonly referred to as jitter, can be determined by several different techniques. The mean and standard deviation of from 50 to 200 consecutive interpotential interval time differences can easily be determined by a computer or a microprocessor which has an internal clock or counter. The clock is triggered by the first potential and is stopped by the second potential. These intervals are subsequently counted. In order to minimize the effect of slow trends, the jitter is better expressed as the Mean of

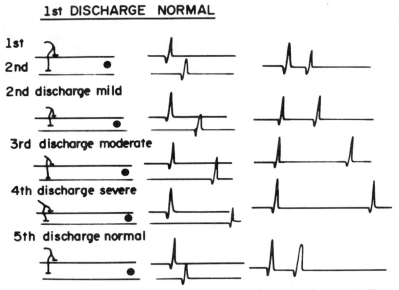

Fig. 12.5. Variation in the interpotential interval of two single muscle fibers with consecutive discharge of the motor unit.

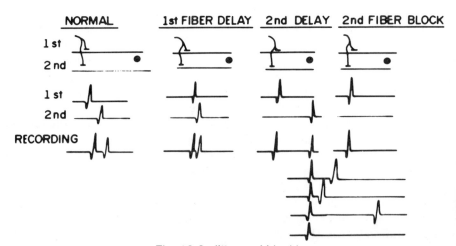

Fig. 12.6. Jitter and blocking.

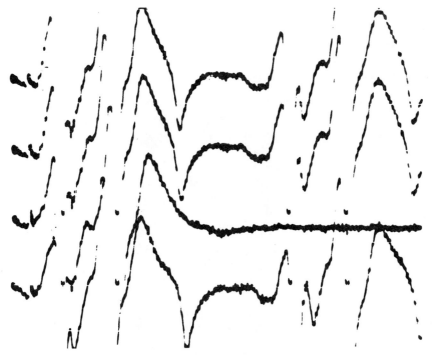

Fig. 12.7. Neurogenic blocking recorded in a patient with amyotrophic lateral sclerosis.

Consecutive Differences of the interspike intervals, or MCD (8). A second method of analysis involves superimposing 10 groups of 5 potentials or 5 groups of 10 potentials that have been recorded on photosensitive paper. The mean range of 10 potentials for the 5 groups, or R10, can be determined as can the mean range of 5 potentials of 10 groups, or R5. The MCD can be calculated from the R5 or R10 by a conversion factor. MCD is equal to R5 × 0.49, and MCD is equal to R10 × 0.37 (Fig. 12.8).

The speed of impulse conduction down a muscle can be varied if a second impulse occurs during the recovery phase of a preceding action potential (4). This change in speed of impulse conduction that results from a preceding condition impulse is referred to as the velocity recovery function, or VRF. If the interval is very short, 3–10 msec, there is a reduction in propagation velocity by up to 20%. If, however, the interval is from 10 to 1000 msec, the propagation velocity can be increased by 10–15%. VRF appears to be related to some, as yet unknown, membrane characteristic.

Velocity recovery function varies from fiber to fiber but appears to be maximum where there is approximately 50 msec between the conditioning response and the second impulse. The super normal velocity then steadily falls to approximately 50% of maximum around 300 msec. In muscular dystrophies, this positive VRF is most pronounced.

Jitter

In jitter determinations, it is important to attempt to maintain a steady rate of voluntary contraction and, thus, the need for a rate meter to give immediate feedback to the patient. For routine clinical work, a frequency of 15–20 Hz seems easiest for jitter determinations.

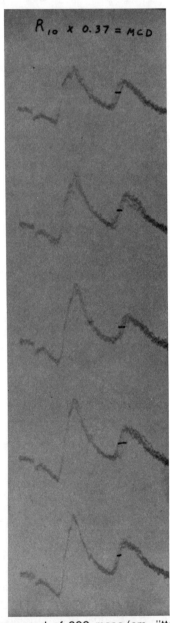

Fig. 12.8. With a paper speed of 200 msec/cm, jitter can be determined by measuring the mean range of 5 groups of 10 superimposed depolarizations.

Variations in voluntary discharge frequency affect jitter determination. This is most noticeable when there is a trend toward increasing discharge frequency with continued voluntary contraction. This results in a decrease in the interpotential interval. In other words, a decrease in the interdischarge interval can result in a decrease in the interpotential interval. VRF is most pronounced in jitter determinations when there is a large interpotential interval of more than 4 msec.

When the frequency of voluntary contraction cannot be maintained, the mean consecutive difference, or MCD, should not be used for jitter determinations. In this instance, the interpotential intervals should be sorted and arranged in decreasing order, and then the mean of the differences calculated. This figure is referred to as the mean sorted difference, or MSD.

In normal instances, the MCD is approximately equal to the MSD. If the MCD is 25% greater than the calculated MSD, then there is felt to be significant variability due to changing interpotential intervals, and the MSD is the more correct jitter value. If, on the other hand, the MCD is 20% lower than the MSD, the MCD value should be used.

Under certain conditions, potentials are recorded with SFEMG techniques that, if used in the analysis of jitter and fiber density, can result in erroneous results. The false double potential, or injured fiber, is one such potential. Frequently a monophasic potential with a longer total duration and slightly prolonged rise time than would be expected for a typical single fiber potential is seen following a triggered potential. When this potential is recorded, it usually demonstrates a large jitter. As the rate of fire of the triggering potential increases, this potential's jitter increases to such an extent that the potential appears to walk off the screen. With subsequent slowing of voluntary contraction, the potential reappears (Fig. 12.9).

On an occasion recording from a single fiber, this potential is seen to walk out of the original potential by minor movements of the electrode. It is for this reason that this second potential is believed to be generated by an injured portion of the triggering muscle fiber. One should be careful that this injured, or false double potential, is not used for jitter determinations and fiber density determinations. These potentials are frequently produced when the electrode tip is not sharp or has a hook on its cutting edge. Careful examination of the electrodes after use, especially when bone is contacted, and subsequent polishing will resolve this problem.

Fibrillation potentials are the spontaneous discharges of single muscle fibers. Fibrillation potentials fire at regular rates. On occasion, two fibrillation potentials can be recorded with single fiber technique and noted to have extremely small jitter values in the range of 5–10 msec. It is felt that since the jitter is less than 10 msec, a myoneural junction is not involved, but the spontaneous discharge of one fiber results in an ephaptic transmission to the second fiber.

Fibrillation potentials can subsequently be time-locked into the discharges of other single fibers in pathologic situations. This results in an increase in the individual fiber number and total duration of the complex. Fibrillation

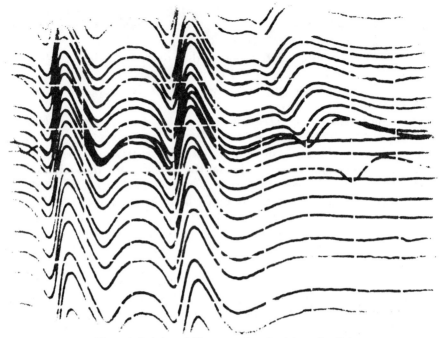

Fig. 12.9. Injured fiber or false double potential.

potentials can be identified from voluntarily activated single fiber potentials merely by stopping voluntary activity and noting the regular continuation of the fibrillation potential.

The fasciculation potentials, when recorded by SFEMG, appear as a series of complex single fibers in most conditions. Their spontaneous irregular firing pattern, however, usually makes confusion with voluntary activity in jitter determinations unlikely.

Bimodal jitter is seen in approximately 1 out of 20 single fiber recordings (Fig. 12.10). This flip-flop phenonomen occurs when the interpotential intervals have a bimodal distribution at consecutive discharges (9). The time interval between the triggering potential and another potential has two mean values, both of which show variability. This flip-flop, or jumping back and forth of the potential, occurs in short jumps or long jumps. Short jumps of less than 250 μsec are frequently seen and occur in normal as well as reinnervated muscle. Longer jumps, 200 μsec to 16 msec, are not seen in normal muscle and are most frequently seen in reinnervation.

The specific etiology of these potentials is unknown. The short flip-flop is felt to be the result of ephaptic transmission. The origin of the long flip-flop is felt to be the result of reinnervation with the irregular impulse conduction in a nerve whose myelin sheath is abnormal. Regardless of their origin, they should not be used for jitter determinations.

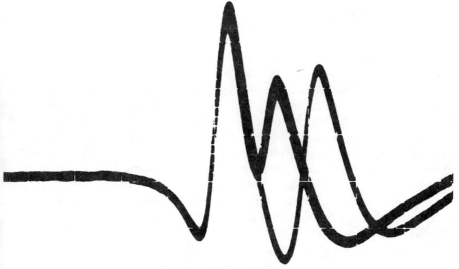

Fig. 12.10. Bimodal jitter.

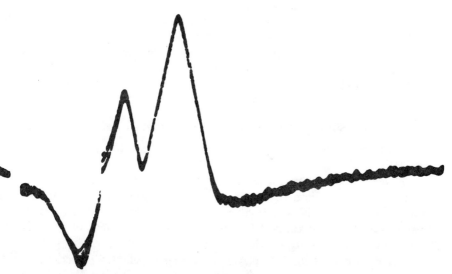

Fig. 12.11. Split fiber.

Two single fiber action potentials can be recorded whose jitter is less than 5 μsec (Fig. 12.11). This variability seems too small for transmission across the myoneural junction. It is, therefore, felt that these potentials most likely represent a single muscle fiber that has split or has a bud. Splitting of muscle fibers is frequently seen in myopathic conditions. These potentials must not be used for jitter determination or fiber density determination.

Fiber Density

The single fiber electrode records from a hemisphere area of approximately 250–350 μ in diameter. Approximately 75% of random electrode insertions result in the recording of one single fiber action potential. In 20% of random insertions, we record from two muscle fibers belonging to the same motor unit that meet the criteria of single fiber action potentials and have an amplitude of more than $200/\mu V$ and a peak-to-peak rise line less than 300/msec. These two fibers are, therefore, within the uptake area of the electrode and less than 350 μ apart. If the single fiber electrode is inserted randomly 20 times into a muscle, the initial potential maximized, and additional fibers searched for that meet the criteria for acceptance, the distribution or density of fibers belonging to the same motor unit in a given muscle could be determined. A mean number of potentials can subsequently be calculated, and fiber densities normally can be established for individual muscles.

Fiber density increases with age and in the lower age ranges below 10 years (10, 11). With reinnervation, there is collateral sprouting of distal axons in an attempt to rescue free fibrillating muscle fibers. The result of reinnervation is that more muscle fibers now belong to the same motor neuron and are grouped together anatomically. Fiber density determinations in such instances are increased. Fiber density would also be increased by extensive fiber splitting or shrinkage of the motor unit. The mean fiber density, or the number of fibers which meet the criteria for single fiber discharges in the pickup area of the single fiber electrode in the extensor digitorum communis, is 1.55 (12).

Single Fiber EMG in Pathological Conditions

Disorders of the myoneural junction are quantitatively studied with SFEMG (5, 13–16).

Routine EMG testing for myasthenia gravis involves recording a decrementing response from the entire muscle with repetitive stimulation pre- and postexercise. If this whole muscle response is negative, single motor unit responses may be examined by following the amplitude of an individual motor unit as it repetitively discharges.

With repetitive stimulation, the presence of blocking occurring at the myoneural junctions of a large number of muscle fibers will be revealed by the composite evoked M response falling in amplitude. The next step is to look at an individual motor unit and watch it discharge with time. If there is significant blocking occurring at one or two fibers of the motor unit action potential, a variation in amplitude with continued contraction will occur. SFEMG moves one step farther. With SFEMG, variation in conduction times across myoneural junctions can be recorded and increased uncertainty (jitter) noted with the presence or absence of blocking. Being able to record increased jitter before the development of blocking permits making the diagnosis prior to the development of significant clinical signs. The frustration of being unable to confirm electrodiagnostically the clinical impression of myasthenia gravis in a patient with facial symptoms only is well known. SFEMG demonstrates an increase in jitter with occasional blocking in some of the fibers of the exterior digitorum communis and also in patients with ocular symptoms.

In a study of the patient with myasthenia gravis, care must be taken that the sample is significant. Twenty endplate pairs should be examined. Typically in patients with myasthenia gravis, a certain percentage of motor endplates are normal. Some will show increased jitter only, and some, depending upon the degree of clinical weakness, will demonstrate impulse blocking with higher jitter values, usually greater than 100 (Fig. 12.12).

In abnormal fibers, as the myoneural junction is stressed at higher frequencies of firing, we see a characteristic increase in jitter and many times blocking (Fig. 12.13). As the frequency of firing is reduced, the high degree of blocking may stop. The jitter will return toward, but not obtain, normality.

Jitter determinations are most frequently performed in the extensor digitorum communis muscle, since this muscle is the one most standardized for SFEMG. A jitter value of greater than 55 μsec is considered abnormal in this muscle. In Dr. Stålberg's (13, 14) and my own experiences, patients with myasthenia gravis, even those with ocular symptoms only, demonstrate abnormalities in jitter of approximately 25% of examined motor endplate pairs, while patients with severe weakness demonstrated marked degree of blocking with high jitter values and relatively few normal endplate pairs. Sometimes all recordings are normal in the forearm muscle in ocular myasthenia, and the investigation should then be made in the facial muscles where abnormalities are likely to be found.

If Tensilon is injected while observing a potential pair with increased jitter and blocking, the blocking will generally stop and the jitter values will return toward, but not reach, normal.

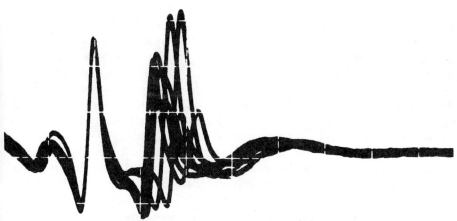

Fig. 12.12. Increased jitter in myasthenia gravis.

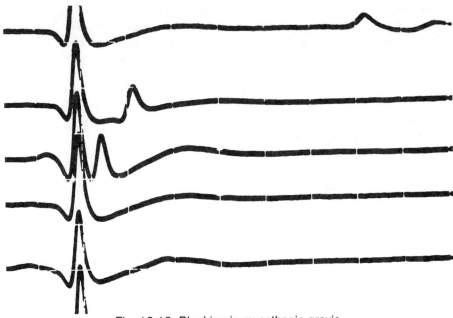

Fig. 12.13. Blocking in myasthenia gravis.

In patients receiving treatment for myasthenia gravis with thymectomy, corticosteroids, and anti-cholinesterase medication, the jitter values return towards, but do not reach, normality (15). Thus, one needs not to stop patient medications prior to SFEMG testing.

Jitter values in the myasthenic syndrome are increased. Some of the highest jitter values have been reported in this syndrome (16, 17). As would be expected, the degree of blocking decreases with an increased rate of fiber discharge, and a larger degree of blocking is noted at lower frequencies.

Neuropathic processes result in a dropout of motor units. Disorders of the nerve cell and axon effect the conduction times through the motor unit. During the process of degradation of the motor unit, SFEMG demonstrates an increase in jitter and blocking. The degradation of the motor unit results in a group of muscle fibers which have lost their nerve supply and trophic influences. These fibers are free to fibrillate. Fibrillation potentials are recorded by SFEMG and, except for their firing characteristics, are no different from the voluntarily evoked single fiber action potentials. Positive sharp waves provoked with standard EMG electrode movement are not directly seen by the typical single fiber electrode because the leadoff surface is some distance from the site of injury. These mechanically provoked potentials, however, can be heard on the audio display. Fasciculation potentials frequently seen in motor neuron disorders are recorded by SFEMG as a complex of individual single fiber discharges. These multispiked discharges are frequently stable and have a normal jitter, while others are quite variable with increased jitter (10).

With axon sprouting and the rescuing of free fibrillating muscle fibers, the process of reinnervation occurs. This process of reinnervation results in fiber grouping and an increase in fiber density noted on SFEMG. Weak points in conduction propagation occur at branching sites of these terminal axon sprouts. The immature terminal axon sprouts and myoneural junctions do not conduct impulses repetitively at a maximum rate. With reinnervation, one will see an increase in jitter and blocking. As these reinnervation structures mature, the degree of jitter and blocking decreases and approaches normal. Fully mature reinnervation motor units may have normal jitter, although some increase in jitter is frequently seen. Because of the weak points in conduction, propagation at the branching sites of the terminal axon sprouts neurogenic blocking is a common finding with reinnervation (Fig. 12.7).

SFEMG can reveal information about the progression of the neurogenic disorder (11). An increase in fiber density suggests reinnervation. Unstable single fiber complexes with increased jitter and a high degree of blocking suggest that the neuropathic process is rapidly occurring. These findings correlate with what one sees in clinical SFEMG examinations. Slowly progressive spinal muscular atrophy patients have very high fiber densities and stable single fiber complexes. Patients with a rapidly progressive course of amyotrophic lateral sclerosis demonstrate an increase in fiber density but unstable single fiber complexes with increased jitter and blocking.

Myopathic processes show us a variety of findings of SFEMG, no doubt due to the variety in the pathophysiology of these disorders. Varying degrees of spontaneous activities are recorded in myopathies with SFEMG. In myopathies as a whole, fiber density is increased, and the amount varies with the specific pathologic process. The single fiber complexes are of long duration with many very late components. With normal rates of voluntary discharge, the single fiber complexes can overlap themselves. One or two completely different single fiber complexes from different motor units occasionally can be recorded from the same electrode position. The degree of jitter and blocking is quite variable but most pronounced in the late components. Due to the VRF of muscle fibers in myopathic conditions, careful attention must be paid to the frequency of discharge during recordings. The MSD should be calculated and compared to the MCD when jitter determinations are being performed in myopathies.

In Duchenne muscular dystrophy, patients reveal an increase in fiber density of two to six times the normal (18). Whether this is a result of reinnervation, shrinkage of motor unit and/or walling off by connective tissue, or variation in conduction down the muscle cell membrane is at the present time still debatable. Recordings may have 10 or more single fiber spike components. The overall duration of these complex single fiber discharges belonging to the same motor unit is increased with occasional blocking (Fig. 12.14).

Limb girdle muscular dystrophy and facioscapulohumeral dystrophy pa-

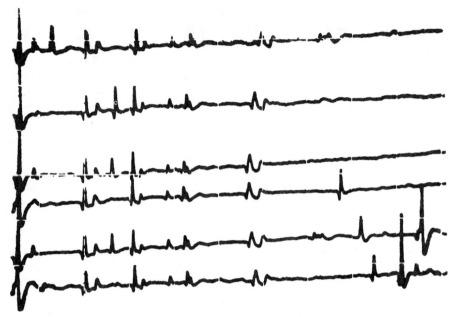

Fig. 12.14. SFEMG recorded in Duchenne muscular dystrophy.

tients have similar SFEMG pictures. There is a mild increase in fiber density. Jitter is slightly increased in about half of the recordings and blocking is uncommon, occurring in only about 10%. The overall duration of single fiber complexes is less than seen in Duchenne muscular dystrophy.

Myotonic dystrophy patients have variable findings on SFEMG in correlation with their clinical variability. Some have an increase in fiber density, others are normal. Jitter is increased in about one-fourth of total recordings (19).

SFEMG in polymyositis varies with the course and state of the disease. Initially, jitter and blocking are markedly increased with a normal or mild increase in fiber density. As the acute stages of the disease subside so does the degree of blocking. During this period, the total duration of spike complexes reduces, as does the jitter. SFEMG may be helpful in following the course of patients with polymyositis (19).

Acknowledgment: Special thanks to my teacher, Dr. Stålberg, for reviewing this chapter.

REFERENCES

1. EKSTEDT, J.: Human single muscle fibre action potentials. *Acta Physiol. Scand., 61 (Suppl. 226):* 1, 1964.
2. EKSTEDT, J., AND STÅLBERG, E.: Single fibre electromyography for the study of the microphysiology of the human muscle. In *New Developments in Electromyography and*

Clinical Neurophysiology, vol. 1, pp. 84–112, ed. by J. E. Desmedt, Basel, Switzerland: Karger, 1973.

3. EKSTEDT, J., AND STÅLBERG, E.: How the size of the needle electrode leading-off surface influences the shape of the single muscle fibre action potential in electromyography. *Comput. Programs Med., 3:* 204, 1973.

4. STÅLBERG, E.: Propagation velocity in human muscle fibers in situ. *Acta Physiol. Scand., 70 (Suppl. 287):* 1, 1966.

5. EKSTEDT, J., AND STÅLBERG, E.: The diagnostic use of single muscle fibre recording and the neuromuscular jitter in myasthenia gravis (abstract). 6th Int. Congr. Electroencephalogr. Clin. Neuophysiol., pp. 669–672, Vienna, 1965.

6. STÅLBERG, E., EKSTEDT, J., AND BROMAN, A.: The electromyographic jitter in normal human muscles. *Electroencephalogr. Clin. Neurophysiol., 31:* 429, 1971.

7. STÅLBERG, E., AND THIELE, B.: Transmission block in terminal nerve twigs. A single fibre electromyographic finding in man. *J. Neurol. Neurosurg. Psychiat., 35:* 52, 1972.

8. EKSTEDT, J., NILSSON, G., AND STÅLBERG, E.: Calculation of the electromyographic jitter. *J. Neurol. Neurosurg. Psychiat., 37:* 526, 1974.

9. THIELE, B., AND STÅLBERG, E.: The bimodal jitter: A single fibre electromyographic finding. *J. Neurol. Neurosurg. Psychiat., 37:* 403, 1974.

10. STÅLBERG, E., AND EKSTEDT, J.: Single fibre EMG and microphysiology of the motor unit in normal and diseased muscle. In *New Developments in Electromyography and Clinical Neurophysiology*, vol. 1, pp. 113–129, ed. by J. E. Desmedt, Basel, Switzerland: Karger, 1973.

11. STÅLBERG, E., SCHWARTZ, M. S., AND TRONTELJ, J. V.: Single fibre electromyography in various processes affecting the anterior horn cell. *J. Neurol. Sci., 24:* 403, 1975.

12. THIELE, B., AND STÅLBERG, E.: Fibre density of the motor unit in the extensor digitorum communis muscles in man. *J. Neurol. Neurosurg. Psychiat., 37:* 874, 1975.

13. EKSTEDT, J., AND STÅLBERG, E.: The effect of non-paralytic doses of D-tubocurarine of individual motor end-plates in man, studied with a new electrophysiological method. *Electroencephalogr. Clin. Neurophysiol., 27:* 557, 1969.

14. DAHLBACK, L., EKSTEDT, J., AND STÅLBERG, E.: Ischemic effects on impulse transmission to muscle fibres in man. *Electroencephalogr. Clin. Neurophysiol., 29:* 579, 1970.

15. STÅLBERG, E., EKSTEDT, J., AND BROMAN, A.: Neuromuscular transmission in myasthenia gravis studied with single fibre electromyography. *J. Neurol. Neurosurg. Psychiat., 37:* 540, 1974.

16. SCHWARTZ, M. S., AND STÅLBERG, E.: Myasthenic syndrome studied with single fibre electromyography. *Arch. Neurol., 12:* 815, 1975.

17. HAKELIUS, L., AND STÅLBERG, E.: Electromyographical studies of free autogenous muscle transplants in man. *Scand. J. Plast. Reconstr. Surg., 8:* 211, 1974.

18. STÅLBERG, E., TRONTELJ, J. V., AND JANKO, M.: Single fibre EMG findings. Findings in muscular dystrophy. Symp. on Structure and Function of Normal and Diseased Muscle and Peripheral Nerve, Kazimierz, Poland, 1972.

19. STÅLBERG, E.: Personal communication.

13

Interpretation and Reporting

ERNEST W. JOHNSON, M.D.
WATSON D. PARKER, M.D.

Demographic data should be included on the EMG report form (for example, name, age, address, referring physician, date, and complaint (Fig. 13.1). The complaint should be summarized as a phrase including the duration of the symptom. For example, limped for 4 months, weakness of the right arm for 6 months, and aching and numbness of the left hand for 4 weeks are typical illustrations (1).

The list of muscles investigated should include the innervation by peripheral nerve and cord levels. If it is important for the localization of the lesion, branches of plexuses or nerves should also be included. Under *no* circumstances should a printed list of muscles or nerves be used on a report form. This tends to stereotype the examination and often restricts or limits the electromyographer's examination, whether consciously or unconsciously.

The evoked muscle action potentials should be described with the amplitude and duration of the negative spike. Distal latencies (with measurements of distances) and conduction velocities should be recorded. The muscle over which the recording electrodes are placed should be specifically identified, in addition to the sites of stimulation.

The neurophysiologic data then should be summarized and translated into a probable clinical diagnosis. This clinical diagnosis must be presented so that the referring physician will be given guidance in the management of the patient. If there is significant difference from the referring diagnosis, a statement may be included that the working diagnosis is ruled out or incompatible with the EMG findings. If the EMG findings are abnormal but inconclusive—so state. You may recommend other diagnostic procedures which may be helpful in clarifying the diagnosis. Also, it is useful to suggest a repeat EMG in several weeks if the conclusions are uncertain.

Know the referring physician! Often he will wish management suggestions. If management directions are crucial and should be immediate, a phone call

FORM 96401 REV. 69

THE OHIO STATE UNIVERSITY HOSPITALS
DEPARTMENT OF PHYSICAL MEDICINE
ELECTROMYOGRAPHIC EXAMINATION

Referring Physician _John Smith MD_

Date _1/29/79_

Problem: _Pain & Weakness (R) arm × 2 wk_

I. M. Neat
20 Public Place

Age 45

MUSCLE	INNERVATION	INSERTIONAL ACTIVITY	FIBRILLATION POTENTIALS	FASCICULATION	MOTOR UNIT ACTION POTENTIALS
Post Neck					
(R) C-3,4,5	Post		○	○	Normal ampl + dur
6,7,8	Primary → pos waves	+			↑ proportion of polyphasics
(L) C-6,7,8	Rami	Normal	○		Normal ampl + dur
(R) Infraspin	C5,6 SS				↓ #, fire rapidly
Teres maj					Normal ampl dur + #
Triceps Br	C7,8 Rad prolonged & occ pos wave				↓ #, fire rapidly
Brach-rad	C5,6 ↓ Normal				
Pron teres	C6,7 med occ pos wave				Normal ampl, dur + #
Flex Dig Sub	C7,8	↓			
1st dorsal Int	C8T1 ul Normal				
abd Poll Br	C8T1 med	↓	↓	↓	↓
abd Dig Q	C8T1 ul				"M"

Nerve Conduction Studies: (R) median N Distal motor 3.9ms   59 M/s   11 K
sensory 3.0ms (30 mV)

Comment: _Normal conduction studies - motor + sensory, (R) median N. Needle EMG exploration reveals EMG abnormalities limited to (R) C-7 distribution. It is a bit early to see max. abnormalities._

Impression: _(R) C-7 radiculopathy - mod. should respond to traction_   E W Johnson

Fig. 13.1. A representative EMG report. Note the recommendation for management—an addition which may be appropriate for certain referring physicians.

may be appreciated. This is also indicated when the diagnostic findings are different from the referring diagnosis or if further diagnostic procedures are indicated on an urgent basis.

The report is both a message to the referring physician and a record of the electrodiagnostic examination. This latter record necessitates sufficient data for comparison with subsequent EMGs as well as serving the requirement of withstanding critical perusal by officers of the court, should that be necessary.

Spontaneous Activity

Under this heading, sufficient room should be available to report number of fibrillation potentials. They are graded from 0 to 4 + (Fig. 13.2). Grading these provides a comparison for subsequent examinations as well as a semiquantitative estimation of the membrane instability at a given evaluation.

Fasciculation potentials should also be graded from 1 to 4 or characterized as being occasional, few, or many. If they are indicated as present, they should be described as simple or complex. Complexity should be further identified as iterative (repetitive discharge) (Fig. 13.3) type or irregularly

O ➡ None Observed

+ ➡ Induced by Electrode Movement

╫ ➡ 1 · 2 Spontaneous Appearance

╫╫ ➡ Many Spontaneous

╫╫╫ ➡ Oscilloscope Screen Filled

Fig. 13.2. Scheme for grading fibrillation potentials.

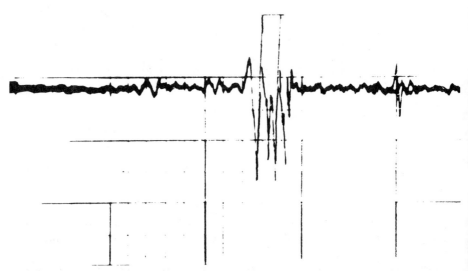

Fig. 13.3. Repetitive discharge potential. Calibration: major horizontal division, 30 msec; major vertical division, 100 μV.

polyphasic. The latter are generally seen in motor unit diseases, while the former are seen in myokymia, alkalotic states, and incipient tetany.

Insertional Activity

If this is characterized as normal, the movement of the needle provokes a burst of injury potentials which stops abruptly. I report it normal when its cessation is "crisp." Note that in the vicinity of endplates it will be prolonged, but this is a normal finding.

An occasional positive wave occurring as the needle movement has stopped may be diagnostically significant. A short train of positive waves are frequently encountered in certain muscles (e.g., paraspinal) without diagnostic significance.

If there is no insertional activity—there is no viable muscle in the area; the exception is in the prolonged contracture of McArdle syndrome, where the muscle fibers fail to repolarize.

Insertional activity may be said to be prolonged in early muscle cell membrane instability. This determination is made on the prolongation of the injury potentials after needle movement stops, *NOT* on the actual

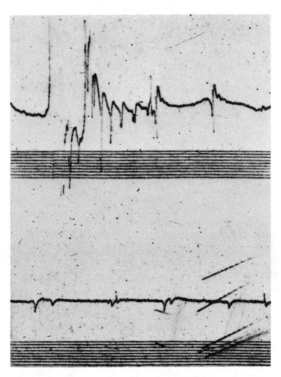

Fig. 13.4. Insertional activity. Note major deflection is positive. Calibration: width of time signal, 200 μV; length, 200 msec.

duration of the burst of injury potentials, a characteristic which is related to the duration and speed of needle electrode movement.

This burst of injury potentials may be said to be reduced in chronic motor unit diseases when fibrosis tissue replaces viable muscle cells. The next characterization about insertional activity is the consequence of the needle movement. This mechanical stimulus will initiate single muscle fiber discharges which will appear as fibrillation potentials and positive sharp waves. Positive waves are reported as occasional, few, many, and trains. The latter should be further described as varying in frequency and amplitude (myotonia).

Note that the burst of injury potentials (insertional activity) may be reduced in chronic motor unit disease, yet positive waves may be present in a substantial number. Incidentally, the major deflection of the burst of injury potentials will be positive so needle electrode movement may be used to check polarity of input leads of preamplifier (Fig. 13.4).

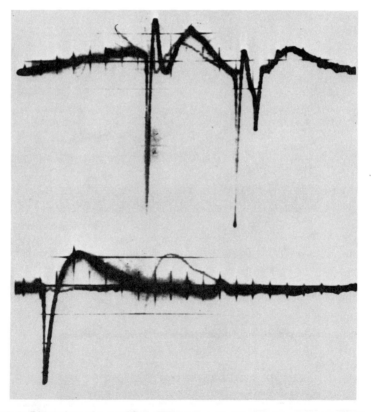

Fig. 13.5. Distortion of a positive sharp wave by interposing a low frequency filter (100 Hz). *Top trace*, filter; *bottom trace*, no filter. Calibration: vertical division, 50 μV; horizontal division, 2 msec.

Reports describing insertional activity may be:
    reduced,
    absent,
    prolonged,
    prolonged with occasional positive wave,
    many positive waves, and
    reduced with occasional positive wave.
Instrumentation manipulation may distort or make unrecognizable fibrillation potentials and positive waves, especially the positive sharp wave (Fig. 13.5).

Motor Unit Potentials

These should be characterized by observing them in step 3, minimal muscle contraction, and step 4, maximal muscle contraction (see Chapter 1).

The motor unit potential should be described in detail, including peak-to-peak amplitude, duration, number of phases, or varying amplitude from moment to moment. If the number of polyphasic units exceed 15%, the motor unit potentials should be described as "increased proportion of polyphasic units."

In neuropathic conditions, the available motor units for recruitment will be reduced so that each firing unit will discharge more rapidly before additional units are recruited (reduced recruitment interval). The sine qua non of neuropathic disease is a reduced number of motor units activated as compared to the strength of contraction, firing rapidly. One should be able to measure the rate of firing before the second motor unit is recruited.

In neuropathic disease, the motor unit potential may be increased in amplitude and duration, especially in chronic states, since sprouting of intact axons will occur to adopt neighboring denervated muscle fibers. Where conduction is slowed down, these immature and incompletely myelinated axons may be late components to the motor unit action potential (Fig. 13.6).

Conversely, in myopathic conditions, since each motor unit will have fewer muscle fibers, the motor unit potential will be lower in amplitude and of shorter duration, with an increased number recruited as compared to the strength of contraction. There will be an increased proportion of polyphasic units of shorter duration (Fig. 13.7). As muscle fibers regenerate, fibrosis occurs and as the architecture of the muscle changes, some of the motor unit potentials may appear "neuropathic." It is axiomatic that *no* electrical activity should be labelled implying diagnostic significance to that activity.

Sample reports:
    "Increased number as compared to strength of contraction; increased
        proportion of polyphasic; amplitude varied from 200 to 500 μV;
        duration from 2 to 5 msec."
    "Reduced number of motor unit potentials as compared to strength of
        contraction; fire rapidly; normal amplitude and duration."

"Normal amplitude, duration, and number."

"Markedly reduced number; fire rapidly. Amplitude to 10 mV and duration to 14 msec."

"Only one motor unit recruited, fired 30/sec. Many phases, duration 16 msec, amplitude less than 200 μV."

"Unable to get maximal contraction; normal amplitude and duration."

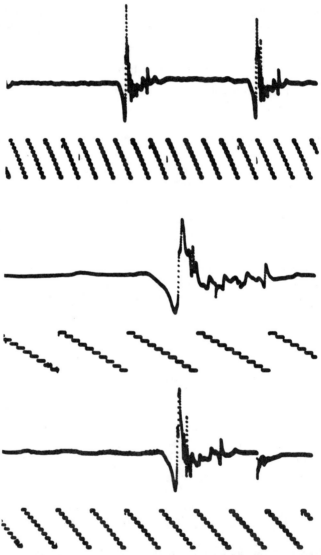

Fig. 13.6. Complex motor unit potential recorded from a reinnervating motor unit. A 52-year-old man with an axillary nerve injury from dislocated shoulder. Note the "late" component. Monopolar needle recording from deltoid. Calibration: width of time signal, 100 μV; each dot, 1 msec. Note middle trace and bottom trace with sweep speed increased.

Distribution of Abnormality

Adequate sampling for identifying the anatomic distribution requires an excellent knowledge of surface and functional anatomy. Report most specific distribution which can be determined.

Errors in Reporting

A survey of 112 EMG reports performed by 112 different electromyographers revealed a substantial number of errors (2) (Fig. 13.8). These were classified as anatomic, terminologic, interpretive, and technical (including inadequate examination or insufficient data) (Fig. 13.9).

Anatomic errors included both incorrect cord levels for the common muscles investigated and indicated nonspecific areas instead of specific muscles (for example, hamstrings, calf, thighs, thenar, hypothenar, etc.). Wrongly assumed location of the needle electrode was a frequent error, for example, listing the posterior tibial muscle when the needle was most likely in the flexor digitorum longus or recording that the opponens muscle was being explored when the needle was in the abductor pollicis brevis.

Terminologic errors abounded (Fig. 13.10). They were counted as errors

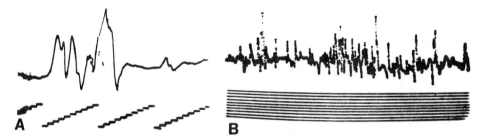

Fig. 13.7. (A) Polyphasic motor unit potential from vastus medialis. Calibration: width, 50 μV; each dot, 0.1 msec. (B) Duchenne muscular dystrophy monopolar electrode recording from vastus medialis. Calibration: width, 100 μV; 200 msec across cathode ray oscilloscope.

112 EMG's FROM 112 EMG'ers

$46/112$ USED FORM

$14/46$ PRINTED MUSCLES

$3/14$ PRINTED NERVES

Fig. 13.8. Survey of forms used by 112 U.S. electromyographers.

when the terminology differed from that recommended by the Pavia Conference 1967 (3). This incorrect usage was generally assigning diagnostic terms to the neurophysiologic phenomenon instead of describing the electrical activity specifically. For example, "denervation" potentials, giant potentials, and myotonic discharges were terms frequently found on the EMG reports. The Pavia Committee recommended that all potentials should be described by their amplitude, duration, shape, and rate of firing, and under no circumstances should the electrical activity be referred to in diagnostic terms or phrases.

Technique errors comprised those errors which were identified from the report as obvious to the reader (for example, distal latencies shorter than residual latencies, motor latencies prolonged with normal sensory latencies in carpal tunnel syndromes, diagnosis of amyotrophic lateral sclerosis without nerve conduction studies recorded) (Fig. 13.11). Incomplete examinations were also included in the technique category.

Errors of interpretation were largely those EMG reports which summa-

ERRORS (112 EMG's)

ANATOMIC	74
TECHNIQUE	41
INCOMPLETE EXAM	36
TERMINOLOGY	31
INTERPRETATION	97

Fig. 13.9. Errors present on 112 EMG reports.

TERMINOLOGY ERRORS

(N = 41)

N = 34	"DENERVATION" POTENTIALS
N = 5	"NASCENT"
N = 6	"GIANT"
N = 4	"MYOTONIC"
N = 3	"MYOPATHIC"

Fig. 13.10. Description of terminologic errors on 41 of 112 EMG reports.

rized data but did not translate the neurophysiologic findings into a clinical diagnosis (Figs. 13.12 and 13.13). Also, the clinical diagnosis was not supported by the data presented. A majority of the reports was determined to lack a probable clinical diagnosis.

How to Report a Normal EMG

While this seems rather simple, there are a number of consequences of writing down the results of the normal EMG, particularly when it has

TECHNIQUE ERRORS

(N = 41)

N =	4	TERMINAL LATENCY TOO SHORT (1.5 ms)
N =	5	DISTANCE NOT RECORDED IN SURAL N. LATENCY
N =	8	MOTOR & SENSORY LATENCIES - INCOMPATIBLE
N =	5	POLARITY-INCONSISTANT ON RECORDS
N =	4	FASCICULATION POTENTIALS -NOT DESCRIBED
N =	7	EVOKED MUS. POTENTIAL (MUS. NOT IDENTIFIED)
N =	31	INSERTIONAL ACTIVITY INAPPROPRIATE

Fig. 13.11. Distribution of 41 technique errors present in 112 EMG reports.

INTERPRETATION ERRORS IV

N =	7	MINIMAL CONTR. "REDUCED INTERFERENCE PATTERN"
N =	6	"DECR. INSERTIONAL ACT." MANY POSITIVE WAVES
N =	2	POSITIVE WAVES DESCRIBED AS VOL. POT.
N =	2	"RECRUITMENT-FAIR MINUS =MYOPATHY POT
N =	4	"INCREASED INTERFERENCE PATTERN"
N =	1	35 $M/_S$ (PERONEAL N) = NORMAL

Fig. 13.12. Sample of interpretive errors found on a majority of Hz EMG reports.

INTERPRETATION ERROR III

(N = 5)

"VULNERABLE" MUSCLES <u>ONLY</u> ABNORMAL

$$
\text{I.M. INJECTIONS} \left\{
\begin{array}{l}
\text{DELTOID} \\
\text{V. LATERALIS} \\
\text{RECTUS FEMORIS} \\
\text{GLUTEUS MAX.}
\end{array}
\right.
$$

EXT. DIG. BR.

Fig. 13.13. Common areas of needle exploration where misleading results may be found of i.m. injections or intrinsic vulnerability, i.e., extensor digitorum brevis.

medical-legal implications. In one study, a third to a half of the EMGs performed were normal. These may be reported in a variety of ways, suggested by the reason for referrals, the referral source, specific diagnoses to be ruled out, medical-legal considerations, and the maturity of the electromyographer. Any or all of these may influence the specific words describing a negative EMG:

> negative EMG;
> normal EMG;
> no EMG abnormality in the areas sampled today;
> no EMG evidence of lower motor neuron or muscle disease or injury;
> no electrodiagnostic abnormality on examination today;
> no EMG evidence of radiculopathy, carpal tunnel syndrome, or whatever the referring diagnosis suggested;
> EMG—OK—today;
> EMG compatible with normalcy;
> EMG does not support the referring diagnosis;
> EMG did not reveal abnormalities in the symptomatic extremities;
> no EMG evidence of motor unit disease;
> no EMG evidence of radiculopathy; and
> carpal tunnel syndrome is ruled out.

I prefer to state that no EMG abnormalities were uncovered in the muscle sampled and that if symptoms continue I would be delighted to repeat the examination.

How to Report an Abnormal but Ambiguous EMG

One can say simply, "EMG is abnormal, but I don't know the diagnosis" and suggest repeating the examination in several weeks.

A single EMG may be compared to a single frame of a motion picture. What may have happened before and what will happen later are assumptions which may be clarified by repeating the EMG or adding additional diagnostic procedures.

Common Mistakes in Performing the EMG

Using a stereotyped set of muscles or nerves—this may mislead the electromyographer. It certainly limits his examination possibilities (Fig. 13.14).

Terminating the examination too soon—this may obscure the diagnosis or may result in reporting a normal examination when in fact motor unit disease is present.

Beginning the examination without a planning history and physical examination—this will prolong the EMG in getting to the diagnosis. Obviously, many unnecessary muscles may be tested or the nerve stimulation studies may be inappropriate or overdone.

Overinterpretation of minor EMG abnormalities (for example, reporting polyphasic motor units and translating them into a clinical diagnosis of radiculopathy)—this may cause unnecessary surgical procedure or other management errors.

Underinterpretation of the EMG—this means reporting abnormal EMG but unable to provide a probable clinical diagnosis or a differential diagnosis. This will only disappoint the referring physician.

Doing an abbreviated EMG and then indicating "compatible with referring diagnosis"—this should be unconscionable and unethical behavior by the electromyographer.

Taking shortcuts (for example, not measuring when doing conduction velocities or terminal delays)—this will mislead the electromyographer.

Improper securing of electrodes—this results in no or unreliable data.

Only exploring one or two muscles instead of seven or eight—this is an incomplete EMG and may miss the essential data.

Prolonging the EMG before technical problems are cleared up—this simply will be a useless and uninterpretable EMG.

Being nonspecific in the diagnosis (for example indicating L4, L5, and S1 radiculopathies when critical analysis of the data would limit the EMG abnormalities to a single root, e.g. S1).

Doing more than is necessary to verify the diagnosis. Consider the patient as well as his pocketbook since most EMGs are billed as "piece work." There are examples of patients who have had two nerves investigated in each of four extremities as well as the muscles of all four extremities when the referring example was a lower extremity radiculopathy and the needle examination confirmed it.

Misinterpretation of the data—this is the most likely error which is committed by the inexperienced electromyographer. The classic example is to recognize positive sharp waves as abnormal when they are simply the result of single fiber discharges provoked by the tip of the needle in the endplate area. This is particularly frequent in the needle exploration of intrinsic hand or foot muscles (Fig. 13.15).

Underinterpretation could be the overlooking of significant subtle abnormalities which have diagnostic importance as root or peripheral nerve

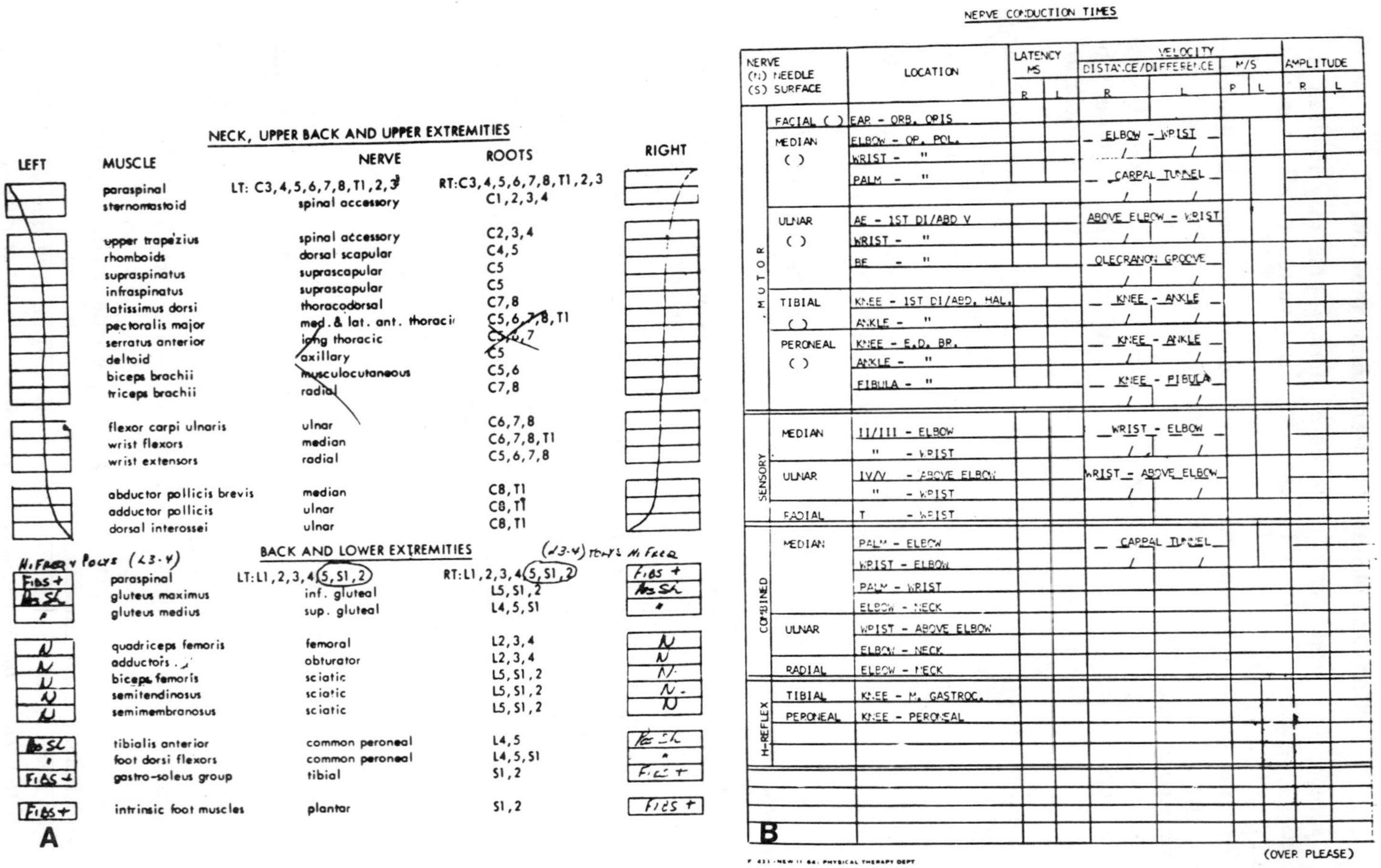

LEFT	MUSCLE	NERVE	ROOTS	RIGHT
		NECK, UPPER BACK AND UPPER EXTREMITIES		
	paraspinal	LT: C3,4,5,6,7,8,T1,2,3	RT:C3,4,5,6,7,8,T1,2,3	
	sternomastoid	spinal accessory	C1,2,3,4	
	upper trapezius	spinal accessory	C2,3,4	
	rhomboids	dorsal scapular	C4,5	
	supraspinatus	suprascapular	C5	
	infraspinatus	suprascapular	C5	
	latissimus dorsi	thoracodorsal	C7,8	
	pectoralis major	med. & lat. ant. thoracic	C5,6,7,8,T1	
	serratus anterior	long thoracic	C5,6,7	
	deltoid	axillary	C5	
	biceps brachii	musculocutaneous	C5,6	
	triceps brachii	radial	C7,8	
	flexor carpi ulnaris	ulnar	C6,7,8	
	wrist flexors	median	C6,7,8,T1	
	wrist extensors	radial	C5,6,7,8	
	abductor pollicis brevis	median	C8,T1	
	adductor pollicis	ulnar	C8,T1	
	dorsal interossei	ulnar	C8,T1	
H. FREQ + POLYS (L3-4)		**BACK AND LOWER EXTREMITIES**	(L3-4) POLYS H. FREQ	
Fibs +	paraspinal	LT:L1,2,3,4,5,S1,2	RT:L1,2,3,4,5,S1,2	Fibs +
Abs SL	gluteus maximus	inf. gluteal	L5,S1,2	Abs SL
"	gluteus medius	sup. gluteal	L4,5,S1	"
N	quadriceps femoris	femoral	L2,3,4	N
N	adductors	obturator	L2,3,4	N
N	biceps femoris	sciatic	L5,S1,2	N
N	semitendinosus	sciatic	L5,S1,2	N
N	semimembranosus	sciatic	L5,S1,2	N
Abs SL	tibialis anterior	common peroneal	L4,5	Abs SL
"	foot dorsi flexors	common peroneal	L4,5,S1	"
Fibs +	gastro-soleus group	tibial	S1,2	Fibs +
Fibs +	intrinsic foot muscles	plantar	S1,2	Fibs +

A

NERVE CONDUCTION TIMES

	NERVE (N) NEEDLE (S) SURFACE	LOCATION	LATENCY MS R	LATENCY MS L	VELOCITY DISTANCE/DIFFERENCE R	VELOCITY DISTANCE/DIFFERENCE L	M/S R	M/S L	AMPLITUDE R	AMPLITUDE L
MOTOR	FACIAL ( )	EAR - ORB. ORIS								
	MEDIAN ( )	ELBOW - OP. POL.			ELBOW - WRIST /	/				
		WRIST - "								
		PALM - "			CARPAL TUNNEL /	/				
	ULNAR ( )	AE - 1ST DI/ABD V			ABOVE ELBOW - WRIST /	/				
		WRIST - "								
		BE - "			OLECRANON GROOVE /	/				
	TIBIAL ( )	KNEE - 1ST DI/ABD. HAL.			KNEE - ANKLE /	/				
		ANKLE - "								
	PERONEAL ( )	KNEE - E.D. BR.			KNEE - ANKLE /	/				
		ANKLE - "								
		FIBULA - "			KNEE - FIBULA /	/				
SENSORY	MEDIAN	II/III - ELBOW			WRIST - ELBOW /	/				
		" - WRIST								
	ULNAR	IV/V - ABOVE ELBOW			WRIST - ABOVE ELBOW /	/				
		" - WRIST								
	RADIAL	T - WRIST								
COMBINED	MEDIAN	PALM - ELBOW			CARPAL TUNNEL /	/				
		WRIST - ELBOW								
		PALM - WRIST								
		ELBOW - NECK								
	ULNAR	WRIST - ABOVE ELBOW								
		ELBOW - NECK								
	RADIAL	ELBOW - NECK								
H-REFLEX	TIBIAL	KNEE - M. GASTROC.								
	PERONEAL	KNEE - PERONEAL								

B

F 431 - NEW 11 64 - PHYSICAL THERAPY DEPT

(OVER PLEASE)

Fig. 13.14. Two sample report which are unsatisfactory (stereotyped list of muscles/nerves without adequate space for description of electrical activity) *distribution* (Fig. 13.16). Also, underinterpretation could be making generalized conclusions when a more precise diagnosis is warranted. An underinterpretation of an obviously abnormal electrodiagnostic examination suggesting motor unit disease instead of a probable amyotrophic lateral sclerosis or perhaps a peripheral neuropathy instead of an entrapment syndrome are examples.

The use of the EMG as a guide for further study is often very helpful; however, it can be misused to recommend unnecessary diagnostic procedures. Occasionally, the step in workup will be indicated, e.g., a myelogram if a tumor is suspected, a spinal fluid examination if a Guillain-Barré is suspected, a CAT (computerized axial tomography) scan or perhaps a muscle biopsy.

The use of the EMG as a response to a referring physician for treatment or for further specialist referral is also helpful. It also could be a misuse of the examination. It is often necessary to say, "I don't know," and a repeat examination in several weeks may clarify the examination.

Another useful technique is to file the questionable examinations in a

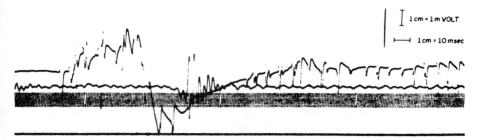

Fig. 13.15. Insertional activity in vicinity of motor point demonstrating endplate spikes changing to positive sharp waves as tip of electrode is advanced.

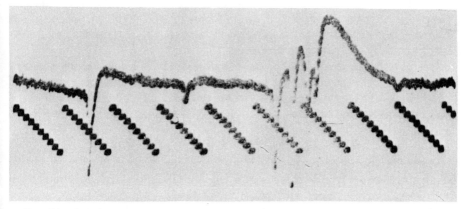

Fig. 13.16. A few positive sharp waves. Calibration: width of time signal, 50 μV; each dot, 1 msec.

special place so that they can be referred to later for verification or followed up so that each EMG examination can be a learning experience for the electromyographer (it ought to be). In my judgment, the use of EMG in its broadest sense will have as its major advantage the improvement of the clinical skills of the electromyographer. This means, when he suspects a radiculopathy but does not find weakness, he may use the EMG to find the abnormality and then return to the patient for reassessment of the physical examination. Using the EMG as immediate feedback may allow the electromyographer to become a better clinician.

Anomalous innervation may be a basis for misinterpretation of EMGs (5, 6). Numerous possibilities of crossover between median and ulnar nerves occur in the forearm and hand (4,7). These must be considered in all patients where the evoked potentials or abnormalities on needle examination do not conform to the suspected clinical syndrome. Remember that all muscles acting on the extremities have motor nerve supply derived from two or more roots (exception, rhomboids C5) (8).

Atrophy of muscle groups secondary to pain, disuse, or joint limitation may be a basis for misinterpretation of minor nonspecific findings.

A tense patient may present with hyperventilation, and repetitive discharge motor unit potentials could mislead the electromyographer. The inability to get complete relaxation of the patient may interfere with accurate diagnosis.

Muscle groups which are areas for intramuscular injections should not be used for exploration (9). Similarly, the extensor digitorum brevis is a muscle which is normally subject to trauma, which may result in the EMG abnormalities (10). Recent popularization of "trigger point" injections also may give spurious and misleading findings on needle exploration.

What Constitutes an Adequate EMG

Clearly, an adequate EMG is one which provides enough data to make the correct diagnosis or at least suggests further diagnostic or management direction. Another definition of a satisfactory EMG is one which rules out the working diagnosis or is incompatible with the differential diagnosis entertained by the referring physician.

It is possible to explore all of the 434 skeletal muscles and study three or four peripheral nerves in each extremity without making clinically useful conclusions. This is especially so when the planning history and physical examination are incomplete.

A Narrative Report

Many electromyographers record the data on worksheets and then dictate a narrative report. While this may be satisfactory, there are objections from both electromyographer and referring physician standpoints. It is more convenient to record data on the report form to avoid transcribing errors and loss of data. Handwritten reports at the time of the EMG ensure accuracy and immediacy of the report. Narrative reports tend to be ambiguous, verbose, imprecise, and they clearly result in stereotyped and solipsistic statements.

For these reasons and the obvious delay introduced by the transcribing typist, I opt for immediate and hardwritten reports on the same forms on which the data is recorded. Multiple, pressure sensitive sheets can provide four or five copies easily.

Recording essential evoked muscle potentials or diagnostic motor unit potentials and then using a copier to provide these data along with the report to the referring physician is both educational and clinically helpful.

How to Bill for an EMG

Philosophically, I believe the patient is paying for a procedure to uncover a diagnosis—that is, he is paying for a diagnosis.

This means the charge should be an overall equitable one, but not for each limb explored or nerve studied. This "piece work" approach tempts abuses which are not in the best interest of either the patient or the electromyographer.

Time ought not to be the variable which dictates the fee either. This rewards the inept poorly trained electromyographer and penalizes the efficient expert one.

Perhaps it is too late to reverse the invidious practice of costing the EMG per muscle and/or nerve studied but I'd like to try. The information obtained from a single muscle or a single nerve (e.g., facial) may be as valuable in the management of a given patient as an afternoon EMG needling of muscles in all extremities.

Conceptually, there should be a charge for an electrodiagnostic examination which leads to a probable diagnosis. Should this be too radical, perhaps two charges, one for a "single" EMG and a higher charge for a more complex study. Even this may be unfair.

An explanation of the EMG may be facilitated by a pamphlet distributed to the patient before the test (Fig. 13.17).

A Final Few Thoughts

Doing EMGs is fun, challenging, and—above all—the practice of medicine. It is the stethoscope of the physiatrist, the head mirror of the neurologist; it must never be removed from the physician-specialist to the technician's domain. The planning of the EMG must await a careful history and physical examination and then be modified as the EMG findings unfold and are interpreted by the physician, all the while considering the list of the differential diagnoses (11).

To keep up with new techniques, each clinical electromyographer should attend a refresher continuing education course every year or two.

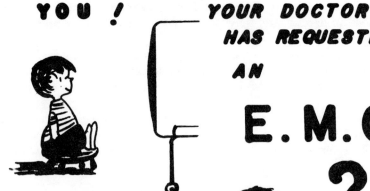

YOU !

SAW YOUR MUSCLES ON TELEVISION.../

YOUR DOCTOR HAS REQUESTED AN E.M.G. ? WHAT'S THAT

What do the letters E.M.G. stand for?
    E. - electro
    M. - myo or muscle
    G. - gram or graph
literally - write muscle electricity
Put them all together and it means: the recording of the electrical activity associated with muscle contraction.

DOES IT HURT?
    A tiny electrode (size of a pin) is inserted through the skin into several muscles. This may be associated with minor discomfort.

WHAT WILL IT TELL?
    The tiny muscle potentials will be changed if there is disease or injury of nerves or muscles.

IS THAT ALL?
    Sometimes, another test is done with the EMG equipment. This requires a small electric shock to be applied on a nerve in the arm or leg. It shows how fast an impulse travels along a nerve.

WILL THERE BE AFTER EFFECTS?
    No, other than occasional minor muscle soreness for a short time after the examination.

WHAT TO TELL YOUR ROOM MATE AND RELATIVES??
    MOUNT CARMEL HOSPITAL
    PHYSICAL MEDICINE DEPARTMENT -over
    WEST STATE STREET
    COLUMBUS 22, OHIO

Fig. 13.17. A sample of handout to be given patients who are to have EMG studies. Upper right, page 1; lower right, page 2; lower left, page 3; upper left, page 4.

REFERENCES

1. JOHNSON, E., ET AL.: Use of electrodiagnostic examination in a university hospital. *Arch. Phys. Med. Rehabil. 46:* 573, 1965.
2. JOHNSON, E., ET AL.: Errors in EMG reporting. *Arch. Phys. Med. Rehabil. 57:* 30, 1976.
3. Report of Terminology Committee, American Association EMG and EDX Newsletter, p. 34, Pavia, Italy, 1967.
4. LUDWIG, G.: Median-ulnar nerve communications and carpal tunnel syndrome. *J. Neurol. Neurosurg. Psychiat., 40:* 982, 1977.

5. LAMBERT, E.: The accessory branch of peroneal nerve. *Neurology, 19:* 1169, 1969.
6. SYS, M. C., AND CHANG, K. S. F.: A study of the radial supply of human brachialis muscle. *Anat. Rec., 162:* 363, 1968.
7. FORREST, W. J.: Motor innervation of human thenar and hypothenar muscles in 25 hands. *Can. J. Surg. 10:* 196, 1967.
8. BRENDLER, S. V.: The human cervical myotomes: Functional anatomy studied at surgery. *J. Neurosurg., 27:* 105, 1968.
9. JOHNSON, E., ET AL.: Electromyographic abnormalities after intramuscular injections. *Arch. Phys. Med. Rehabil., 52:* 250, 1971.
10. WIECHERS, D., ET AL.: Electromyographic findings in the extensor digitorum brevis in a normal population. *Arch. Phys. Med. Rehabil., 57:* 84, 1976.
11. LAMBERT, E.: Electrodiagnosis of neuromuscular disease. *Pediatrics, 34:* 599, 1964.

14

Traditional Electrodiagnosis

JOSEPH B. ROGOFF, M.D.

As noted in Chapter 17, the use of galvanic and faradic current in determining the integrity of the lower motor neuron and in distinguishing diseases of the lower motor neuron from diseases of the muscle itself dates back to about the midpart of the 19th century. This very simple qualitative method, requiring very minimal apparatus, was the only electrical test available for testing the lower motor neuron until the early part of the 20th century. At that time, the work of the Lapicques (1) in defining chronaxy and strength duration relationship and the work of Bourguignon (2) in introducing chronaxy into the clinical armamentarium led to the use of this more sophisticated and quantitative measurement, which remains useful in spite of the availability of today's more sophisticated methods.

The Reaction of Degeneration

The type of electrical current produced by a battery—an electrical current which does not change in direction or intensity during the time it is used—is called direct current. In medical usage, however, this type of current is called galvanic current. It is, of course, the type of electricity which was first discovered by Galvani (3) and which was correctly noted to be of chemical origin by Volta.

Faradic current was the type of electrical current produced by a special electromagnetic generator called a faradic stimulator (4) (also Ruhmkorff coil, DuBois-Reymond's coil, and others) (Fig. 14.1).

This apparatus produced a very short pulse of electrical current, approximately 1 msec in duration, repeating about 50 or 100 times per second. This current is now produced electronically and usually consists of trains of 1-msec square wave pulses, repeating about 100 per second. In the same manner, it is not necessary to use a chemical battery for the production of galvanic current. A source of rectified alternating current of long duration

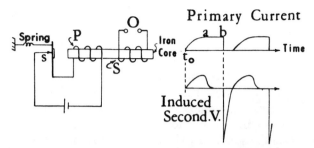

Fig. 14.1. Representation of a faradic coil. (*P*) is primary coil; (*S*) is secondary coil. When primary current is broken at (*b*), secondary current has sharp rise.

(at least 100 msec) can be used effectively. However, a small 90 V battery with a rheostat to control the intensity, using a stimulator electrode with a switch to control the duration, is quite adequate and can be usefully employed as a simple testing method.

A source of galvanic and faradic current being available, a patient is tested as follows: The large area dispersive electrode and the small area testing or stimulating electrode must be well soaked in conductive water (Fig. 14.2). (In most cases, it is not necessary to add any salt to ordinary tap water.) The dispersive electrode is placed over any portion of the patient's body but is most usefully placed in proximity and usually not over the muscle to be tested. The stimulating electrode is then applied to the surface of the muscle to be tested. These are both connected to a source of galvanic current. The duration of current flow usually is determined by a switch on the handle of the testing electrode. The duration of current flow determined in this manner is not less than about 1/10 of a second and is usually nearer to 1 or 2 sec.

When the muscle being tested is a normally innervated muscle, the following will be found:

1. There is a limited area of the muscle where the largest contraction will be obtained with the smallest amount of electrical current. This area corresponds to the loci of motor endplates (5), in proximity to the area where the motor nerve enters the muscle. It is known as the motor point.

2. The best contraction with the least amount of current will be produced if the stimulating electrode is connected to the negative or cathode pole of the source of galvanic current.

3. Although it is possible to obtain a contraction at the moment the circuit is opened, the best contraction using the least amount of current is produced at the moment of establishing contact.

One can thus establish a hierarchy of the ease with which the stimulus can produce an electrical contraction with the least amount of current. This hierarchy is abbreviated "CCC" (Closing Contraction using the Cathode). In the same manner it will be found that the anode closing contraction

(ACC) will require a small additional current. The anode opening contraction (AOC) will require still more current, and the cathode opening contraction (COC) will require the greatest amount of current. Thus, the polar formula is established as CCC> ACC> AOC> COC.

This formula, first established by Erb (6), was described in the past as important and always altered during denervation. However, the alteration of the "polar formula" in denervation is not consistent and is now known to have no importance in the reaction of degeneration.

The contraction produced by the galvanic current in normally innervated muscles is a brisk contraction. The muscle relaxes immediately, even though the current continues to flow. It is thus possible to characterize the galvanic stimulation of normal muscle as "quick twitch" (QT) at the "motor point" (MP) with "cathode closing contraction" (CCC) or "QT at MP with CCC."

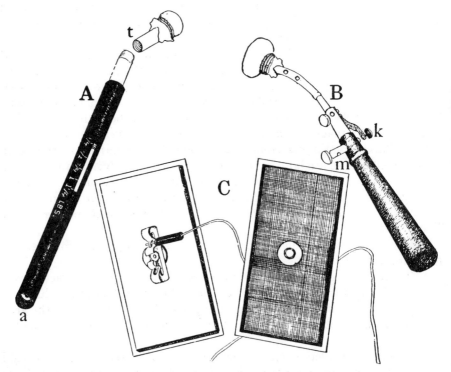

Fig. 14.2. Testing electrodes. (A) An active electrode with an internal spring which makes it possible to determine pressure applied to skin. The tip (t) unscrews so that the cylindrical well may be filled with water which feeds the cloth tip through a very small opening in the terminal ball. At (a) is a jack to receive the lead from the stimulating generator. (B) A standard electrode with wooden or plastic handle. If connection is made at m, current is transmitted manually by closing key (k). If other binding post is used, current will flow as delivered by generator. (C) A standard dispersive electrode. At left, back view with clip to receive plug from generator; at right, obverse view showing wire mesh depression in which soaked pad is set. (In *Electrodiagnosis and Electromyography*, 3rd ed., ch. 8.)

When the faradic current is used to stimulate normally innervated muscle, it is also applied at the motor point and results in a continued tetanic contraction of the muscle. It is obvious that at a rate of 100 pulses/sec, the muscle cannot contract and relax but has a sustained contraction.

When denervation occurs (whether due to anterior horn cell, root, or motor nerve involvement) and when Wallerian degeneration is complete, the following events take place: with the loss of nerve conduction, the motor point is no longer present; stimulation at its former location is no longer the best point for stimulating the muscle; and the greatest contraction with the least current occurs when the current flows through as much muscle tissue as possible. To accomplish this, the dispersive electrode should be placed at the origin of the muscle and the stimulating electrode at the insertion. This flow of electricity through the entire muscle is termed "longitudinal stimulation." The denervated muscle still contracts to galvanic current, but the contraction is now a slow worm-like or vermicular contraction. Its character is easily distinguished from the brisk contraction which occurs in normally innervated muscle. Faradic current at tolerable intensities no longer results in any contraction of the denervated muscle.

Stimulation of normally innervated muscle thus always occurs through stimulation of the nerve (or the motor endplates;) while in denervation, the muscle is directly stimulated.

The combination of the disappearance of the motor point, longitudinal stimulation, vermicular contraction, and failure to contract to faradic current is called the "RD." This is usually considered to mean "Reaction of Degeneration" but can also be translated as "Reaction of Denervation." The test is a simple one requiring only the most primitive apparatus, as described. It can frequently be used to distinguish upper from lower motor neuron involvement or lower motor neuron involvement from myopathy. Indeed, galvanic-faradic testing was the only form of electrodiagnosis available up until the eve of World War I, when this qualitative method was partially displaced by the use of chronaxy and strength-duration curves.

Certain aspects of the RD which were considered important in the past are no longer considered useful. The change in the polar formula (as indicated above) is one. Another which was frequently described was that of the partial RD. The definition of partial RD varied with the authors and was quite inconsistent. Some definitions of the partial RD described the disappearance of the motor point and vermicular contraction with galvanic current, but with some contraction to faradic current. Usually these situations arose when some innervated muscle was present together with the denervated portions.

Chronaxy and Strength-Duration Relationship

Attempts at converting the reaction of degeneration to a quantitative one were made in the latter half of the 19th century. DuBois-Reymond was one of the first to do so. The effect of DuBois-Reymond's "law" upon neurophysiological investigations directed towards quantitating the galvanic-faradic test is described under The Time Factor, Chapter 17. DuBois-Reymond attempted to determine the relationship between the intensity of the galvanic current required for a minimal contraction and the duration of this galvanic current flow. His unsophisticated method of producing short duration current flow was to control it by means of the hand-operated switch. The shortest duration which can be obtained in this manner is no less that about 100 msec. In view of the utilization time of normally innervated muscle, it is not surprising that DuBois-Reymond, using this method, found that the amount of current necessary for minimal contraction did not vary with the duration of current flow.

A period of almost 50 years elapsed between the enunciation of DuBois-Reymond's "law" in 1848 to the early part of the 20th century, when M. and Mme. Lapicque (1) finally defined the relationship between duration and intensity. If a graph is established comparing the intensity of galvanic current required for a minimal contraction with the duration of this same current flow, the curve thus obtained is called a "strength duration curve." When long duration currents are used (usually in excess of 100 msec) the intensity of the current required for a minimal contraction was called the basal flow or "rheobase" by the Lapicques.

As the duration of the current flow is shortened, a point is finally reached at which rheobase intensity is no longer adequate, and the intensity must be slightly increased to produce the minimal contraction. The exact point at which this occurs is quite difficult to determine since the curve begins to rise very gradually. The duration of current flow at this point was called by the Lapicques "temps utile" (1). This term, which means "useful time" in French has been called in English "utilization time." It was considered by the Lapicques the only useful portion of the current flow necessary to produce the rheobase contraction or (if called utilization time) the only portion of the current flow which is actually used for the contraction. The remainder of the current flow would then be described as useless or unnecessary. Thus, if the utilization time of each muscle were known in advance, the rheobase could be determined using no more current duration than the utilization time. In order to make sure that the utilization time is always included in the rheobase determination, a much longer duration must, therefore, be used.

Lapicque (1) called the duration of current flow necessary to produce a minimal contraction at twice rheobasic strength chronaxy. The mathematical reasoning used by the Lapicques for using this point on the strength-duration curve is not generally accepted. However, if one inspects the strength-duration curve, the chronaxy point usually occurs in a portion of the strength-duration curve which is changing rapidly in direction. It is, therefore, relatively easy to determine it with exactitude.

When Wallerian degeneration is complete, the entire strength-duration curve shifts to the right. This shift almost always results in an increase in the chronaxy. The chronaxy in denervated muscle is usually about 50-100 times greater than normal. There is, therefore, a clear difference between the chronaxy of normally innervated muscle and that of denervated muscle. However, some authorities consider that the establishment of the entire strength-duration curve is always more useful than only measuring chronaxy (7, 8).

Determining chronaxy values is simple and rapid with modern chronaxy apparatus. These machines usually have two settings, one marked "rheobase" and the other marked "chronaxy." After determining the rheobase, the operator changes this setting from rheobase to chronaxy. This automatically doubles the current which had previously been determined as the rheobase, and one can now determine the duration of current flow which produces the same minimal contraction as the rheobase. This is the chronaxy.

Bourguignon (2), by very meticulous testing, established the range of normal chronaxy values in man. The apparatus used by Bourguignon was a condenser discharge apparatus with characteristics more like the current stabilized generator than the voltage stabilized generator (9). The current stabilized generator gives chronaxy values which are greater than those produced by the voltage stabilized generator. In addition, the strength duration curve is steeper with the voltage stabilized generator and differences between normal chronaxies of various muscle groups are much smaller. Many British investigators, however, prefer the voltage stabilized stimulator, since they find it less painful than the current stabilized stimulator (8). In my experience, this difference is slight. The short chronaxy values obtained with the voltage stabilized stimulator may be less useful than those obtained with the current stabilized stimulator.

Bourguignon's (2) values for normal chronaxies were all less than 1 msec. He divided the muscles generally into three groups. The proximal flexors (for example, biceps) have the shortest chronaxies, between 0.07 and 0.15 msec. The second group consists of the proximal extensors and distal flexors (for example triceps, wrist flexors). These have a chronaxy approximately double those of the first group, chronaxies between 0.15 and 0.35. Group three includes the distal extensors (wrist extensors) and have chronaxies about double those of the previous group, that is, 0.35-0.7. No normal chronaxy should exceed 0.7 according to Bourguignon. As stated above, the limit of msec is accepted as normal chronaxy; chronaxies above 1 should be considered as abnormal. However, chronaxies as high as 2 or 3 may sometimes be found in normal individuals when the motor point is not accurately determined. This is also true in some myopathies where chronaxy values of 2 or 3 may be noted without indicating the presence of denervation. Increased rheobase is also frequently found in myopathies. Truly abnormal chronaxies in the denervated range usually are above 10 and more frequently between 20 and 30.

Phillipe Bauwens (10) devised an interesting variation of chronaxy measurement which gives adequate information in a simplified form. With Bauwens' method it is not necessary to have a chronaximeter. A stabilized current generator capable of producing various durations from 0.01 msec to 100 msec (without the necessity for doubling the intensity) is adequate and is included in some EMG apparatus. This generator can be used for establishing the complete strength-duration curve. However, Bauwens showed that determining only two points on the strength-duration curve (at 100 and at 1 msec) was adequate to establish the normality of chronaxy. It is evident that, if the amount of current used for determining the rheobase (at 100 msec) is less than twice the amount of current needed for a similar contraction at 1 msec then the chronaxy must in that case be less than 1. Of course, chronaxy determination also determines two points and is similar; these two points on the strength-duration curve are the rheobase and the chronaxy point itself (Fig. 14.3).

Rheobase alone cannot be used as characteristic of the state of innervation of a muscle. In the first place, the apparent rheobase (that is the amount of current actually being used to stimulate the muscle at the motor point) cannot really be determined when testing at the skin surface, since the amount of current which actually reaches the motor point of the muscle is a small and undetermined proportion of the amount of current actually used at the surface of the skin. The proportion of current which actually stimu-

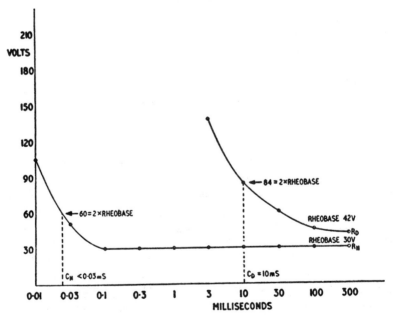

Fig. 14.3. Left hand curve, normal innervation; right hand, denervated. This shows deviation of chronaxy values from the strength-duration curve. (In *Electrodiagnosis and Electromyography*, 3rd ed., ch. 10.)

lates the muscle will necessarily vary with the skin resistance, the amount of subcutaneous tissue, the amount of fibrosis present, etc. It is usually found that in the early stages of denervation, the rheobase may be much shorter than that found in symmetrically noninvolved muscles. As time goes on, edema and fibrosis develop and the rheobase will vary, either increasing or remaining low. Thus, the rheobase cannot be used to determine the presence or absence of denervation.

The entire strength-duration curve unquestionably has advantages over chronaxy determination alone, especially in cases of partial denervation. This difference is clearly demonstrated during reinnervation. At that time, the strength-duration curve shows "breaks" in its form. These breaks are due to the presence of partially reinnervated areas which now have normal strength duration curves. However, these breaks cannot be made visible unless the rheobase of the denervated portion is lower than the rheobase of

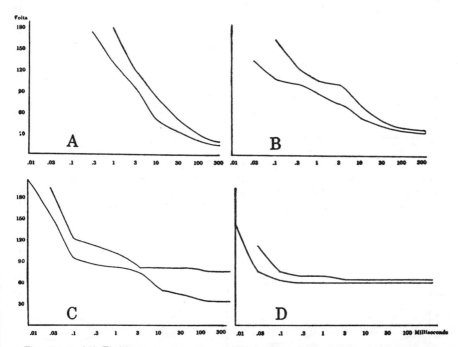

Fig. 14.4. (A) Eighteen weeks after nerve suture, upper curve. Lower curve, 2 weeks later showing discontinuity between 10 and 3 msec and appearance of a new point on curve at 0.3 msec. (B) Upper curve 4 months later showing two distinct curves. The part between 3 and 0.1 msec represents response of reinnervated fibers. Lower curve 2 weeks later showing lowered slope and new point at 0.03 msec. (C) Upper curve 1 week later showing pronounced flattening between 300 and 3 msec. Threshold doubled; if rheobase is reduced to unity, general slope less steep. Lower curve 1 week later shows new point at 0.01 msec. (D) Upper curve 1 week later shows fall in slope and no response at 0.01 due to threshold rise. Lower curve 3 weeks later; now normal. (In *Electrodiagnosis and Electromyography*, 3rd ed., ch. 10.)

the innervated portion (11). Where the rheobase of the innervated portion is lower than that of the innervated portion, this is seen first; the denervated rheobase can only be revealed at a higher value and is masked by the normal rheobase.

Because of the interest of these breaks, and also because he has noted cases with normal chronaxies and abnormal strength duration curves, Wynn Parry (8) feels that chronaxy should not be used, but that the full strength-duration curve should always be described. Examples of the interest of breaks can be seen in Figures 14.4–14.6.

Chronaxy and strength-duration curve determination are not as sensitive as EMG in determining small or localized areas of denervation. Further, myopathies have normal or almost normal chronaxies and strength duration

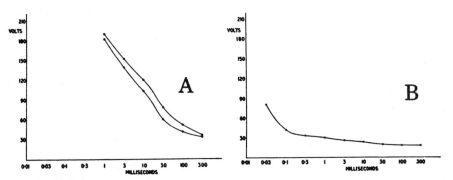

Fig. 14.5. (*A*) Two curves taken at 8 months' interval showing slight recovery in abductor digiti minimi following ulnar nerve suture. Upper curve taken 7 months after suture at wrist. (*B*) Unsutured radial nerve palsy; muscle power graded 5 when curve was taken. (In *Electrodiagnosis and Electromyography*, 3rd ed., ch. 10.)

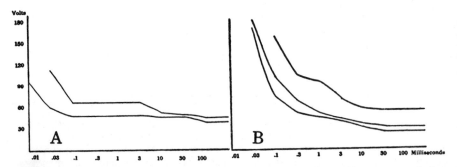

Fig. 14.6. (*A*) Ulnar neuritis following old fracture of elbow. Upper curve before transposition showing partial denervation; lower, 1 month later showing almost complete recovery. (*B*) Poliomyelitis of quadriceps; middle curve 10 months after onset; upper curve 4 weeks later; lower curve 14 weeks later. Curves almost identical except for absence of point at 0.03 msec in upper curve due to higher rheobase. No difference in clinical power in 18-week interval. (In *Electrodiagnosis and Electromyography*, 3rd ed., ch. 10.)

curves and thus cannot be clearly characterized by this method. EMG, on the other hand, can frequently characterize these involvements positively.

Clear changes characteristic of denervation or reinnervation can be appreciated at an earlier stage by chronaxy or strength-duration curve testing than with EMG. Rising chronaxies appear as early as the 6th day following acute denervation. The presence of breaks in strength-duration curves also appear earlier than characteristic EMG changes indicative of reinnervation. In doubtful cases where rest activity or voluntary activity is difficult or impossible to obtain, the presence of normal or abnormal chronaxies can be of distinct aid in determining the type of condition present. It is also useful to have chronaxy/strength-duration curve measurements as confirmation of abnormal EMG findings. For example, in the case of the EMG abnormalities (fibrillations) noted in early cerebral or spinal cord upper motor neuron involvement, chronaxies and strength-duration curves remain steadfastly normal, thus indicating that these EMG findings are probably not indicative of lower motor neuron involvement.

Excitability

There are certain cases where the comparison of threshold currents can be very useful. This is especially so in Bell's palsy (12). Here the comparison of the current necessary for producing a minimal contraction on the involved and noninvolved sides can be the earliest change to be noted. The method used is to stimulate the facial nerve at the tragus with a 1-msec pulse and to observe the amount of current needed to produce similar minimal contractions. This current, usually in the neighborhood of 4 or 5 mA, remains normal for at least 3 days after the onset of the facial palsy in all cases. However, if Wallerian degeneration is proceeding, the nerve gets less excitable starting at about 3½ days, and an increasing current strength will be required; after about 8 or 9 days, the involved nerve may no longer be excitable, and no contraction can be obtained. Usually a difference of 1 or 2 mA between the normal and involved sides can be significant. When the involvement is mainly neurapraxia, no change occurs in the excitability.

Galvanic-Tetanus Ratio

It is possible to obtain a short tetanic contraction with galvanic current if the intensity is sufficiently increased. In normally innervated muscle, the amount of current required for this galvanic tetanus is about six times the intensity of current required for a threshold contraction. Needless to say, this can be extremely painful. For denervated muscle, the quantity required is much less and is usually 1–1½ times the intensity required for threshold contraction. This is to say, that the vermicular contraction itself is almost in the nature of a galvanic tetanus. Thus, the relation between the amount of current needed to produce a galvanic tetanus in normal and in denervated muscle is about 6:1. During reinnervation, the amount of current needed to produce a galvanic tetanus may rise very high, perhaps as much as four times the amount of current required to produce a galvanic tetanus in normally innervated muscle; reinnervation is thus characterized by an increasing galvanic-tetanus ratio.

While the galvanic-tetanus ratio might appear a simple method for determining the presence of denervation and of reinnervation, it is little used. It is quite painful and rather difficult to determine accurately. The galvanic-tetanus threshold is not as definite as the above description would seem to indicate and has been generally abandoned.

Strength-Frequency Curves (*Fig. 14.7*)

Attempts have been made in the past to use strength-frequency curves as a means of testing for the presence of denervation. C. B. Wynn Parry (8), in the 3rd edition of *Electrodiagnosis and Electromyography* writes as follows:

"The method is based on the fact that denervated muscle and innervated muscle each have different optimum frequencies to which they respond . . . .

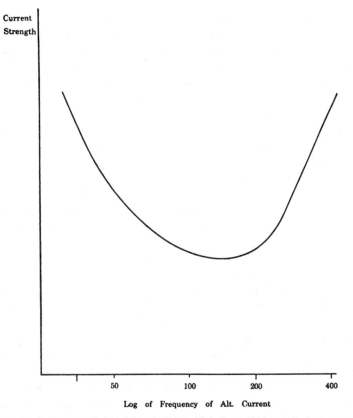

Fig. 14.7. Threshold voltages for alternating currents (schematic representation). (In *Electrodiagnosis and Electromyography*, 3rd ed., ch. 11.)

"Pollock (indicates that) during degeneration of a peripheral nerve, the muscle shows an increase in threshold amperages at all frequencies from 20 cycles per second and discontinuities in the curve appear. As many as three discontinuities in the curve have been seen, the most common ranges occurring between 20 to 100, 100 to 300, and 3000 to 7000 cycles per second.

"During denervation, the threshold amperage for higher frequencies is high but diminishes very much with low frequencies. During regeneration, there is a diminution in threshold amperage from 5000 to 20 cycles per second, the threshold amperage is high and increases steeply as the frequency is diminished.

"The salient features of the curve during recovery are the appearance of discontinuities, a drop in the threshold or acuteness of the curve, and gradual return of the muscle response to its optimum frequency . . . .

"Ritchie (states that) the threshold usually varies only 20 per cent between 20 and 100 cycles per second (and) this seems too narrow a margin for accuracy and tetanus can develop so gradually that it is difficult to assess . . . ."

REFERENCES

1. LAPICQUE, L: La Chronaxie et ses applications physiologiques. *Compt. Rend. Soc. Biol., 1:* 615, 1907.
2. BOURGUIGNON, G.: *La Chronaxie Chez L'Homme,* Paris, 1923.
3. GALVANI, L.: *De Viribus Electricitatis.* Translation by R. Green, Cambridge, Mass.: E. Licht, 1953.
4. LIEBIG, G. A., AND ROHE, G. H.: Induction coils. In *The Practical Application of Electricity in Medicine and Surgery,* Philadelphia: F. A. Davis, 1890.
5. COERS, C., AND WOOLF, A. L.: *The Innervation of Muscle. A Biopsy Study,* Springfield, Ill.: Charles C Thomas 1959.
6. ERB, W.: *Handbook of Electrotherapy,* New York, 1883.
7. HARRIS, R.: Chronaxy. In *Electrodiagnosis and Electromyography,* 3rd ed., ch. 9, New Haven, Conn.: E. Licht, 1971.
8. PARRY, C. B. W.: Strength-duration curves. In *Electrodiagnosis and Electromyography,* 3rd ed., ch. 10, New Haven, Conn.: E. Licht, 1971.
9. ROGOFF, J. B., AND REINER, S.: Electrodiagnostic apparatus. In *Electrodiagnosis and Electromyography,* 3rd ed., ch. 3, New Haven, Conn.: E. Licht, 1971.
10. BAUWENS, P.: Introduction to electrodiagnostic procedures. In *Electrodiagnosis and Electromyography,* 3rd ed., ch. 7, p. 174, New Haven, Conn.: E. Licht, 1971.
11. LIBERSON, W. T.: Electrodiagnosis. In *Encyclopedia Electrodiagnosis Chemistry,* edited by A. Hampel, pp. 440-447, Reinhold Publishing Co., 1964.
12. CAMPBELL, E. D., ET AL.: Value of nerve excitability measurements in prognosis of Bell's Palsy, *Br. Med. J.,* 2:7, 1962.

15

Instrumentation

STUART REINER, M.E.E.
JOSEPH B. ROGOFF, M.D.

EMG examinations include recording of the electrical activity of voluntary muscles and motor and sensory nerves at rest, during volitional activity, and while subjected to electrical and mechanical stimuli. EMG potentials are recorded with metal needle and skin surface electrodes. Similar electrodes are also used to apply the electrical stimuli used. These techniques impose different performance requirements on the EMG system.

The wide anatomical range of structures dealt with in clinical EMG, coupled with the broad spectrum of clinical objectives preclude rote methods in most of the procedures. EMG examinations are not laboratory tests but rather are an extension of the clinical examination.

The electrical potentials recorded range from fractions of microvolts (μV, 10^{-6} V, millionths of a volt) when recording action potentials of some of the sensory nerves to about 50 mV (mV, 10^{-3} V, thousandths of a volt) encountered in some muscle action potential recording. Time resolution in the order of tens or hundreds microseconds (μsec, 10^{-6} sec, millionths of a second) is required when recording fibrillation potentials and in single fiber EMG (SFEMG), while epochs as long as seconds are studied in the evaluation of interference patterns associated with strong muscle contraction.

In addition, electrical stimulation is required for many important evaluations performed by the electromyographer. The apparatus used in modern EMG must, therefore, be adjustable over a wide range of sensitivity and time scales and be capable of a number of modes of operation. Since the electromyographer must contend with this equipment to carry out his objectives, we will attempt in simple terms, as far as possible, to describe the technical features involved, making sure to include those which can significantly effect the results obtained so that the equipment can be used with confidence and facility and with appreciation of its limitations. The advent of the commercially designed EMG systems has freed the electromyographer from the many technical details of instrumentation and the problems of interconnection of a number of separate pieces of apparatus.

A background in basic electricity and in simple direct and alternating current circuits will facilitate the understanding of the electrophysiological concepts in practial EMG and in discussion of instrumentation which follows. The reader is referred to the references at the end of this chapter for this material (1–6). These concepts have great generality, but this chapter will emphasize in practical terms those ideas that specifically relate to EMG instrumentation, its use, and its limitations.

EMGs range from one channel instruments which incorporate the necessary facilities for performing the basic clinical tests to equipment permitting simultaneous recording of two or more channels of EMG and the electrical activity concurrent with force, displacement, acceleration, etc., and the output of electronic analyzers.

Special purpose limited performance EMG equipment is available, designed to respond primarily to gross myoelectric activity which finds application in muscle re-education and in biofeedback. Similarily, multichannel systems have been built to record the presence or absence of EMG activity simultaneously in many muscles for studies in kinesiology. This equipment is not used in diagnostic EMG nor in the measurement of nerve conduction velocity since it does not have the sensitivity, dynamic response, and measurement facility necessary.

The Basic EMG System

The functional elements that comprise a basic single-channel EMG system are shown diagramatically in Figure 15.1. Brief descriptions of these elements follow; later sections provide more elaboration. These blocks, electrodes, preamplifier, amplifier, cathode ray tube display, and stimulator represent functional components and are not necessarily actual interconnections of unique electronic circuits or devices. In practice, the EMG is a unique system designed as a whole, with considerable interrelation between circuit functions and with a number of common power supply and control circuits (7).

ELECTRODES

The choice of recording electrodes, their location relative to the anatomical structures being studied, and their state of cleanliness and repair have the dominant effect on the observed potentials. The electrodes are the critical link in the EMG system. They function to convert the varying ion currents moving within the body in response to the nerve and muscle activity to varying electrical currents in wires which are connected to the amplifier. The electrical interface between the metal recording electrodes and the body tissues and fluid is complex and variable and strongly effects the nature of the tiny recorded potentials.

This electrical contact at the interface is a poor one, particularly in small area needle electrodes. It is at this point of tenuous electrical contact that the ubiquitous technical problem of EMG appears, namely the recording of

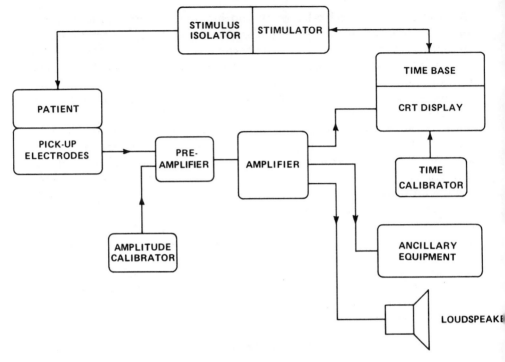

Fig. 15.1. Block diagram of a single channel EMG.

microvolt potentials at an imperfect electrical contact (the needle tip) in the presence of often large electrical interference. These are induced into the patient from surrounding electrical influences, e.g., electric power wiring, lighting and appliances, unwanted potentials originating from bioelectric sources within the patient, and the direct effect of electrical stimulation applied to the patient. These external electrical interference problems are usually resolved satisfactorily by properly connecting the apparatus to a good electrical ground (usually accomplished by a grounding connection in the power cable); applying a ground or a zero potential electrode to the patient; observing some simple electrical environment precautions, which includes disconnecting nearby electrical appliances or removing them and their power cables from proximity to the patients; by good electrode technique; and by the design of the EMG preamplifier to which the electrodes are connected.

PREAMPLIFIER

The preamplifier increases the magnitude and the power of the potentials picked up by the electrodes so that they can be conducted to the amplifier without being influenced by unwanted electrical effects which would cause distortion and error or would add spurious potentials. They are further amplified and manipulated by the amplifier until they are of sufficient voltage and power to be applied to the cathode ray display system, loudspeaker, and other devices used to display, monitor, record, and further process the EMG signal.

The preamplifier must be electrically compatible with the electrodes used and must process the smallest biological potentials encountered in the EMG system. It, therefore, must meet stringent requirements. It is often located in a remote box connected to the main EMG system by a cable. This arrangement permits the preamplifier to be placed close to the electrodes to which it is directly connected by relatively short cables in order to minimize interference.

The three primary factors that electrically characterize the preamplifier are: a) internal noise level, b) input impedance, and c) differential amplification, parameters which will be discussed later. These characteristics essentially determine the performance of the EMG System.

Noise

Briefly, all electrical circuits containing resistors and amplifiers generate thermal and amplifier internal "noise," i.e., unwanted electrical signals. The term noise is not used only in its accoustical sense; any interfering unwanted influence may be termed noise. Internal noise originates from sources within the system. Other sources of noise are external to the instrument system. These external sources, also termed interference or artifact, include unwanted bioelectric potentials and electrical sources such as power wiring in the building, the major source of interference requiring care in equipment and patient grounding. Broadcast transmitters and other radio frequency generators also originate interference.

Internal equipment noise extends over a wide spectrum of frequencies and is due mainly to random electrode and amplifier fluctuations. These noise potentials usually can be ignored in most electrical signal transmission systems when they are very small with respect to the signal amplitudes encountered. When dealing with electrical potentials in the low microvolt range and maximum amplification is required, the noise potentials are amplified along with the desired potentials and contaminate the resulting records. This internal noise appears as random irregular fluctuations in the baseline, fuzzy thickening of the trace and hissing and rumbling over the loudspeaker. Care in the design of the preamplifier minimizes such degrading effects on the EMG potentials. [When recording small evoked nerve potentials (neurograms) less than a few microvolts in amplitude, ancillary signal averaging devices are used to process potentials after amplification, so as to further minimize the effects of random noise potentials on the desired response waves.] When the EMG potentials leave the preamplifier and pass on to the main amplifier, they are of sufficient amplitude and power level so as not to be further influenced by external or internal electrical noise potentials in subsequent properly designed amplifiers and other system elements. The preamplifier, therefore, essentially determines the internal noise of the system.

Input Impedance

The input impedance of the preamplifier must be designed to be compatible with the electrical properties of the metal-electrolyte interface of the electrodes used in EMG. Input impedance describes the resistance and capacitance of the input circuit of the preamplifier to which the electrodes are connected and has a major influence on the effectiveness of the electrodes in conveying information from the patient to the amplifier.

The term impedance refers to the resistance which represents the energy dissipated by electrons as they move through the atomic structure of a conductor, to the capacitance which measures the energy stored in the electric field that surrounds a conductor, the inductance which measures the energy stored in the magnetic field set up by an electric current, and the effect of these three parameters on electrical potentials and currents in circuits. Impedance is an inevitable property of all electric circuits. When dealing with direct current (DC) circuits having no fluctuations, impedance effects simplify to resistance only and capacitance and inductance do not mediate the current flow. The resistance only determines the hinderance to current flow. Its effect is described by Ohms Law, $E=IR$ or $I=E/R$, where E is voltage (or potential), I is current flow, and R is resistance. The higher the resistance, the smaller will be the current flow.

When dealing with fluctuating and alternating voltage and currents (AC) such as EMG signals, circuit impedance which includes capacitance and inductance, as well as resistance, must be dealt with. Determining the hinderance on current flow of capacitance and inductance is more complex because the effect of these parameters depends upon the rate-of-change of voltage and current not upon their magnitude, as does resistance. The total impedance effect of all three parameters on current flow is somewhat similar to the Ohms Law effect of resistance in direct current circuits, namely, current flow in an AC circuit is equal to applied voltage divided by impedance, $I=E/Z$ where Z is impedance.

Impedance may be stated in ohms only when calculated for an applied sine wave voltage at a particular frequency. Impedance is, therefore, stated with more generality by specifying its resistance, capacitance, and inductance. This permits its effects to be calculated for an applied voltage at any frequency and for any waveform.

Resistance and capacitance effects predominate in the electrode-preamplifier input impedance circuit; inductive effects are insignificant and can be ignored. The input impedance of the preamplifier appears as a shunting effect at its input terminals. This impedance must, therefore, be high, so as to receive the potentials from the small area needle electrode, which themselves are characterized by a series impedance, with minimum loss of amplitude and minimum distortion. (Ideally, the electrodes would have zero impedance and the input impedance of the preamplifier would be infinitely high.) High input impedance additionally enhances preamplifier performance for reasons to be discussed later. High impedance is characterized by high resistance and small capacitance.

Differential Amplification

The third special characteristic of the preamplifier is its differential amplification property. This permits selective amplification of potentials originating near the two recording electrodes required with differential amplifiers while discriminating against interference, i.e., unwanted potentials originating at a distance and presenting at both electrodes. The interfering potentials are rejected by the mechanism of the differential amplifier to the extent that the interference equally influences the two recording electrodes (the exploring and reference electrodes). The differential amplifier, therefore, permits substantially interference-free recording of small potentials picked up by the recording electrodes while these electrodes are being influenced by often larger interference potentials from external sources, so long as the interference has mostly equal effect on the recording electrodes. Interference that does not impinge equally on both electrodes will not be rejected. *Note:* Ideally the exploring and reference electrodes should be of similar dimensions.

The differential preamplifier has three terminals: two recording electrode terminals, an exploring (or active) electrode terminal and a reference electrode terminal; and a third ground, zero potential, shield or guard electrode. The recording electrodes are placed as close as possible to the structures whose electrical activity is being studied (the exploring electrode being closer when feasible), while the ground electrode is placed on the body surface at some distance over an area of little electrical activity.

Amplitude Calibration

The amplitude calibrator is a source of electrical potential of known amplitude which can be selectively switched to the input terminal of the preamplifier to provide a test signal to verify the performance of the EMG system. The calibration voltage is specifically arranged to be applied at the electrode-input terminals to ensure that it is influenced by all parts of the EMG system. Amplitude calibration voltages of 10 μV, 100 μV, and sometimes more are usually provided. The wave shape of the calibration voltage is usually rectangular so as to provide additional information about the dynamic response of the EMG system, which can be obtained by observing the shape of these waves after passing through the system.

AMPLIFIER

The amplifier which follows the preamplifier usually contains the sensitivity control calibrated in units of microvolts per unit vertical deflection of the trace on the cathode ray display screen. This permits the operator to select a sensitivity that will be in accordance with the expected EMG potential amplitudes.

Frequency Response - Filter Controls

In order to most effectively accommodate the slow waves of some tests and the rapid waves of others and to minimize noise obvious in some test conditions and base line wander encountered in others, a means for adjusting EMG dynamic performance is provided to optimize results for various tests. These controls usually associated with the amplifier are termed variously, high and low frequency limit controls, frequency response controls, filter controls, or time constant controls. They limit the response of the system to the most rapid potential fluctuations on one hand and to the slowest fluctuations on the other, so as to enhance the shape of the desired potentials by eliminating unwanted rapid or slow fluctuations in the recorded wave form. A number of different settings of the high and low frequency filter controls may be selected depending on the special requirements of needle EMG, motor nerve conduction tests, electroneurography, and other tests. The function of these filter controls is analogous to the base and treble controls of a music reproduction system.

The output of the EMG amplifier is a filtered representation of the potentials picked up by the electrodes adjusted so that they are of suitable amplitude and of sufficient power level to drive the various display devices and to provide the output to drive ancillary equipment which might be used to further process the EMG signals.

CATHODE RAY TUBE DISPLAY

The cathode ray tube (CRT) display permits visualization of the transient action potentials by presenting them as dynamic amplitude versus time graphs on the fluorescent screen of the cathode ray tube. The patterns on the screen are drawn by an inertialess beam of electrons, which result in a spot of light when they impinge on the phosphor-coated screen. The traces are formed by uniform motion of the beam from left to right on the screen (X axis) generated by the time base, or sweep, circuits, while simultaneously being deflected up and down (Y axis) in response to the output potentials of the EMG amplifier. When the motion is sufficiently rapid, the observer sees continuous curves. Uninterrupted monitoring is achieved by repetition of this action. The amplifier sensitivity control selects the vertical scale of the display, and the time base control or sweep control selects the horizontal scale of the display.

Time Base - Time Calibration

Accuracy of time measurements made on the screen of the CRT will depend on the accuracy of the time base circuits which control the uniform left-to-right movement of the beam on the CRT. Time calibration means independence of the time base circuits is required. This is usually an independent signal of accurately known timing that can be displayed on the screen to verify the X axis calibration by comparing the timing of the calibration signal wave with the settings of the time base controls.

STIMULATOR

The stimulator applies electrical pulses to the patient to elicit muscle and nerve action potentials in motor and sensory nerve conduction tests. A principal objective of these tests is to measure the elapsed time or latency between the application of the stimulus and the appearance of evoked action potentials, under nearby recording electrodes. The sweep generator is arranged to start, or trigger, the left-to-right excursion of the beam on the CRT screen only when a stimulus is applied. This stimulus triggered sweep has the effect of making the stimulus and response waves each to appear at the same points on the screen every time a stimulus is applied. This results in superimposed response waves on the screen, which greatly facilitates recognition and measurement.

The stimulus, which can be a brief shock, 150 V or more in amplitude, is applied to the patient, in some cases, a few centimeters away from recording electrodes. These electrodes are connected to the preamplifier, which is arranged to record a few microvolts. This situation would normally cause overwhelming stimulus artifact currents to be conducted directly into the preamplifier via the patient and common EMG power supply circuits. This, in turn would result in electrical overload of the preamplifier and render it inoperative during the time it is required to record the evoked action potentials. This overwhelming stimulus artifact is eliminated or reduced to acceptable proportions by providing the stimulator with electrically isolated stimulus output circuits. These stimulus isolation circuits render the output portion of the stimulator that makes contact with the patient, free of any electrical connection to any of the circuits that are in common with the remainder of the EMG system.

LOUDSPEAKER

While obviously no sound is associated with the action potentials of EMG, the potentials recorded do produce audible sounds when applied to a loudspeaker because EMG potentials have components that fall within the audible spectrum. Audio monitoring has been a valuable adjunct since the earliest days of clinical EMG because many changes in the motor unit action potentials and their firing patterns produce characteristic alterations in the sounds they generate, often before changes are obvious in the visual patterns on the CRT screen.

ANCILLARY EQUIPMENT

Since the events that appear on the face of the CRT are brief and transient, all but the simplest EMG apparatus is equipped with some means for retaining the graphic images that appear on the face of the CRT. This permits visualization, analysis, and measurement, an increasingly important part of modern EMG. This can be done simply by adding an instant photography camera arranged to properly frame and focus on the CRT screen. It is used with the shutter open and the CRT in the triggered sweep mode or with the sweep start synchronized with operation of the shutter to ensure that only one sweep is recorded.

More facility is achieved by providing a storage display facility which instantly and electronically retains a trace (or a number of traces) on a CRT screen for analysis and more leisurely photography. It is then erased or updated with new information. Most flexibility and graphic records are achieved by special high speed graphic recorders that not only permit rapid visualization of the trace, but provide continuous sequences of traces allowing many potentials to be seen and in context as well.

A number of additional ancillary devices have become associated with the basic EMG equipment to aid in interpretation and analysis. These include magnetic tape recorders which record and play back the potentials observed on screen. Various special purpose computers process the EMG activity to extract potentials hidden in noise, modify the form of the data to enhance certain characteristics (integrators, action potential counters, etc.), or statistically display various parameters of the action potentials (a wide range of so-called EMG analyzers).

EMG Electrodes

The potential changes recorded in EMG originate as the moving depolarization—repolarization waves along muscle and nerve cell membranes, termed action potentials. The ion movement which constitutes this activity (which differs somewhat in muscles and nerves) is an electric current in the extracellular fluid and gives rise to the transient (approximately 110 mV) change in transmembrane potential. This lasts less than 1 msec and can be recorded with tiny intracellular electrodes, a process with little application in the clinical laboratory due to the fragile electrodes and the meticulous electrode fixation required.

Instead, recordings are made with large (with respect to muscle and nerve fiber size) metal needle electrodes which record a measure of the activity of many fibers (motor unit) and at a distance, except where extracellular recordings from single fibers are made in SFEMG. The moving action potentials spread within the extracellular fluid, a good electrolytic conductor, in three dimensions, a process termed volume conduction. The resultant motor unit action potentials recorded from the clinical needle electrode are more than 10 times smaller and three to five times longer in duration than the intracellular single fiber action potentials. This is due to the larger surface area of the clinical needle electrode which averages the activity from all the tissues it contacts, the attenuating effect of volume conduction (which reduces the voltage at least as the inverse square of the distance), the asynchronous arrival at the recording electrode of the individual action potentials, and the electrical properties of the metal-electrolyte interface at the tip of the needle. When surface electrodes are used, the increased distance from the origin of the action potentials, the wide range of potentials that influence the electrode which are then integrated by it, the complicating effect of the various tissue components such as skin, fat, muscle, connective tissue and blood vessels, all of which further attenuate the amplitude of the recorded potentials, slow their rapidly changing components and increase their apparent duration. Surface electrodes are, therefore, not useful in recording details of motor unit activity and are relegated to recording gross EMG activity and compound nerve and muscle potentials resulting from nerve stimulation. Surface electrodes are used as ground and reference electrodes.

ELECTRICAL PROPERTIES OF METAL ELECTRODES

The transmission of action potential waves across the metal-electrolyte interface which exists at the active surface of the recording electrodes where it contacts body tissues and fluids depends on combination of ions in the extracellular fluids with the electrode and discharge of ions from the electrode into solution. This complex electrochemical process can be described in simplified form as resulting in the formation of a charge gradient at the electrode surface. This can be visualized as two parallel layers of charge of opposite polarity. The electrical equivalent of this resembles a resistance, a capacitance, and a battery. The value of these elements is variable and unstable and depends upon the kind of metal, the electrolyte and its concentration, and the nature of the electric current being passed through the interface, among other factors (8).

The resistance and capacitance portion of the interface (which is in a circuit that is completed by the input impedance of the preamplifier) causes reduction in the amplitude and distortion in the slow portion of the recorded action potentials respectively, especially when small area needle electrodes are used. These effects are minimized by high input impedance preamplifiers.

Electrode offset potential (or polarization voltage), the voltage generated at the interface, may be in the order of 600 mV. This is usually not of any consequence since EMG equipment is designed to ignore fixed resting potentials because they are not components of the clinically recorded waves. However, these potentials are large and unstable, and when electrodes move, large abrupt changes in polarization voltage occur. This is a major source of artifact in EMG, because these transient *changes* in potential are amplified and appear as spike waves or discontinuities in the base line.

SURFACE ELECTRODES

A remarkably wide range of skin surface electrodes has been used to perform clinically useful EMG. The electrodes establish the ground (or zero reference potential) connection to the patient required to reduce externally induced electrical artifact as well as stimulus artifact. Surface electrodes are used for stimulation of peripheral nerves, for recording compound muscle action potentials in motor nerve conduction tests, for recording compound nerve action potentials, and as reference electrodes with monopolar needle electrodes. They are not used for studies of motor unit potentials.

The skin surface should be cleaned to remove perspiration, which is electrically conductive, from the general area of recording or stimulation. When stimulating, this reduces the possibility of conducting a portion of the large stimulating voltage to the nearby recording electrodes. During recording, this cleansing aids in reducing the area of recording and avoids reduction of action potential amplitudes by shunting effects. When recording low amplitude potentials, improved results can often be achieved by lightly abrading the skin under the electrodes to remove some of the high resistance superficial skin layers.

Bare metal electrode contact is made to the skin via electrically conductive electrode paste which reduces contact resistance, improves recording, and permits stimulation with less stimulus intensity, thus improving patient tolerance and reducing artifact. Excessive electrode paste on the skin surfaces should be avoided for the reasons mentioned above.

Surface electrodes may be discs, or rectangular or strip forms, of various size, with larger sizes used as ground electrodes. These electrodes, sometimes mounted as a pair on an insulating holder, are held in place with adhesive tape, straps, or with double faced adhesive tape die cut in a ring shape ("adhesive collars"). Small noose shape electrodes made of short lengths of coiled metal wire spring, for flexibility, designed to be slipped over the fingers or toes and then drawn tight, can be used for stimulation and recording. Finger electrodes made of short lengths of curved metal strips attached to each of the jaws of a common spring loaded "alligator" electrical clips are also used for recording or stimulation. Dual prong metal electrodes mounted in a plastic handle are used for stimulation; the stimulus intensity control may be located, as a convenience, in the handle (Fig. 15.2).

When mechanical movement occurs during a test, artifact is generated due to transient changes in the recording electrode metal-electrolyte interface. To minimize this effect, surface electrodes have been devised that remove the metal-electrolyte interface which is close to the metal surface from proximity to the skin surface. Contact between the metal and the skin is made solely via electrode paste that fills an insulating collar in the electrode (recessed electrodes), or by saline-saturated felt plugs that project from cup-shaped electrodes. Most movement, presumably, will then occur between the electrolyte and the skin surface, with minimum mechanical effect on the metal-electrolyte interface which is close to the metal surface (9).

A variant of this type of electrode utilizes metal discs with a domed impression in the center to retain electrode paste. These electrodes are

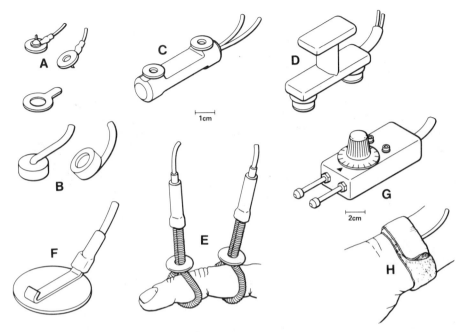

Fig. 15.2. Some surface electrodes. (A) Metal discs, shown with doublefaced adhesive collar sometimes used for attachment to skin; (B) metal discs with insulating collar uses electrode paste for contact to skin; (C) dual electrode for direct contact; (D) dual electrode utilizing saline saturated felt contacts; (E) spring ring electrode, moveable collar tightens noose; (F) typical metal disc ground electrode; (G) bipolar stimulating electrode with intensity control; and (H) wrap-around saline saturated fabric covered flexible metal electrode.

applied to the skin by means of double-sided adhesive tape rings without electrode paste, which would interfere with adhesion; the paste is then added after the electrodes are firmly in place, by means of a hypodermic syringe with a blunted needle via a hole in the domed center of the disc.

Metal electrodes covered with fabric or felt which must be soaked in saline before use are also used as ground and stimulating electrodes. A thin metal strip is stitched between two strips of velcro and wrapped around the extremity being tested and functions as a self-retaining ground electrode. A miniature version is used for stimulation of the fingers or toes. Stimulating electrodes comprising pairs of metal cups containing felt plugs which contact the skin are also used after soaking in saline. The metal used in these electrodes include silver, stainless steel, lead, tin, nickel, and German silver (alloy of nickel, copper, and zinc, also termed nickel silver).

NEEDLE ELECTRODES

Needle electrodes are used when activity of individual motor units or muscle fibers are studied since they permit a relatively small exploring surface which discriminates against distant activity to be placed near the

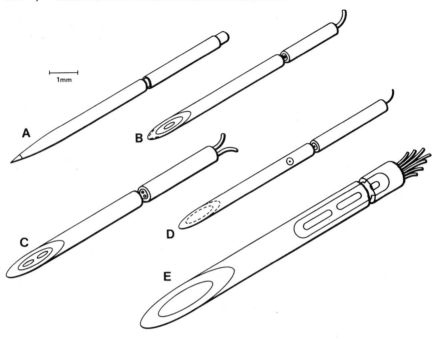

Fig. 15.3. Needle electrodes. (A) Monopolar needle electrode; (B) concentric needle electrodes, dashed lines show alternate point shape; (C) bipolar needle electrode; (D) single fiber needle electrode; and (E) multielectrode.

active tissue. Needle electrodes are also used for nerve stimulation, allowing the use of smaller stimulus intensity than is required for surface stimulation; a larger tip area than used for recording should be considered for needle electrodes used this way, to minimize high current density at the active surface (Fig. 15.3).

The monopolar electrode used by Jasper and Ballum in 1949 (10) is the simplest needle electrode. In current use it is a stainless steel needle properly tempered for strength and point stability, yet not brittle, approximately 0.4 mm in diameter coated with an insulating film of Teflon except at the very tip. While stainless steel is a poor electrode material, especially when used as a small area contact, it is almost universally used for monopolar needle electrodes because of its mechanical properties. A surface, bare subdermal needle or another monopolar needle reference electrode must be used, located near the monopolar recording electrode.

Advantages include simple relatively inexpensive construction and more uniform recorded potentials due to symmetrical nondirectional pickup pattern. Also, insertion and movement is well tolerated by the patient because of small diameter and anti-friction properties for Teflon coating. Disadvantages include the difficulty of standardizing the tip area; the exposed area increases with use because of the poor mechanical properties of the Teflon coating. The fragile coating is also easily susceptible to damage along the length of a needle and is nonrepairable. Also, a reference electrode in addition to a ground electrode is required. Tip area of 0.14 to 0.20 mm^2 is typical but may vary widely with manufacturer and will increase with use, causing reduction in amplitudes and, to some extent, in the sharpness of the recorded potentials.

Concentric needle electrodes described by Adrian and Bronk in 1929 (11) are comprised of a stainless steel hypodermic needle with an insulated wire (platinum, nichrome, or silver) within the lumen. The active electrode area is the bare surface of the wire where it emerges at the 15°, typical, bevel at the tip of the needle. The bare stainless steel cannula is the reference electrode. A separate ground electrode is required. Tubing diameters typically range from 23 to 28 hypodermic gauge. The exposed surface area of the active inner conductor ranges from 0.015 to 0.07 mm^2.

The advantages of the concentric electrode include the easily standardized exposed surface of the active electrode which remains constant with use. For this reason, the concentric (or coaxial) electrode has been used for many years in quantitative EMG studies (i.e., amplitude and duration measurement of motor unit potentials). No reference electrode is required. This electrode is not easily subject to damage and the tip is able to be resharpened. (Somewhat restricted pickup area and directional properties may be of use when searching.) Disadvantages include the directional property of the bevel, and less patient comfort than with the monopolar needle. Recent studies suggest positive waves may be more easily provoked with the monopolar needle.

The bipolar needle electrode is similar to the concentric electrode except that two insulated wires are placed within the cannula. Here the active areas (or the "active" and the "reference" electrodes) are the exposed surfaces of these wires at the bevel at the tip of the needle. This electrode has no polarity sense since both exposed recording surfaces are equal in area and symmetrical. Neither can really be termed exploring or reference.

The outer surface of the cannula is the ground or zero potential electrode connection to the patient. The connecting cable to this electrode is identified by its three terminals, the two active recording terminals and the ground terminal.

Advantages are that the recording range is most restricted and somewhat directional and isolated motor unit activity can sometimes be seen during strong contraction. Electrical symmetry of the recording surfaces makes this electrode least susceptible to electrical artifact since it permits the differential amplifier properties of the EMG to be most effective. No additional patient electrodes are required; all three required contacts are self-contained. The major disadvantage is that the recording range is too restricted for routine EMG. Recorded potentials appear smaller (due to close spacing of the recording surfaces) and of shorter duration than those recorded with other needle electrodes. Tubing diameters used in the construction of this electrode must of necessity be somewhat larger than with other electrodes.

Many electromyographers do not consider a single type of electrode to be ideal for all of their work and use monopolar and concentric electrodes, taking advantage of each to achieve their desired objectives (12). When quantitative EMG studies are reported, the materials and dimensions of the needle tip should be noted, since these parameters can significantly effect the results.

Other more special purpose needle electrodes include the needle multi-electrode, which is constructed of hypodermic tubing approximately 1 mm in diameter with a number of recording surfaces brought out flush with the tubing surface through an opening along the length of the needle. Fourteen such surfaces are typically used (13). The known spacing between the recording surfaces makes it possible to use this electrode to determine motor unit territory by recording the electrical activity of the same motor unit from the various recording surfaces.

Flexible wire electrodes are useful in kinesiological studies and in other studies where rigid needle electrodes would interfere in the relative sliding motion of overlaying muscles. These electrodes consist of fine insulated wires which are inserted singly or in pairs by first threading them through a hypodermic needle, hooking the exposed end of the wires around the tip of the needle, and then leaving the wires in place within the muscle by withdrawing the hypodermic needle after properly localizing the wire ends within the muscle (14). Other techniques do not thread the wire through the needle but merely hook the ends of the wire which are outside the needle around the tip of the needle a short distance into the lumen. It is then inserted into the muscle, drawing the wire within the muscle along the outside of the needle, which is then withdrawn leaving the wire in place.

A variant of the concentric needle electrode is used to study the activity of single muscle fibers of the motor unit (SFEMG). This electrode utilizes a (one or more) small area, 25 μ diameter recording surface which is brought out to the surface of the needle via a small hole drilled through the wall of the hypodermic tubing a short distance from the tip (15, 16). The small recording surface, which is small relative to the average muscle fiber diameter, is flush with the outer smooth surface of the tubing wall, permitting recording from uninjured single muscle fibers. Its restricted pickup area and very directional properties permit this electrode to pick up single fiber action potentials from uninjured fibers when sufficient care and patience is utilized in localizing the electrode. Similar designs have also been described utilizing a number of recording surfaces brought out through the side wall of the needle, extending the scope of single fiber recording. Recording from these small areas, high impedance electrodes requires high impedance amplifiers (in the order of 100 megohms).

SUMMARY OF ELECTRODE PERFORMANCE FACTORS

Location

The shape and amplitude of the recorded potentials depend entirely upon the location of the electrodes relative to the source of the potentials. The amplitude of the recorded motor unit action potential will decrease exponentially with the distance between the needle tip and source of electrical activity. In addition, the high frequency components (that is, the sharp rapidly changing portions of the action potential wave), will be lost as the distance increases. Motor units recorded at a distance will then have a low thudding sound compared to the sharp "ticking" sibilant sound made by motor unit activity close to the needle tip. For this reason, the search with the needle within the muscle is of vital importance in obtaining truly characteristic motor unit activity.

The location of the surface electrodes in recording the compound action potential in motor nerve conduction time testing will determine the shape and polarity of the recorded waves. In duplicating standard technique, attention should be paid to this factor, the most common location being one electrode over the motor point or the muscle belly, the other near the distal tendon. Some techniques, however, call out particular spacing, usually in the order of 3 or 4 cm between the two surface recording electrodes.

When separate connectors are provided on the EMG amplifier for use as the active and reference input terminals, the user can establish the EMG trace deflection polarity sense (negative up or positive up) of his choosing for concentric electrodes by first determining from the manufacturer the deflection polarity sense, on the CRT screen, of the two terminals. They are electrically symmetrical, a negative voltage into one terminal will deflect the trace up while a positive voltage into the same terminal will deflect the trace down, the opposite obtained with the other terminal. Obtaining the desired polarity sense simply requires that the active electrode wire be connected consistently to the desired terminal. When a single multipin polarized input connector is used, the polarity sense is established by the internal connector wiring when using concentric electrodes.

The patient ground electrode should not be placed over a muscle. A location over a bony or tendonous area will minimize pickup of unwanted muscle activity by this electrode.

Area

The variations in area of surface electrodes used in clinical EMG are of little significance. Variations in the smaller areas encountered in needle electrodes greatly effect the recorded waves. When recording near the action potential source, the amplitude and sharpness of the recorded wave will be higher with small area needle electrodes than with larger area electrodes. As the recording surface area gets smaller and approaches the size of the source of potentials, a maximal difference in potential will be recorded between it and the reference electrode. On the other hand, larger tip surfaces will be in contact with a greater area of tissue, some of which is inactive, and the resulting signal, which will be an average, will have lower amplitude. If the larger area tip is within the area of influence of two sources, the resultant of the two sources will be recorded. Large area needles will, therefore, tend to record more polyphasic activity. These points are exemplified by the small area single fiber electrode which records potentials of high amplitude.

It should be noted that needle electrodes with very small exposed area have very high metal-electrolyte interface impedances, that is, they are characterized by high series resistance and small series capacitance. As a consequence of this, they must be connected to amplifiers with high input impedance to avoid serious reduction in recorded amplitudes and distortion in the recorded waves. The input impedance of these preamplifiers should also have low shunt capacitance components to minimize loss of high frequency information from the high impedance small area needle electrodes. Large area surface electrodes put much less constraint on the input impedance requirements of the preamplifier, provided proper contact is made with the skin surface. Large area electrodes also generate less electrical noise than small area needle electrodes.

Shape

The symmetrical conical shape of the monopolar needle electrode has Omni directional recording properties, of value in a searching electrode. The bevel of the recording surface of the concentric electrodes gives them directional properties. From an electrical standpoint, symmetrical recording surfaces of equal area are desirable (when possible) to minimize artifact pickup by maximizing the differential amplifier performance of the system.

Materials, Sterilization

The materials used in electrode construction are chosen to meet some obvious mechanical strength requirements (especially in the needle electrodes) and to be relatively chemically inactive. Metals used for the inner core of concentric electrodes include platinum, silver and nickel-chromium alloy (nichrome). Electrolytic etching of platinum core concentric electrodes (by passing current through the electrode while immersed in a saline solution) has been recommended to reduce electrode impedance and noise and improve fidelity.

Metals and plastics used in some needle electrode construction will withstand the time and temperatures involved in steam autoclaving. Some needle electrode lead wires and connectors are not autoclavable. Those that are not are sometimes arranged to be disconnected from the autoclavable needle. Autoclaving time and pressure instructions provided by the electrode manufacturer should be carefully followed to ensure adequate electrode service life. [One hour autoclaving has been recommended to avoid transmission of certain slow viruses (17)].

A number of laboratories are successfully using gas sterilization; however, some plastics might be sensitive to some of the gas sterilizing agents. Electrodes should be thoroughly outgassed after gas sterilization because of the tendency of plastic materials to retain the sterilizing agent.

When possible, especially when attempting to record very small potentials, the electrodes in contact with the patient should be of the same metal. Silver surface electrodes provide less noise and the greatest stability and, in some cases, reduce stimulus artifact. Each electrode should be designed so that dissimilar metals do not contact the patient or the electrode paste since the electrochemical activity between the dissimilar metals and the electrode paste might cause artifact. For this reason, when a solder joint is made between a lead wire and a surface electrode, this contact should be electrically insulated or care should be exercised to avoid simultaneous contact between the electrode paste, the solder, and the metal electrode.

Maintenance

Electrode and electrode lead wire movement are insidious sources of artifact which often mimic action potentials. It is, therefore, important to stabilize both the lead wire and the electrode during examinations. All electrodes and lead wires should be carefully inspected and cleaned after every use, since foreign matter can be a significant source of noise in both needles and surface electrodes.

Visual and electrical inspection of needle electrodes should be carried out after each use before autoclaving. This should include visual inspection (using at least a 6× loupe or preferably a low power binocular dissecting microscope) and testing for electrical continuity and insulation. The visual inspection should note the condition of the point. Monopolar needles cannot be resharpened; broken or bent points must result in discarding the needle. Also, note the amount of needle tip exposed. Discard the electrode when the distance from tip to the Teflon coating becomes greater than the diameter of the needle. This process is accelerated by contact with bone tendon and fibrotic tissue. Since punctures and tears in the Teflon coating cannot be repaired, monopolar needles should be handled carefully to protect the relatively soft coating.

Concentric needles with bent or broken points can be resharpened on a fine hypodermic needle sharpening stone or 400–600 grit wet-grinding paper. The concentric needle should also be inspected to determine that the inner conductor is present and clean, since this inner conductor can be corroded during use.

Electrical inspection requires the use of an ohmmeter, a commonly available inexpensive meter. The other materials required are normal saline solution and hydrophilic cotton or sponges.

Note: The following tests indicate gross faults in electrode insulation and electrical continuity; other more complex measurements are required to determine impedance and other quantitative electrical characteristics of electrodes.

Monopolar needles are electrically inspected or tested to determine the electrical continuity of the plug, lead wire, and needle point and to rule out the presence of holes in the Teflon coating. Connect the needle plug to one terminal of the ohmmeter and use an ohmmeter test lead covered with saline-saturated cotton or sponge as the other terminal (Fig. 15.4). When the point of the monopolar needle is applied to the saturated cotton covered lead, a reading of less than a few thousand ohms should be noted, indicating electrical continuity. No reading (very high resistance) should be obtained when the needle is touched elsewhere upon its length (except possibly a few millimeters from the handle), indicating the Teflon insulation is intact.

The testing for concentric needles is more simple (Fig. 15.4). Connect *both* terminals of the needle to the ohmmeter. No reading, very high resistance, should result, demonstrating that no short circuit exists. Dip the needle into a container continuing the saline solution; a reading of less than a few thousand ohms should result. This indicates intact connection between

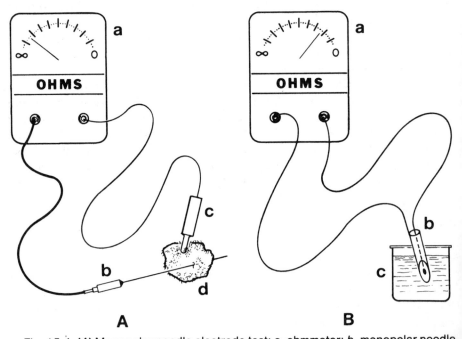

Fig. 15.4. (*A*) Monopolar needle electrode test: *a*, ohmmeter; *b*, monopolar needle electrode connected to ohmmeter; *c*, test lead with probe; *d*, saline saturated cotton or sponge covering the probe tip. Meter shows high resistance when saline soaked cotton is in contact with intact insulating coating—a defect in the coating would cause the meter to read low resistance. The reading should be less than a few thousand ohms when the cotton is in contact with exposed tip (and also perhaps within a few millimeters of the handle). A high reading in this second test indicates an occluded tip or broken lead wire or plug connection. (*B*) Concentric needle electrode test: *a*, ohmmeter; *b*, concentric needle electrode connected to ohmmeter; *c*, container with saline solution. Meter shows low resistance when tip is immersed in saline solution, indicating electrical continuity and properly exposed tip. A high resistance reading obtained with the electrode tip dry indicates that no short circuit exists.

plugs, connecting wires, and electrodes. When the tip of the needle is wiped dry, the reading should increase to at least many megohms. Electrolytic activity will cause meter readings to drift in these tests.

Needle electrodes should not be immersed in saline solution while connected to the ohmmeter for unnecessary long periods in order to avoid electrolytic changes which occur due to the current flow through the solution from the battery in the meter. In these tests, it would be preferable that the negative ohmmeter terminal be connected to the monopolar needle or inner conductor lead wire, with the positive ohmmeter terminal connected to the saturated cotton or the cannular lead wire. This precaution will further minimize the effects of electrolysis on the electrodes. A voltmeter would then be required to determine the polarity of the ohmmeter terminals.

A remarkably common source of noisy or distorted recordings is a fault in the connection somewhere between the preamplifier terminal and the electrical contact at the patient in the active, reference, or ground electrode path. This can sometimes be overlooked because a record, albeit poor, is often still obtained even in the absence of the requisite three connections. The fault may be within the connecting wires, at the connection with the electrical connectors, or between the connecting wires and the electrodes. Considerable stress and flexing at these points can result in a break or intermittent failure of the wires within the insulation at these points. These faults can be detected with an ohmmeter by flexing and stressing the wire at these points while making the measurement.

The EMG Amplifier System

INPUT IMPEDANCE

The input impedance of modern EMG preamplifiers can be represented by a resistance of from 10 to 100 megohms (1 megohm, 10^6 ohms or 1,000,000 ohms) shunted by a capacitor of 10 to 100 pF (1 pF, 10^{-12} F or one millionth of a microfarad). This impedance is in series with the metal-electrolyte junction impedances at the electrode tip, and together they form a voltage divider. This voltage divider effect reduces the amplitude of the action potentials that appear at the input terminals of the preamplifier and somewhat distorts them (18). These undesirable effects are minimized by making the input impedance many times higher than the highest anticipated electrode impedance (especially important in SFEMG where small area, high impedance electrodes must be used). The electrode impedance is difficult to state and measure since it is a function of voltage, current, and test signal frequency used to measure it. Nonetheless, the capacitative portion of this impedance causes the electrode to conduct rapid changes in wave forms better than slower ones. High input impedance also enhances the interference rejection properties of the differential amplifier, which would otherwise be degraded when using recording electrodes which substantially differ in area (e.g., concentric needle electrodes).

The high resistance portion of the input impedance (50–100 megohms is easily achieved with modern semiconductor amplifiers) also minimizes the amplitude loss by voltage divider action with the resistance portion of the electrode impedance. The capacitative portion of the input impedance should be as small as possible, since a large capacitance (large capacitance results in *low* impedance) here would shunt high frequencies or rapid changes in the action potentials and not permit them to be amplified by the preamplifier. The minimum value of capacitance is limited by the physical presence of conductors in the input circuit. Electrostatic shielding* to minimize extraneous pickup serves to increase this capacitance. The capacitative portion in the input impedance ranges from 20 to 100 pE in clinical EMG amplifiers. (Where long shielded leads are required, the driven shield method involving additional circuitry achieves the effects of shielding with minimal additional increase in shunt capacitance.)

Since the differential amplifier has two recording electrode terminals and a common ground or zero potential terminal, input impedance measured between the input terminals is often specified as the differential or balanced input impedance, and the impedance measured between the input terminals and the common terminal is often also specified as the common mode input impedance.

DIFFERENTIAL AMPLIFIER

A conventional amplifier has two input terminals and amplifies potentials that appear between them. The differential amplifier has three input terminals, two recording electrode input terminals and a ground or zero potential terminal. The differential amplifier amplifies potentials that appear as difference-potentials between the two input terminals and discriminates against potentials that appear equally at both of the input terminals when measured to the ground terminal. The recording electrodes connected to the input terminals of the differential amplifier used in EMG are connected to the patient in such a way so that the potential to be amplified appears between them. The body is a relatively uniformly good conductor of electricity and, therefore, interference potentials (coupled to the patient from the power wiring and electrical appliances in the examining room) will appear almost uniformly at both recording electrodes, which are close to each other, but relatively distant from the source of interference. Interfer-

---

* Electrostatic shielding refers to an electrically conductive sheath or enclosure surrounding circuits or devices. The shield is connected to ground and acts to prevent undesirable capacitive coupling of external voltages to the elements within the shield. Where the elements within the shield are the source of undesirable potentials, the shielding prevents coupling to external circuits and devices. Cables are shielded, for example, by enclosing them in braided flexible metallic sleeves that are insulated from the conductors and grounded. The shield can add significant capacitance from the conductors to ground, reducing impedance and possibly compromising high frequency performance. (Where magnetic fields cause problems, iron or magnetically permeable alloys are used as the shield materials.)

ence potentials measured on a typical patient can be much greater than the action potentials to be recorded in EMG.

The operation of the differential amplifier may be understood by considering it to be made up of two conventional amplifiers, each with a single input terminal and a common ground terminal, the only difference being that the output of one of the amplifiers is always exactly of opposite polarity to the other. These amplifiers are then connected to a summing circuit which provides an output signal equal to the sum of the outputs of each of the amplifiers.

Consider the output that will result when the following input voltages are applied to the two input terminals of the differential amplifier for two input situations: a) identical inputs, b) differing inputs. In case a), the output of the summing circuit will be zero if the inputs to the amplifiers are identical (identical inputs result in two signals of opposite polarity which cancel each other in the summing circuit). In case b), the output will be proportional to the difference in potential that exists between the input terminals of each amplifier. This is the performance we desire from the differential amplifier. The input terminal of each amplifier comprise the two recording electrode connections of the differential amplifier. Interference potentials in common on both input terminals are cancelled and action potentials which appear as a voltage difference between the recording electrodes are amplified (Fig. 15.5).

The interference is usually externally induced power line interference potential. It could just as well be a stimulus artifact; the stimulus would have to be at a sufficient distance from the recording electrodes and arranged symmetrically with respect to them so that the stimulus artifact impinged on both recording electrodes equally, permitting the differential cancelling effect to take place. The desired signal (action potential) is termed the differential signal or the difference mode signal. The undesired signal (interference potential), which is cancelled by the differential action of the differential amplifier, is termed the common mode signal.

Under idealized conditions, the common mode signal is totally cancelled and disappears from the output. In practice, however, the common mode signal is not totally cancelled for a number of reasons. It is not possible to build the differential amplifier so that the signal applied to each input terminal is amplified exactly equal, especially at all frequencies; also the common mode signal does not always appear at the input terminals of the amplifier at exactly the same amplitude. Obviously, when using a concentric needle electrode, for example, one recording electrode is the tiny tip of the inner conductor while the other recording electrode is the large surface area of the stainless steel cannula. This means that the impedance of one electrode will be much higher than the impedance of the other electrode. Consequently, when a common mode signal reaches the concentric electrode, these two impedances, which form a voltage divider with the input impedance of each half of the differential amplifier, will cause the common signal to appear at different amplitudes at the inputs of the differential amplifier, and they will, therefore, not be cancelled. This effect, whereby unequal electrode impedances permit common mode interfering signals to defeat the common mode rejection properties of the differential amplifier, is minimized by making the input impedance of the preamplifier high, since this high input impedance minimizes the difference in voltage divider action resulting from differences in electrode contact impedance.

Common Mode Rejection Ratio

A technical measure of the ability of a differential amplifier to discriminate against common mode signals is called its common mode rejection ratio (CMRR). The common mode rejection ratio is determined by measuring the differential amplification of a differential amplifier by connecting a test signal generator between its active input terminals (a differential input signal) and then measuring the common mode amplification of the amplifier by connecting a test signal to the two active input terminals, shorted together as a common point with the other terminal of the generator connected to the common ground connection of the amplifier (common mode signal). Obviously, the differential amplifier will exhibit much less amplification when driven with a common mode signal (the second case) because of the cancellation effect described earlier than it will when it is driven in its differential mode (in the first case). The common mode rejection ratio is the ratio of the differential amplification to the amplification in the common mode case (Fig. 15.6).

Common mode rejection ratios achievable in the laboratory by careful adjustments to each of the two halves of the differential amplifier are in the order of many hundreds of thousands to one at a particular test frequency. Maintenance of high common mode rejection ratio is difficult over a wide range of test frequencies. When practical needle electrodes are used, unequal electrode interface impedances are connected to the input terminals. This reduces common mode rejection ratios to less than 100:1 over a range of frequencies.

A method of measurement of the actual common mode rejection ratio of an amplifier with a concentric needle electrode in situ, as described in a report by Guld, Rosenfalck, and Willison (19), would provide actual values (and provides a check on seriously increased electrode impedance as well), since this test accounts for all major parameters, e.g., needle interface impedance, cable shield capacitance, amplifier input impedances, and amplifier common mode rejection; it would be valid only at the sine wave frequencies tested. Fortunately, as a practical matter, adequate common mode rejection is usually available to permit satisfactory clinical EMG under most conductions.

FREQUENCY RESPONSE

The wave shapes encountered in EMG range from the relatively slowly changing compound muscle action potential wave of motor nerve conduction tests (which can have duration of many tens of milliseconds) to the rapid

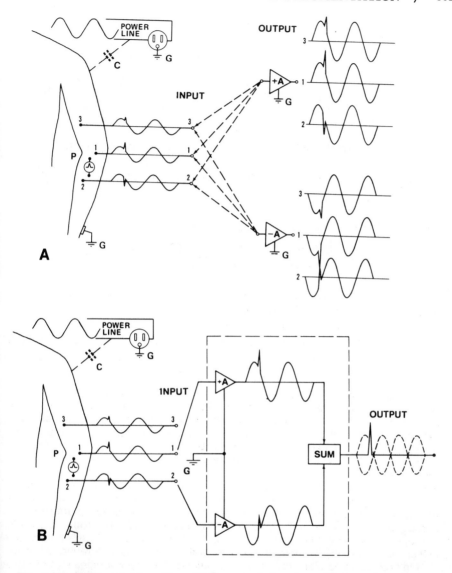

Fig. 15.5. Differential Amplifier. (A) Two single input amplifiers, +A and −A, are connected to electrodes in various locations with respect to action potential generator P in subject influenced by 60 Hz power line interference. The outputs of each amplifier for three electrode locations are shown. Each amplifier and the subject are connected to a common ground G. Amplifier +A and amplifier −A are conventional amplifiers having two input terminals, one connected to the signal source and the other a ground connection to complete the input circuit. Amplifier −A is identical to amplifier +A except for the fact that its output potentials always have the opposite polarity as its input. The power line is inducing sinusoidal power line interference into the subject by capacitance effects C. Each amplifier is connected in turn to electrode location 1, 2, and 3 where the input voltages are as shown. The output of each amplifier, shown appropriately larger because of the amplification effects, is also shown for each of the electrode locations tested, which are also labelled 1, 2,

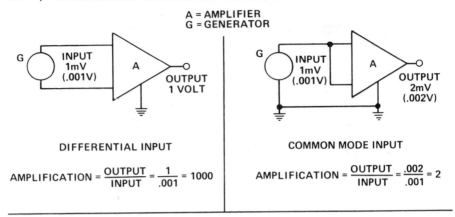

Fig. 15.6. Common mode rejection ratio (CMRR).

$$\text{CMRR} = \frac{\text{DIFFERENTIAL AMPLIFICATION}}{\text{COMMON MODE AMPLIFICATION}} = \frac{1000}{2} = 500.$$

0.1 msec positive-to-negative transition phase of a motor unit action potential recorded with needle electrodes.

The shape of these waves as seen on the CRT screen depends upon electrode configuration and their location and is mediated by factors which

3. The sine wave interference is about the same for each electrode location. The induced interference affects the body essentially uniformly and the electrode locations are in close proximity to each other relative to the interference source. The action potential, which is severely contaminated by interference, has a polarity that is dependent on the electrode location relative to the source of the action potential P. Location 3 has the smallest action potential because it is at the greatest distance. Locations 1 and 2 have opposite polarity because they are nearest opposite terminals of the hypothetical action potential generator P. When the outputs are examined, note that the amplified interference wave at the output of $-A$ amplifier is always the opposite polarity image of the sine wave interference portion of the output of the $+A$ amplifier. The action potential, however, at the output of $+A$, electrode location 1 is the same polarity as the output of $-A$, electrode location 2. This property is used in the differential amplifier (Fig. 15.5B). (B) The two separate amplifiers in 15.5A are combined into a hypothetical single differential amplifier (which in fact contains elements of two amplifiers). The input terminals of the two amplifiers are arranged so that they share a common ground terminal. The active input terminal of each of the two amplifiers become the two active inputs that characterize the differential amplifier. The 1 and 2 electrodes are used because electrode 3 is too distant from P. The outputs of amplifiers A and $-A$ are added or summed to produce the output of the differential amplifier. With the inputs connected to the 1 and 2 electrode locations as shown, the sine wave interference portion of the outputs are of opposite polarity so that they cancel each other when they are summed. However the action potential portions are of the same polarity and reinforce each other when they are summed. The differential amplifier has thus rejected the interference wave and amplified the action potential. (Total cancellation of the interference in this idealized example assumes exact symmetry of electrodes, volume conductor paths and amplifiers, conditions not realized in practice.)

include a) the electrical impedance (series resistance and capacitance) of the electrode-electrolyte interface at the needle tip, b) the EMG amplifier input impedance (shunt resistance and shunt capacitance, including shunt capacitance of the electrode cable shield), and c) the frequency response properties of the EMG amplifier.

Amplifiers can be designed so that their output responds to static values of input potentials, e.g., resting potential or potentials that do not change continuously (or that change very slowly) with time. These are called DC Amplifiers. Amplifiers can, as well, permit response to potentials which change much faster than the fastest biological potentials.

If the response of the EMG amplifier encompasses the slowest and fastest components of waves to be encountered, it will not materially distort the recorded waves. An amplifier's ability to respond to fast and slow changes can be expressed in a number of ways. One method involves application of a step wave or a square wave to the input of the amplifier and then notation of the rise time and droop or decay time of the output wave, which will not have the instantaneous rise nor the perfectly flat top of the test input wave (Fig. 15.9, see step wave bottom trace A, B, C).

A more common method is to apply sine wave test signals of various frequencies but of equal amplitude to the input terminals and then to plot, versus frequency, the relative amplitude of the sine waves at the output for the various test frequencies. This plot, termed a "frequency response curve," will appear for a simple amplifier, as shown in Figure 15.7. It will show decreasing output voltage for sine waves below some frequency f_l and above some frequency f_h. The output voltage for sine waves between f_l and f_h will be more or less uniform. The range of frequencies between f_l and f_h is the "bandwidth" or "passband" of the EMG amplifier. This band extends from 2 Hz to 10 kHz for clinical EMG systems. The frequencies f_h and f_l and the frequency response curve of the amplifier can be mathematically related to the rise and decay time of the amplifiers, respectively; either can be used to predict or specify amplifier dynamic performance.

Sine waves are used in calculating the impedance of resistor capacitor circuits as well in determining the bandwidth of amplifiers, since they are the only wave forms which pass through these frequency response determining circuits without change in shape, the only effect being relative change in amplitude (and phase) with change in frequency.

The sine wave bandwidth of an amplifier can be used to predict its response to other nonsinusoidal input wave forms even EMG potentials, because nonsinusoidal time varying waves can be analyzed in terms of sine waves by the technique of harmonic analysis. The harmonic analysis method describes a nonsinusoidal wave as a sum of sine waves of various frequencies and amplitudes. These sine waves, termed harmonics, when added together, will form the original nonsinusoidal wave. Thus, the stated bandwidth requirements, 2 Hz to 10 kHz, of a clinical EMG amplifier mean that there are no harmonics of significance expected above or below the stated band-

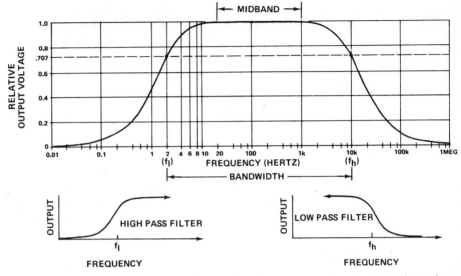

Fig. 15.7. Frequency response curve. The frequency response curve shows how the output of an amplifier will change when constant voltage sine waves of various frequencies are applied to the input. Frequency is plotted on a logarithmic horizontal axis. Relative output voltage is on the vertical axis. (Relative output voltage is obtained by dividing the actual output by the midband output voltage. This makes the midband relative output voltage 1, thus simplifying the notation.) The bandwidth of the amplifier is that range of frequencies over which the relative output voltage is more than 0.707 and is defined on the graph by f_l and f_h, the low and high cutoff frequencies. Stated another way, one might say that the amplification of the amplifier is uniform for all frequencies within its bandwidth to within 0.707 of its midband value. (The relative output voltage is often expressed in decibels (dB), an engineering notation that derives from the logarithm of the ratio of two voltages. The voltage ratio of 0.707 is −3dB in decibel rotation. $dB = 20 \log \frac{V1}{V2}$.) The bandwidth of the amplifier is adjusted by setting high pass and low pass filters in the amplifier. The high pass filter passes all frequencies above f_l, thus establishing the low frequency limit of the amplifier. The low pass filter passes all frequencies below f_h, setting the high frequency limit of the amplifier as shown in the frequency response curves for typical filters. Together they establish the bandwidth of the system. The shape of the frequency response curves shown is typical for many amplifiers. However, filter designs used to achieve special noise performance effects result in more rapid falloff of the curves outside of the midband region. Specification of f_l and f_h and the performance of the amplifier may be modified in these cases.

width limits in the EMG waves being recorded. The low frequency harmonics relate to the slowly changing portion of the waves while the high frequency harmonics relate to the rapid changes in the waves.

Filters

The frequency response of the EMG amplifier is intentionally limited to the harmonics of the waves being studied and does not extend appreciably above or below them for the following reasons. Extending the low frequency response materially below 2 Hz would permit slow artifact potentials originating from electrode polarization potentials and from electrode or lead wire movements to cause the base line of the EMG trace to wander excessively. If the high frequency response extends substantially above 10 kHz, high frequency resistance thermal noise and amplifier noise which appear as a thickening of the base line and hissing noises in the loudspeaker would excessively contaminate the results. The bandwidth of the amplifier is adjusted to encompass only the significant harmonics of the potentials being recorded, thus excluding noise and artifact frequencies that fall above and below the bandwidth limits.

High and low frequency response limits are selectively reduced by means of filters, to reduce the high and low frequency noise in the system when performing certain tests where the full bandwidth of the system is not required. High and low pass filters are frequency selective, usually resistance-capacitance circuits, that shape the high and low limits of the frequency response curve of the amplifier (Fig. 15.7).

For example, in routine needle EMG where long duration slowly changing waves are not encountered, the low frequency response limit can be moved from 2 Hz to 20 Hz, thus additionally reducing base line wander; the high frequency setting should be set at maximum so as not to distort the fibrillation potentials and rapid transition portions of motor unit action potentials. (In SFEMG where base line stability is of paramount importance and low frequency components are of no concern, the low frequency response limit is moved to 500 Hz.)

Conversely, the high frequency limit can be reduced, if desired, from 10 kHz to 3 or 4 kHz in electroneurography, thus materially reducing the high frequency noise which becomes obvious at the sensitivity setting required to record small nerve potentials (Fig. 15.8). The reduced high frequency response can be tolerated here because the neurograms do not usually contain rapid deflections, and the primary object of the test is to record a latency. In addition, the low frequency response can be decreased in these tests from 2 Hz to 20 or 50 Hz to reduce base line fluctuations.

When performing motor nerve conduction tests when the duration and amplitude of the compound motor action potential wave is to be measured (in addition to the more common latency measurement), the low frequency limit should be set to 2 Hz to accommodate the slow portions of the recorded waves without distortion. Figure 15.9 shows the effects of limiting the high and low frequency settings on records and their effects on a step calibration wave.

AMPLIFIER NOISE MEASUREMENT

The noise originating within the amplifier should be measured by observing the screen at maximum amplification with the input terminals shorted (this is accomplished by setting the EMG to the "calibrate" setting in many

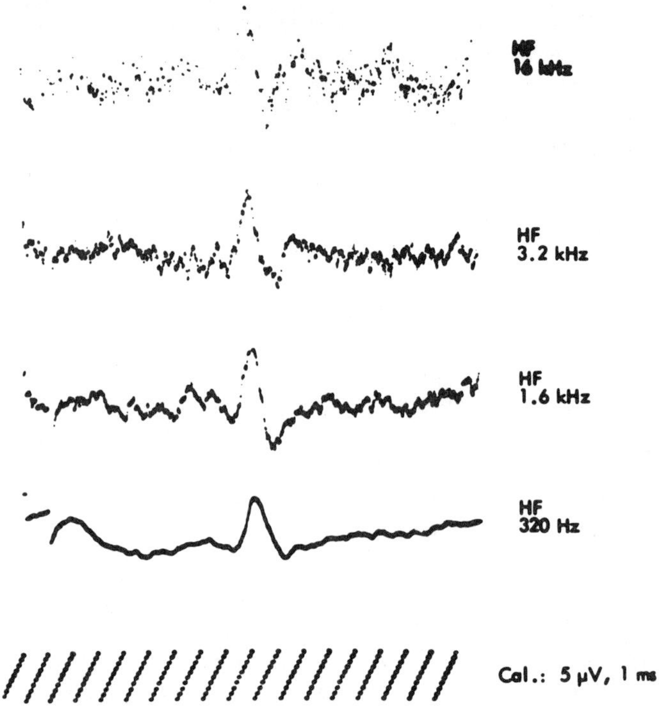

Fig. 15.8. Neurograms recorded with various high frequency bandwidth limits. Records were made by stimulating the finger and recording over the ulnar nerve at the elbow with surface electrodes. The high frequency response of the amplifier was progressively reduced from the top trace down. The bottom calibration trace is 5 μV and time between peaks in 1 msec. The low frequency limit was 32 Hz for all records. The high frequency limit was reduced from 16 kHz for the top record to 3.2 kHz, 1.6 kHz and to 320 Hz for the lowest record. The top record shows all the effects of system, electrode, and bioelectric noise. The noise was effectively filtered in the third record (1.6 kHz); however, the fourth record (320 Hz), which is cosmetically cleanest, shows the effects of excessive filtering which introduces error by reducing the apparent peak-to-peak amplitude of the recorded potential.

instruments) and with the filters set for maximum bandwidth (which should be stated for the noise measurement to be valid). The internal noise then appears as irregular fluctuations in the base line and as fuzzy thickening of the trace and is heard on the loudspeaker as hissing and rumbling. The apparent noise increases as the bandwidth of the amplifier is increased. (Any resistance larger than a short circuit connected across the input terminals will also increase the apparent internal noise.) Peak-to-peak noise measurements on screen require estimation of the "thickness" of the base line trace and are quite subjective due to the random nature of the noise.

High impedance EMG amplifiers designed for needle electrodes exhibit random peak-to-peak noise of from 5 to 10 μV when set for 2 Hz to 10 kHz bandwidth (shorted input). These measurements require estimation due to

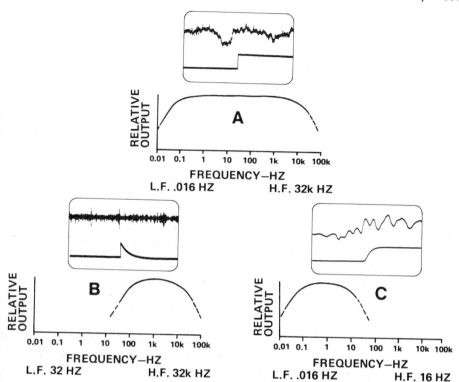

Fig. 15.9. Demonstrating the effect of filter settings on recorded action potentials and a step wave calibration signal. Frequency response curves are shown below the potentials for each of the three sets of filter settings. (A) Records were made with the amplifier set for maximum high and low frequency response, .016 Hz to 32 kHz. The upper trace shows rapid high frequency activity as well as slow baseline excursions. The step calibration wave below shows a rapid rise due to the extended high frequency response. This is followed by a steady deflection with no droop, the result of extended low frequency response. (B) The high frequency limit remains unchanged, but the low frequency filter setting has been moved up to 32 Hz. The high frequency information in the upper trace remains but the slow variations have been filtered out. The portion of the step wave following the rapid rise shows considerable decay due to reduction in low frequency response. (C) The low frequency setting is .016 Hz, as in A, but the high frequency filter setting is lowered to 16 Hz. All the high frequency variations in the upper trace have been filtered, leaving the slowly changing potentials. The step wave now has a slow rise because of severely reduced high frequency response, followed by a steady deflection with no decay, the result of the extended low frequency response. *Note*: The settings shown are not used in routine EMG. They were chosen to be most effective for demonstration.

the random nature of the noise and depend, among other factors, upon sweep speed and beam intensity used to observe the noise and observer bias which make peak-to-peak noise measurement ambiguous. A method called tangential noise measurement reduces the ambiguity of noise measurement from the screen to about 20% (20); it results in noise voltages one-third the peak-to-peak estimates and requires some additional equipment.

Noise voltages are sometimes measured in microvolts root mean square (RMS) with a meter instead of peak-to-peak values obtained from observing the CRT screen. A meter measurement of an alternating current presents problems because current flows equally in both directions, and the meter may be used for measurement of current of various waveshapes. When any alternating current of a given RMS magnitude is applied to a resistor, it will cause the same heating in the resistor as a DC of the same magnitude applied to the same resistance. For cyclic waveforms, e.g., sine or square waves, a simple relationship exists between the peak value of the AC observed on a CRT and its RMS value. (Power line voltage is specified as an RMS voltage and is 0.707 times the sine wave peak value of the voltage.) However, when RMS values of amplifier random noise voltages are specified, there is no simple relationship to the random peaks observed on the CRT screen. In practice, peak-to-peak values from observation of the screen will be approximately five or six times the RMS voltage obtained by RMS meter measurement. The conditions and methods of measurement must be specified before careful comparisons of any of the amplifier parameters can be made.

When an electrode position in tissue is changed or when the needle electrode is initially inserted, transient changes in electrode polarization voltage appear which may be hundreds of times greater than the action potentials the amplifier is adjusted to record. These large voltage changes "overload" the amplifier for a period of time, during which potentials cannot be recorded with acceptable fidelity. This time, termed "blocking time," should be less than 1 sec in a clinical EMG, since insertion potentials which occur after needle movement are of clinical interest. Smaller overloads originating from bioelectric sources should not result in blocking, so as to permit observation of small sensory potentials in the presence of large motor potentials.

The EMG Display

The cathode ray tube, which permits visualization of the EMG potentials, consists of an evacuated funnel shaped envelope with a source of electrons at the small end and a glass face coated on the inside with a screen material which fluoresces upon being struck by electrons, called a "phosphor," at the large end. The electrons are released from the electrically heated cathode into the vacuum surrounding it. They are then formed into a narrow beam and accelerated toward the screen by a series of electrodes maintained at a potential positive with respect to the cathode. This positive potential attracts electrons and accelerates them toward the screen. The beam-forming electrodes are shaped and maintained at relative potentials to each other so as to form lens-like electrostatic fields which form and focus the electrons into a sharply collimated beam. This assembly is the electron gun.

The positive accelerating potentials of many thousands of volts cause the electrons to hit the flourescent screen with sufficient energy to generate a bright spot of visible light on the screen. The color and persistence, or afterglow, of the light after extinguishing the electron beam is determined by the formulation of the phosphor and the beam accelerating potential. The accelerated beam, after leaving the electron gun, passes between two sets of deflecting plates within the tube, one set arranged horizontally and the other vertically. The negatively charged particles (electrons) comprising the beam can be attracted or repelled by voltages applied to these deflecting plates. Applying appropriate applied voltages to these plates can deflect the beam as it passes between them, causing the spot of impact at the screen to move vertically in response to the voltage applied to the vertical (Y) deflection plates and horizontally in response to the voltage applied to the horizontal (X) deflection plates. (This beam deflection method is termed electrostatic deflection.) The EMG potential is applied to the Y plates, and the time base, or sweep signal, which is a sawtooth wave, is applied to the X plates. The sawtooth wave voltage increases uniformly with time, then returns very quickly to its starting value and repeats. This uniformly changing voltage moves the spot from left to right at constant velocity across the screen and returns it rapidly to the left, repeating continuously. The result is a repetitive voltage-time graph of the EMG waveform. Total sweep times are adjustable from 2 msec to 5 sec in most EMG equipment. Faster sweep speeds are provided for SFEMG (Fig 15.10).

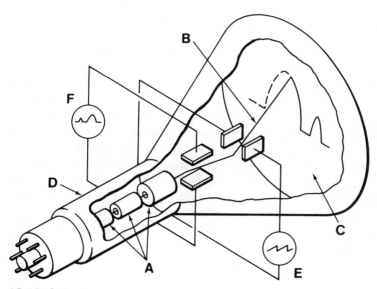

Fig. 15.10. Cathode ray tube. (A) Electron gun; (B) electron beam; (C) phosphor-coated screen inside faceplate; (D) evacuated envelope; (E) sawtooth sweep voltage source connected to horizontal deflection plates; and (F) signal voltage source connected to vertical deflection plates.

Another means of CRT beam movement, magnetic deflection, utilizes magnetic coils placed outside the tube around its narrow portion, to deflect the beam in the X and Y direction by magnetic effects on the beam. Magnetic deflection CRTs are commonly used in television, in radar in computer terminals, and in some EMG systems where the patterns are generated by causing the whole screen to be covered uniformly by the beam which draws a raster, a closely spaced series of parallel lines from the top of the screen to the bottom. The picture or wave form information is generated by turning the beam on or off or varying its intensity as the raster is drawn, so as to generate the desired pattern from discrete elements rather than by a moving point of light. Magnetic deflection systems permit economies where information is available in discrete form, such as the output of digital systems, and when many channels are simultaneously displayed.

TIME BASE, TRIGGERED

In conventional motor unit studies, the time base is free-running, i.e., the beam cyclically sweeps across the screen and randomly occurring action potentials appear at various locations along the base line, since these potentials are not synchronous with the time base. However, when an action potential is expected in response to a known event, such as an electrical stimulus to a nerve or mechanical impact of a percussion hammer on a tendon, the free-running sweep is interrupted and a sweep is released only in response to the initiating event. In this stimulus "triggered sweep" mode, the response wave, having a fixed latency with respect to the initiating event, will always appear at the same location on screen. With repeated stimuli, the response wave will superimpose and appear as a standing pattern on screen, facilitating identification, measurement, and detection of change.

The triggered sweep mode can be used in some apparatuses to observe randomly occurring action potentials ("signal triggered" sweep) if they are consistently larger than the other simultaneously occurring activity. The sweep triggers (starts) only when potentials appear that exceed an adjustable "triggering level" voltage and are of selected polarity (slope). The selected motor unit waves will, when they occur, appear superimposed at one location on screen. Since other smaller distant potentials that do not exceed the triggering level voltage will not cause the sweep to start, and they will not be seen, only the selected waves will appear as a steady repeating image. More elaborate triggering modes and use of the delay line with signal triggered sweep will be described later.

TIME SCALES

The accuracy with which time measurements can be made on the EMG screen depends on the time accuracy and linearity of the time base sawtooth wave generator, the linearity of the deflection amplifier that drives the CRT deflection circuits and the linearity of deflection of the CRT itself. (Nonlinearity results in nonuniform speed of the trace across the screen, causing time calibration to be different at various points along the trace.) These errors should not result in on-screen timing error of more than a few percent. Thus, time measurements of EMG potentials can usually be read from lines on a transparent panel (called a graticule) superimposed on the face of the CRT. The sweep or time base switch settings in milliseconds per division on the graticule permit timing of events on the CRT screen.

Some EMGs are also equipped with a second time reference trace which can display a known accurate series of pulses or steps representing, for example, 0.1, 1 or 10 msec. Since all traces are influenced by the same X axis deflection mechanism, this time reference trace permits accurate time measurement unaffected by any errors in the time base or X deflection system nonlinearities. A time reference trace has the further advantage of providing at all times a known time reference on screen (and on photographs) without reference to the time base or sweep dial settings.

When triggered sweep is used, a moveable electronic time index is generated on many EMGs in synchronism with the start of each sweep or with the initiation of a stimulus. This index, which appears variously as a step, pulse, vertical line, or bright portion of the trace on the CRT screen, is under the control of a knob with an indicator calibrated in whole and decimal parts of milliseconds. Latency from the sweep start or from the stimulus to a desired point on the evoked response is measured by turning the index dial until the index mark is at the desired point on the wave on screen and then reading the calibrated dial, usually to an accuracy greater than could be obtained from the fleeting wave on the screen.

TIME CALIBRATION

A convenient, accurate method for verifying the time accuracy of an EMG time base, CRT deflection system, time reference, and index, utilizes the commercial power line frequency timing which is more than sufficiently accurate for EMG. Introducing some power line signal is easily done by bringing a subject connected to the EMG input near an insulated appliance power cable (a common cause of power line artifact). (Under no circumstances should any attempt be made to make an electrical connection to the power line, since a lethal shock hazard could exist.) The resulting cyclic power line induced artifact waves on screen (with sweep set to show 100 or 200 msec full screen) will have a one-cycle period of 16.7 msec, and three cycles will represent 50 msec in 60 Hz power areas (20 msec/cycle in 50 Hz power areas). The time scales on the EMG should agree with the power line derived waves in timing to within 3-5%. (Some EMGs will display the induced power line waves as standing patterns or have provision to lock the sweep to the power line frequency for test purposes.)

MULTICHANNEL DISPLAY

When more than one trace of information is to be displayed simultaneously on the EMG screen, special cathode ray tubes containing two independent electron guns and deflection systems have been used. Careful adjustment is required to obtain accurate time coincidence in both sweeps. To obviate this, dual beam CRTs with common X deflection and independent Y deflection systems have sometimes been used. These methods for two or more trace displays have been superseded by electronic switching (or chopped display), a method that utilizes a conventional single beam CRT. The single beam rapidly (at least 100,000 times per second) moves from its first location, writing a dot forming a portion of the first trace to its second location, writing a dot forming a portion of the second trace, as it sweeps from left to right across the screen. The result is two series of closely spaced dots across the screen, each series forming one of the two traces. The two traces could typically be made up of 10,000 dots when the sweep duration is 100 msec (a spacing of 0.01 mm between dots on a 10-cm long screen), resulting in two traces that appear continuous. (The beam is turned off during the brief period when it is moving from one trace to the other to avoid smearing effects between the traces). The two traces are essentially coincident in time. This method applies as well to simultaneous display of additional traces.

Magnetic deflection cathode ray tubes using television-like raster displays have been used to provide multichannel displays. These methods are somewhat limited in maximum display speed.

STORAGE DISPLAY

The phosphors used on the screen of conventional cathode ray tubes usually retain the image for fractions of a second. Persistence of a few seconds can be provided, but this may interfere with the writing of a new information. Special storage display cathode ray tubes can retain information written on their screens, with the sweep off, for hours or longer and can be electronically erased rapidly at will. These CRTs, which have a capacitative mosaic storage surface behind or on the screen, can also be used in a nonstorage mode as conventional short persistence display tubes. They have obvious advantages in EMG since evoked potentials as well as transient motor unit activity can be stored on screen for study, measurement, and photography.

Since a confusion of EMG traces will result if more than one sweep is written, the storage display CRT sometimes has additional automatic circuitry for writing multiple sweep without superimposition. One method stacks multiple sweeps so that after one sweep is completed, the beam automatically moves to a new base line location, permitting the next sweep to be written on an unused portion of the screen. This can be repeated a number of times so that many "stacked" traces of EMG can be observed simultaneously, permitting motor unit activity to be studied in context. Automatic erasure then permits the process to be repeated unless inhibited when further study or photography is desired.

EMG traces may be retained on the screen of a conventional CRT by electronically recording the potential and then repetitively playing back the recorded trace on screen synchronously with the sweep. The result is a standing pattern on screen similar in appearance to the pattern observed on a storage CRT. This has been done by storing the potentials on a continuous loop of magnetic tape arranged for repetitive playback. A more flexible method converts the potentials to digital form, stores them in digital memory circuits of the type used in digital computers, and then repetitively reads out and converts them to original form for display on a conventional CRT. These methods require additional complexity and a separate storage channel for each trace stored simultaneously, while a storage CRT can store any number of traces for simultaneous viewing or recording, the limitation being screen resolution. The digital storage methods can erase and update very rapidly, however, permitting sweep-by-sweep updating with new information and even updating during the course of a sweep.

SPECIAL SIGNAL TRIGGERING

When signal triggered sweep is used, the sweep on the CRT starts only when potentials exceeding a triggering level voltage occur. The triggering level is set by the operator sufficiently high so as to permit only the desired nearby potentials to appear on screen. Action potential criteria other than largest amplitude can be used in more elaborate systems for triggering the sweep; for example, "window" triggering can be used, which requires that the selected waves be greater than one triggering level voltage but *less* than a second higher level (the window is the region between the two voltage levels). This permits the selection of potentials that are smaller than nearby larger ones.

A time window may be used for triggering, e.g., triggers will occur only when the selected wave exceeds a set level and then goes through the base line (zero amplitude) a proscribed number of milliseconds later. This discriminates against long duration waves. These more elaborate triggering methods are more difficult to use but can be useful in appropriate conditions.

DELAY LINE

When signal triggering is ued, it is often supplemented by a delay line. This device permits the portion of the potential wave that just precedes the triggering point to be seen on screen. Obviously, without the delay line, if the sweep does not start until the wave reaches the selected triggering level, the initial portion (below the triggering level) of the action potential which caused the sweep to start will be not be seen on screen.

When the delay line is used, the potentials displayed on screen are not those occuring in "real" time. They are stored instead in an electronic storage device and played back or "read out" for display many milliseconds later (the delay time). The potentials on screen, therefore, are those that have occurred earlier. Thus, when the triggered sweep starts, in real time, as the rising part of the selected wave exceeds the triggering level, the initial portion of the sweep at the left edge of the screen does not show this rising part of the wave; instead, the earlier parts of the wave appear, which preceded the triggering point, followed by the complete wave (Fig. 15.11). The wave which triggered the sweep is, therefore, seen in its entirety.

Large storage capability is not required in the delay line since it is constantly being read out and loaded with new material not more than 10 or 20 msec after being recorded. Delay has been accomplished by recording and then delayed reading and erasing of a continuously moving endless loop of magnetic tape. More commonly now, the signals are converted to digital form and circulated through a digital memory for the delay time, and then converted back to original form for display. (The word *line* in "delay line" derives from the early use of transmission lines or equivalent cascaded filters to achieve signal delays (21). This method, and others using delay of ultrasonic signals, provided only short delay for their bulk and were not easily adjustable in delay time.)

The unique ability of the signal triggered sweep and delay line to capture transient spontaneous activity enables large numbers of samples of the desired potentials to be collected quickly for motor unit duration measurement collection of denervation potentials, fasciculation, and polyphasic

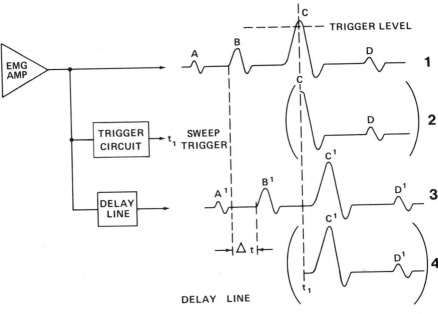

Fig. 15.11. Delay line. (*1*) EMG waves *A*, *B*, and *D* do not reach triggering level. Wave *C* exceeds triggering level at time t_1, causing a sweep on screen to start at t_1 resulting in trace (2). (*2*) Displayed trace with triggered sweep, no delay line. Note initial portion of wave *C* is lost on screen. (*3*) EMG waves delayed Δt in time at output of delay line (storage) circuit with waveshapes unchanged. (*4*) Delayed wave C^1 displayed on screen with sweep triggered by undelayed wave *C* at time t_1. Note complete wave C^1 is seen on screen, permitting visualization of portion of wave that occurred before t_1.

potentials, either for direct observation or for selective synchronized graphic recording.

The EMG Stimulator

The EMG stimulator is provided (as stated earlier) with an electrically isolated, ground free, output circuit to prevent electrical conduction of a large stimulus artifact to the preamplifier input. Artifact would otherwise occur via a circuit path comprised of the stimulator, patient, preamplifier input, and the EMG ground circuit, using the common ground for the stimulator, the amplifier, and their common power supplies. The path for conduction of artifact with a nonisolated stimulator is through the patient to the amplifier input then back through the common ground connection to the stimulator (Fig. 15.12). (All circuits in the system usually share common power supplies, and by virtue of their usual interconnection means, they all have a common ground circuit.) In the isolated stimulator, the common path between stimulator and amplifier is broken by the isolating device.

The isolator is commonly a transformer (other means are available). A transformer consists of two coils of wire, primary and secondary coils, in close proximity so that they share a common magnetic field. The stimulus current pulse generated by the grounded stimulator circuits flows in the primary coil and generates a pulsed magnetic field which induces a pulse of current in the ungrounded secondary coil of the transformer by the process of electromagnetic induction. The secondary current stimulates the subject. Since there is no electric current path between the primary and secondary windings, the artifact path through the common ground is broken. The isolation transformer breaks this path by converting the electrical output of the stimulator to magnetic energy and then back into electrical current flow in the secondary circuit.

In practice, total isolation is not achieved because of unequal capacitance effects from each output terminal to ground. Shielded stimulator output cables are not used because they would permit paths to ground via the capacitance of the shield. The isolator does not reduce the shock or artifact component that is directly conducted through the patient to the recording electrodes.

Poor electrode technique can defeat stimulus isolation, with resultant large shock artifact. Locating one of the stimulus electrodes closer to the ground electrode (or recording electrodes) than the other or, worse still, allowing a current path from a stimulating electrode over the skin surface to the ground electrode (or recording electrodes) via a bridge of electrode paste or perspiration are errors to be avoided.

STIMULUS OUTPUT

The EMG stimulator usually provides rectangular pulses with duration adjustable from 0.05 to about 1 msec; output pulse voltage should be adjustable to approximately 300 V maximum. The high voltage and long

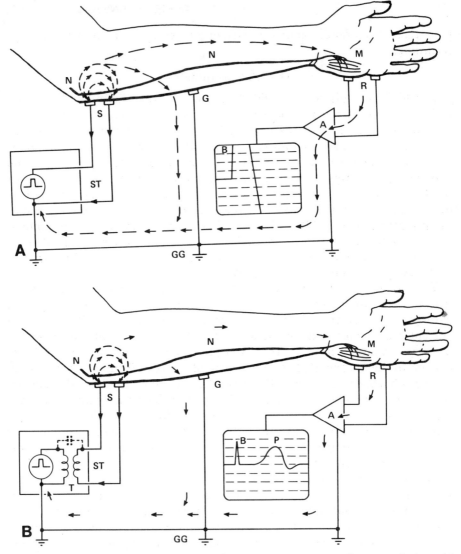

Fig. 15.12. Isolated stimulator. (*A*) Stimulating electrodes *S* are applied to skin over nerve *N*. A nonisolated conventional stimulator *ST*, which has one output terminal connected to the common system ground *GG* is shown in *A*. Stimulating current (arrows) flows between the electrodes *S* exciting the nerve. Some of the current flows through the patient to the ground electrode *G* and the recording electrodes *R* connected to EMG amplifier *A* because both have paths through the common ground back to the stimulator. This stimulus current flowing to the amplifier results in unacceptably large stimulus artifact *B*, which makes recording of the compound muscle action potential from muscle *M* very difficult. (*B*) The stimulator is equipped with an isolating transformer *T* which effectively disconnects the stimulating electrodes from the common system ground circuit. The stimulus current path through the patient to the amplifier has been substantially interrupted since no easy common path through the system ground is now available. Stimulus artifact *B* is, therefore, substantially reduced and compound muscle action potential *P* is recorded.

duration pulses are used when required to excite nerves with high threshold or those that are deeply located. The amount of current which stimulates the nerve is a small fraction of what actually is applied to the patient. This fraction varies with depth of the nerve from the surface and the conductivity of intervening tissues.

Most stimulators permit adjustment of pulse *voltage* amplitude; the resulting pulse *current* which flows depends in amplitude and shape on the electrical load (subject resistance and capacitance) at the electrodes. For a given output setting, the actual *voltage* at the electrodes will usually be somewhat reduced, depending on the stimulator design, when more current flows due to lower resistance at the electrodes.

A stabilized voltage stimulator, however, provides adjustable rectangular voltage stimulus pulses unaffected by variations in electrical load at the electrodes over its design range. Current flow and wave shape will depend on the electrical load.

A stabilized current stimulator permits the intensity of rectangular pulse current flow through the electrodes to be set, unaffected by variations in load within its design range. The output voltage amplitude and wave shape of this type of stimulator will be dependent on load. Although stabilized output stimulators are not required for conventional latency measurements, they do permit quantitative studies where control of stimulus is of interest.

The stabilized voltage and stabilized current types each have their advocates, but, in any case, it is difficult to predict or control the actual path of stimulus energy within the volume conductor (represented by the tissues of the patient) after the current leaves the stimulating electrodes.

Delayed Stimulus

Some stimulators include a control which delays the application of the stimulus a millisecond or so after the trigger that starts the sweep. This moves the stimulus artifact, which would otherwise appear at the extreme left start of the trace, slightly to the right, a distance proportional to the delay time setting, so that the whole of the artifact may be observed.

Recording the EMG

Graphic records permit documentation, measurement, and verification of transient potentials and are an important part of the modern EMG examination. Conventional polygraphic recorders utilizing mechanical writing means do not have the requisite writing speed to directly record action potentials. In addition, recorders which use paper or chart motion as the time base are hard pressed to move paper sufficiently fast to resolve the 1 msec/cm (10 m/sec) useful in some latency and motor unit measurements. (See Digital Storage Time Transformation Recorders.)

INSTANT PHOTOGRAPHY

Instant photography of the CRT is widely used to record nerve conduction tests by either electrically synchronizing the camera shutter with the stimulator and sweep or by opening the shutter just before the sweep starts and closing it before the next sweep. Free running sweeps in EMG must be interrupted to avoid unwanted superimposed traces on the photograph, a consequence of a number of sweeps occurring while the shutter is open. This is done automatically in some EMGs by utilizing shutter contacts to interrupt the sweep.

When the EMG is equipped with a storage display CRT, photography is greatly simplified since the storage traces are static, no sweep is required for viewing, and there is no synchronization problem. It is important to mark the photographic records with time and amplitude information if not already shown on the CRT screen.

CRT RECORDERS

A motor driven camera photographing a separate monitor CRT provides greater recording capability since, in addition to single sweep recording, it can operate in the raster mode, which permits sweep after sweep to be recorded so that information can be seen in context. In this mode, the recording paper of film moves slowly in direction perpendicular to the sweep, so that each sweep writes across the width of the moving paper. The subsequent sweeps appear as parallel records across the width of the record. These modes have no mechanical speed limitations since recording in both X (time) and Y (signal) axes are electronic and do not depend on paper movement.

Continuous records can also be made in a manner similar to a polygraph where high time resolution is not required. The sweep is turned off and the beam deflection, in response to the EMG signal, is retained along one axis. The movement of the recording medium serves as the time axis; continuous records along the long axis of the record results.

FIBER OPTIC RECORDER

Fiber optic recording provides all the advantages of single sweep superimposed sweep, raster, and continuous recording, along with the advantage of immediate access to the record. It utilizes a special cathode ray tube with a faceplate comprised of millions of micron-sized fiber optic light pipes. The fiber optic faceplate has the special property of transferring the traces that are formed in the phosphor on the surface of the faceplate inside the evacuated CRT to the outside surface of the faceplate without the optical dispersion that would occur if a conventional faceplate were used. The light efficiency, which is higher than even a large aperture lens, permits direct recording on to special sensitized recording paper in contact with the faceplate. The fastest EMG potentials are recorded by this high optical sensitivity system. The recording paper develops a visible, permanent image a few seconds after emerging from the recorder into a lighted room (Fig. 15.13).

DIGITAL STORAGE TIME TRANSFORMATION RECORDERS

The CRT display and the fiber optic recorder have no speed limitation in EMG recording because they are inertialess in the time (X) as well as the signal (Y) axis. The limitations on other recorders that rely on recording paper movement for the time axis, described earlier, can be obviated by a time transformation technique. The information to be recorded is first stored electrically and then played back slowly at a speed that provides the desired time resolution compatible with reasonable paper speed. (For example: 1 msec/cm time resolution in real time requires unreasonably high 1,000 cm/sec paper speed; an electrically stored signal played back at 1/20 speed would provide 1 msec/cm resolution at an acceptable paper speed of 50 cm/sec). Magnetic tape storage with slow speed playback has been used as the storage medium. More recently, EMG signals converted into digital form and stored in digital computer memory, in real time, are read out of memory at reduced speed, decoded or converted into original form, and then mechanically and graphically recorded on moving recording paper.

An inertialess spark recorder utilizing high contrast metallized paper and having a linear array of 256 fixed recorder points has been applied to EMG recording. It utilizes the slow read-from-memory time transformation technique just described for recording on moving paper in the time axis. Conventional ink or hot stylus graphic recorders can also be used in this slow read-out time transformation technique. The limitations of digital storage recorders include memory speed and memory capacity and writing time.

MAGNETIC RECORDING

EMG potentials may be recorded for later playback on a magnetic tape recorder permitting future visualization, graphic recording, and analysis. The common "analog" or "direct" magnetic recorder, used for speech and music, records on the tape patterns of magnetization that are analogous to the signals being recorded. The magnetic patterns on the tape are converted to electrical signals in the playback process. It has adequate high frequency response to reproduce EMG waves, but the 40 or 50 Hz low frequency response limit is inadequate for accurate reproduction of the slow components of long duration action potentials and positive sharp waves. (These slow components are contaminated by their first derivative by the playback process and, therefore, appear more polyphasic.) Some improvement in performance is obtained by using equipment modified to extend the low frequency response to 20 or 15 Hz.

Instrumentation tape recorders utilize modulation methods whereby the

EMG signals cause the frequency of a locally generated constant amplitude alternating voltage to fluctuate. This constant amplitude fluctuating frequency voltage is then recorded magnetically. The information is carried as frequency variations rather than intensity variations of the recorded magnetization patterns on the tape. On playback, these frequency variations are converted to electrical signals. (Pulse-code or pulse-time modulation techniques which are similar are also used.) This system, termed Frequency Modulation (FM) recording, has no low frequency limitation (it can record unvarying DC potentials) but has limited high frequency performance which can be extended, however, by utilizing higher tape speeds. They can provide good fidelity EMG recordings. FM recorders are more complex and expensive than analog types.

When recording, a sample of known calibration voltage should always be included and noted each time the EMG sensitivity is changed. This will permit adjustment of amplitude to known values on playback. An additional speech channel permits recording simultaneous detailed notes during EMG, quite necessary for interpreting potentials during playback.

Noise and Interference

When small amplitude signals are encountered in EMG, their detection and measurement becomes difficult because of the obscuring effect of noise. The interfering noise falls into three classes: a) bioelectric noise, b) equipment noise, and c) external noise.

Bioelectric noise, which includes potentials generated within the patient as part of life functions, includes distant muscle activity, e.g., respiration, cardiac, and other sympathetic functions (also distant skeletal activity due to incomplete relaxation or placement of the patient ground or zero potential electrode over a muscle rather than over a tendon or bony area). These can often be detected by their cyclic nature and minimized somewhat by proper electrode location.

Equipment noise, as discussed earlier, originates in electrodes, movement of lead wires and electrodes, amplifiers, and stimulator (shock artifact). These are minimized by use of proper electrodes, maintaining them and their connectors, and proper electrode technique. This source of noise is also minimized by use of filter settings on the amplifier. Also important are the ground-free (isolation) properties of the stimulator, patient preparation, and electrode technique in stimulation.

External noise sources (interference) include a wide range of electrical and electromagnetic influences, the most common being electrostatic induction of power line energy into the patient, by capacitance effect, from the power cords of appliances or from building power wiring. This appears as periodic waves, pulses, or spikes with 16.7 msec (in 60 Hz power areas and 20 msec in 50 Hz areas) periodicities in the EMG record. After making the basic checks for proper equipment grounding and patient ground (or zero potential) electrode connection, the most effective cure is to unplug the offending appliance at the wall outlet. Turning the appliance off does not

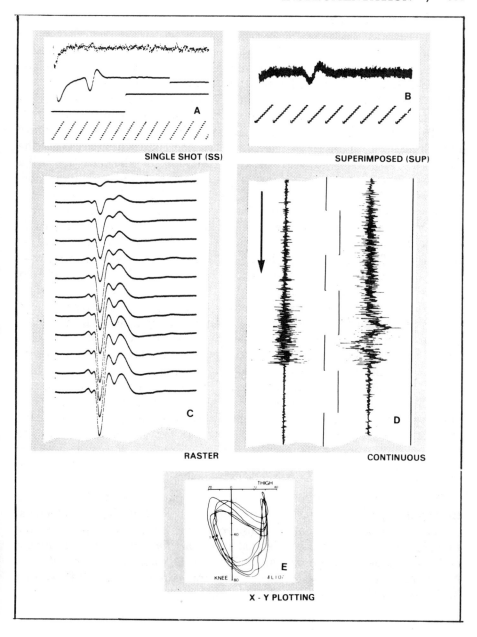

Fig. 15.13. Some recording modes possible with CRT or Fiber Optic Recorders are shown. (A) Single shot record, showing four channels recorded simultaneously. The paper is advanced after each sweep in preparation for the next record. (B) Superimposed record, showing two channels. The recording paper remains stationary; any desired number of sweeps are superimposed on the record. (C) Raster record, showing a single channel. The paper is moved as each subsequent sweep is recorded, showing progressive change in the recorded potential. (D) Continuous record, showing three channels. No electronic sweep is used, continuous movement

remove the offending power line voltage from its power cable. All building wiring in the vincinity of the patient should be within grounded metal conduit (required by most electrical codes). This shields the conductors within, substantially eliminating external electrostatic effects which might otherwise induce power line interference into the patient.

Radio frequency (rf) sources are a particularly insidious form of interference. They include entertainment broadcast transmitters in the AM, FM, and TV bands; public service and CB transmitters; some paging systems; and therapeutic diathermy. These sources can induce potentials in the patient and electrodes which are often much larger than the potentials being recorded. The best defense against these sources is distance. The quasioptical nature of rf waves also makes changes in location in the building useful; a move to a location opposite from the offending transmitter can sometimes help. Interposing grounded metal or mesh screening between the patient and the transmitter can sometimes help, especially if the interference is not too serious. The placement of the ground screen is sometimes capricious—occasionally a shield under and insulated from the patient can be of help.

A six-sided screened enclosure for the EMG, patient, and examiner might be required in serious power line and rf interference situations. Such enclosures should be constructed in a manner totally isolated from ground and then electrically grounded to the power line ground at only one point. This avoids circulating ground currents in the conductive shielding, which can result if multiple contacts are made to various grounded objects which are often at slightly different potentials. These circulating ground currents in the screening can result in serious power line interference. Power lines entering such a shielded enclosure might require radio frequency filters, since rf energy can sometimes travel along power wiring. All wiring and lights within the enclosure must, of course, be shielded. Nearby powerful rf sources make the design of the screened enclosure more difficult and exacting.

The extent to which all sources of noise can be minimized will determine the smallest potential that can be reliably recorded. Filtering as a means of reducing noise is limited only to those sources of noise that do not have the same harmonic content as the desired potentials. Only noise that has higher or lower frequency components than the EMG potentials can be filtered. Noise components having the same harmonic content as the EMG cannot be filtered without distorting the EMG wave.

---

of the record in the direction of the arrow provides the time axis. (E) X-Y recording, one channel of information is applied to one axis of deflection while a second related channel is applied to the other. No sweep or time axis is used. Relationships between the signals appear as characteristic looped patterns. These patterns, sometimes called Lissajous patterns, are useful in identifying relationships between related signals. Here the angle of the knee is plotted simultaneously against the angle of the thigh. Five trials are superimposed.

Signal Averaging

When very small responses to stimuli are recorded in the presence of random noise, it is possible to detect these responses, even when each response wave is obscured by noise which has the same harmonic content as the response, by the method of signal averaging. Such noise problems occur when recording stimulus-evoked neurograms from deep lying nerves in the presence of pathology and from poorly relaxed patients (also, when recording stimulus-evoked potentials from the cortex or brainstem via scalp electrodes; here the spontaneous EEG, in addition to system noise, obscures the response).

A simple early method utilized stimuli repeated as many as 50 times with responses superimposed and photographed from the CRT screen (22). Superimposition may also be done on a display storage CRT or on a fiber optic recorder. The effect of superimposition is to enhance the response wave (Fig. 15.14).

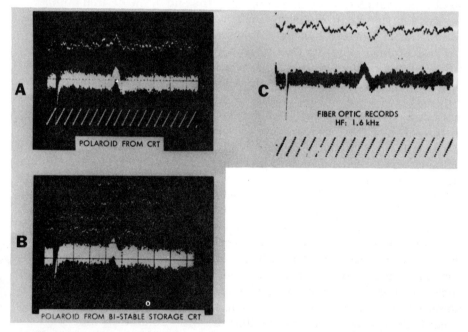

Fig. 15.14. Superimposed records. Records were made by stimulating the finger and recording over the ulnar nerve at the elbow with surface electrodes. The downward-going spike wave near the left end of the traces is the stimulus artifact. Amplifier bandwidth is 32 Hz to 3.2 kHz. Calibration waves at the bottom of each record are 5 μV, 1 msec between peaks. Upper traces are single sweeps; action potentials are difficult to discern from noise. The action potentials are obvious in the lower traces, made by superimposing 25 sweeps. (A) A Polaroid photograph from a conventional CRT, the camera shutter was held open during the 25 sweeps; (B) superimposition was done on the screen of a storage CRT and then photographed; (C) record from a fiber optic recorder in the superimposed mode.

A more powerful method, which permits recording and detecting of regularly occurring responses to stimuli more completely obscured by random noise fluctuations, involves adding corresponding time segments of the records of repeated stimuli instead of superimposing them (23). This technique, termed variously averaging, signal averaging, evoked response averaging, and ensemble averaging, utilizes a method of summing many repetitive trials that has been long known in other applications to detect systematic fluctuations obscured by larger irregular ones.

Signal averaging is accomplished by dividing each response sweep into a predetermined number of small contiguous samples in time termed "ordinates" or "words." (A sufficiently large number of samples is chosen so as to adequately describe the shape of the expected response.) The instantaneous amplitude of the signal in each time sample is stored in separate storage elements equal in number to the samples (ordinates). Each store is related to the same time sample in each sweep. As subsequent sweeps are recorded, each storage element accumulates the algebriac sum of the signal amplitudes sampled at its unique time. At the end of the desired number of sweeps, the summed contents of each storage element is read in sequence and the resulting wave is displayed on screen.

Those storage elements that summed ordinates in time that were only influenced by random noise will have received potentials of random amplitude and polarity, while those storage elements that received inputs from ordinates that were located in time so as to be influenced by the response wave and random noise will have received nonrandom potentials reflecting the presence of the response wave potential. The storage elements for the response wave will have significantly greater sums relative to the storage elements influenced by random noise potentials only. When the storage elements are read out in sequence on screen, the resulting response wave will be larger in porportion to the noise by a factor equal to the square root of the number of samples averaged (Fig. 15.15). The response wave obscured by noise on any one sweep will now be visible.

This technique permits visualization of potentials, fractions of a microvolt in amplitude obscured by microvolts of noise. In this form, it can only enhance stimulus-evoked potentials, not random spontaneously occurring ones (the stimulus may occur randomly). It will only discriminate against noise potentials that occur randomly in time with respect to the stimulus.

Artifact or system fluctuations that are synchronized in time with the stimulus should carefully be avoided because they will be enhanced. Even when these flucutations are very tiny and not obvious, they will appear after averaging along with the desired physiological response potential, if any. For these reasons, stimulation should not occur snychronized with the power line frequency, and the patient should avoid proximity with the CRT to obviate artifact pickup synchronized with the sweep traversing the screen.

While many technical approaches have been successfully used in the design of averagers, present equipment utilizes electronic sampling and

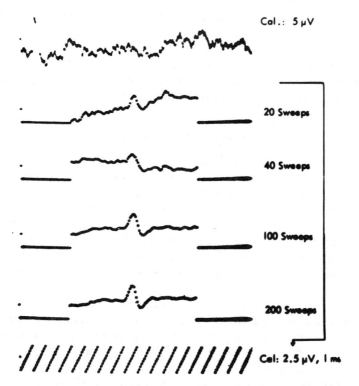

Cal.: 5 µV

20 Sweeps

40 Sweeps

100 Sweeps

200 Sweeps

Cal: 2.5 µV, 1 ms

Fig. 15.15. Averaged neurograms. The top trace was made by stimulating the finger and recording over the ulnar nerve at the elbow with surface electrodes. Amplifier bandwidth was 32 Hz to 1.6 kHz. Calibration trace at the bottom is 5 µV for the top trace and 2.5 µV for the others. Time is 1 msec between peaks. Spike wave near left end of top trace is the stimulus artifact. The nerve action potential is not discernable in the top trace because of system, external, and bioelectric noise. The lower traces were made by repeated stimulation and signal averaging, 20, 40, 100, and 200 times from the top down, in a 100-ordinate averager. Note the improvement in the response wave as the number of stimuli is initially increased. Less improvement results when stimuli are increased from 100 to 200.

digital techniques for storage, addition, and system control. As few as 100 ordinates are adequate to resolve response waves in many studies; 1,000 ordinates or more are often available to provide additional capability. Ordinate duration is adjustable and should be as short as 10 µsec to resolve the fastest potentials. Averagers are often provided with artifact rejection capability that will reject a sweep containing a gross artifact potential such as patient movement that would unnecessarily disturb the summation. In addition, sweep counters and indicators monitor the progress of the test and can terminate stimulation at a preset count. Calibrated output is available which normalizes the summing process so that the actual amplitude of the response can be read from the record without calculation. The output averaged wave can, in some units, be multiplied or divided in amplitude or expanded or contracted in time for detailed examination.

Since the averager inherently incorporates storage elements, the output may be read repeatedly and sufficiently frequent, so as to present a flicker-free stored trace on screen. It may, therefore, be arranged as a single sweep storage device to display random transient action potentials on a conventional nonstorage CRT.

Digital Processing

The action potentials which are picked up by the electrodes and then amplified are represented by electrical fluctuations in the EMG apparatus. These continually varying electric currents, capable of an infinite number of values, change in time and amplitude exactly in proportion to the action potentials themselves (within the finite limits of system performance). The electric currents and voltages in the amplifier representing the action potentials are, thus, analogs of the original quantities. The amplifier is then termed an analog signal processing device, as is a telephone connecting two parties by wire.

Signals can also be transmitted between two points by first coding them into a form that has a finite number of values and then transmitting the code in a form that is not analogous to the signal; finally, at the receiver, the code is converted back to a recognizable analog signal.

Morse code telegraphic transmission of information is an example of a coded transmission process. Digital processing of EMG signals is also a coded processing system. Here the continuously varying signal is first fragmented in time into a series of closely spaced contiguous samples of voltage, each sample being an analog representation of the signal amplitude at an instant in time. The samples are then coded, transmitted (or processed), and then decoded. The decoded series of time samples are then recognizable analog representations of the original signal. They may then be smoothed, if required, to convert the discrete series of time samples into a smooth-appearing continuous wave.

The primary advantage of digital systems, in common with telegraphy, is that the code used can be represented by only two voltage states in the system, e.g., on or off. Signal and logic circuits are reduced to a collection of the equivalent of on-off switches and simple circuits to detect the on-off condition. In contrast, an analog circuit must respond linearly to every subtle change in amplitude of the signal. Noise in an analog system contaminates the signal and establishes the minimum useful signal level. A two-state digital coded system is indifferent to significant amounts of noise so long as the on and off states can be unambiguously detected. Considerable signal processing and manipulation can be done without degenerating the signal in coded systems; this is in contrast to analog systems where each step in signal processing tends to add its toll of system noise.

Quantities can be expressed to a very high resolution, over a wide range, by merely increasing the number of code elements (bits) used to represent them in digital form. This is difficult in analog systems because of the limits imposed by noise and limitations of maximum permissible signal size.

Digital systems are physically more complex than analog systems, especially where long codes of many bits grouped into "words" are required to represent signals to high resolution. The sampling process also puts limitations of speed on the signals that can be represented.

Since each element of the code contains so little information (on-off, yes-no, etc.), many coded elements must be transmitted or manipulated in order to represent magnitudes (numbers) of useful size. This takes time, which becomes a problem when samples occurring as rapidly as 100,000 times a second (as is required to represent a rapidly changing action potential) are to be handled. Therefore, instead of handling the information serially (in sequence) on a single pair of wires, as in analog systems, each element (on-off channel) of the code is handled by its own path in the system and is transmitted and processed simultaneously in most parts of the system. This simultaneous multipath (parallel) processing contributes to the physical complexity of high speed coded systems.

In order to be processed in a digital system, an analog signal must be first sampled repetitively at frequent intervals. The magnitude of each sample is converted to a digital code. The process is called "analog to digital conversion" (A-D conversion). The digital code used must have the capability of representing sufficient discrete voltage levels (quantization levels) in the sampling process to provide the desired accuracy and resolution. At each sample time, the analog signal voltage is measured and represented by the discrete quantization voltage nearest the actual analog voltage at the time of sampling (Fig. 15.16).

The effectiveness of the A-D conversion process depends upon the sampling interval being sufficiently short (sampling *rate* sufficiently high) and the quantization levels being sufficiently small and adequate in number (adequate word length) so as to accurately represent the time and amplitude fluctuations of the analog signal. These digital system parameters (sampling rate and word size) must be considered when applying digital systems to EMG potentials.

The quantization levels shown as decimal voltage in Figure 15.16 are converted to a binary code, a numbering system based on two states, represented by zero and 1 in the figure. A four digit (bit) binary code or word which can represent 16 decimal numbers is shown.

The decimal value of each bit is determined by its location in the 4 bit number, just as the value of each digit in the decimal system is determined by its location in the decimal number (units, tens, hundreds, etc.). The bottom bit of the code in the figure, and when more commonly written horizontally, the right hand bit (least significant bit) has the decimal value

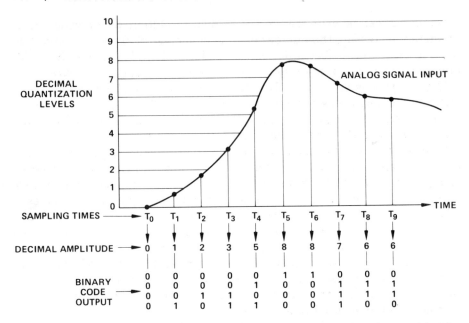

Fig. 15.16. Analog to digital conversion. The Analog signal represented by the curve varies continuously in time and can assume a potentially infinite number of values. When converted to digital form, the curve is represented by a sequence of digital numbers that can assume a specified limited number of values. These values or quantization levels are represented here, in decimal form, by the numbers along the ordinate. The instantaneous amplitude of the signal is sampled (measured) repetitively at T_0, T_1, T_2. . . . in time, at a rate sufficiently rapid so as to follow the fastest anticipated changes in the signal with adequate time resolution. Since the amplitude of the signal at each sample can only be represented by one of the discrete quantization levels, the decimal amplitudes shown for the T_1, T_2, T_5, etc., samples represent rounded-off approximations of the signal amplitudes to the nearest quantization level (quantization error). The amplitude value for each sample is then converted to its equivalent binary number for subsequent digital processing. The number of levels which determine the amplitude resolution of the system is determined by the number of bits or word length that characterizes the digital system (see Fig. 15.17). The 4-bit binary numbers shown can represent only 16 quantization levels. Eight-bit systems capable of 256 levels are often used to represent EMG waves in digital systems.

of 0 or 1 (equivalent to 2^0); the next has a value of 0 or 2 (equivalent to 2^1); the third, 0 or 4 (2^2); and the fourth (most significant bit), 0 or 8 (2^4).

A binary number may be converted to its decimal value by adding the decimal values of each bit that is in the "one" condition. Thus the 4 bit binary number 0101 has a decimal value of $0 + 4 + 0 + 1 = 5$.

EMG potentials can be adequately represented by 8 bit binary numbers (also termed binary word length) which provide a resolution of 256 levels (Fig 15.17). Sampling rate should be about 100,000/sec or 10 μsec per sample

Number of Binary Bits	Amplitude Resolution[a]	% Full Scale Error[b]
4	16	6.3
5	32	3.1
6	64	1.6
7	128	0.78
8	256	0.39
9	512	0.20
10	1,024	0.10
11	2,048	0.050
12	4,096	0.024
13	8,192	0.012
14	16,384	0.0061
15	32,768	0.0031
16	65,536	0.0015
17	131,072	0.00076
18	262,144	0.00038

[a] Maximum resolution for a binary coded digital system utilizing numbers (words) of binary bit length shown in first column.

[b] Maximum accuracy of such systems expressed as percentage of full scale.

Fig. 15.17. Binary word length and amplitude resolution.

to ensure an adequate number of samples during rapid positive-to-negative transitions of action potentials which might occur within 100 μsec. The number of words that can be stored depends upon the application. However, devices utilizing as little as 100 words (samples) have been used. The falling cost of digital memory has made 1,000 words and more increasingly common in dedicated EMG devices. General purpose computers are provided with fast access memories of tens or hundreds of thousands of words.

Solid State Digital Devices

The advent of transistors and solid state technology has permitted the large number of digital switches called gates, which are major components of digital systems, to be densely packed into compact circuits. The process of large scale integration (LSI), which permits thousands of these circuits to be photographically constructed on chips of silicon only a few millimeters square, permits even more functions to be built in compact form and at reduced cost. The commercial pressures generated by the poliferation of minicomputers which this technology made possible have made available a growing host of sophisticated economically attractive digital circuit elements. While analog methods might be simpler and more direct in concept and circuitry in certain operations because of the economy, compactness, noise immunity, and precision possible with these devices, digital techniques are increasingly used for signal manipulation, system control and logic operations, mathematical operations on signals, and short term signal storage.

The microprocessor is a recent class of LSI digital circuit elements that permits flexibility and economy in the design of digital devices. Conventional design and construction of digital devices utilizes basic gate and other logic elements uniquely wired into complex circuits to perform the job at hand. The microprocessor, which is a relatively inexpensive subminiature microcomputer, utilizes stored instructions (program) which cause the desired operations to be executed and permit many functions to be accomplished without time consuming unique physical circuit design layout and construction. Modifications and changes are easy and inexpensive since they are usually accomplished by simple stored program changes. They are used in processing and control functions in home appliances and automobiles and are finding applications in instruments and in EMG equipment.

Electrical Safety

All electrically operated devices present a potential electrical shock hazard. This hazard is minimal when the device is designed to eliminate the possibility of unwanted electrical currents, termed leakage currents, from being unintentionally applied to the patient or operator (stimulation currents are not leakage currents) who contacts the metal case or recording electrodes of the device. This is accomplished by providing adequate insulation between the current carrying parts of the device and those portions of the device the patient and operator can contact. Active circuits in the device are also designed so that a component failure will not cause leakage current to flow of sufficient magnitude to cause injury. Allowable leakage current and specific measurement methods are specified or are being studied by international standards groups, National Government Standards groups, professional societies, and private testing laboratories (24–31). Smaller leakage currents are specified for equipment designed and labelled for use on so-called electrically sensitive patients, those that have electrodes or catheters with direct electrical paths to the heart, rather than equipment that only makes contact to non-electrically sensitive patients.

Modern building power wiring, according to code and practice in many countries, has one of the two current carrying wires in the power circuit connected to ground. The ground connection is, in fact, at earth potential, as is (or should be) the metal structure of the building, plumbing, air handling ducts, most metal panels and trim, and all other electrically conductive mechanical parts of the building. This means that the full power voltage (110 volts 60 Hz in the U.S., parts of South and Central America and some other areas; 220 volts 50 Hz in England and parts of Europe and Africa, as well as parts of South and Central America) is available to anyone coming in simultaneous contact with one conductor of the power line and any of the above grounded objects, a potentially lethal situation. This is not likely to occur in a well designed and maintained appliance. However, due

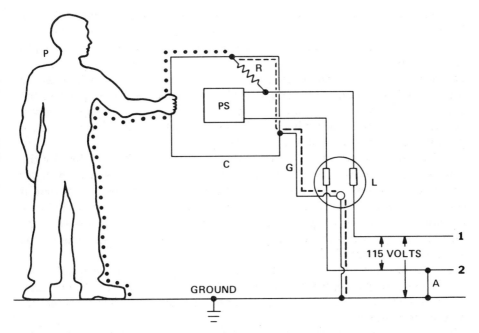

Fig. 15.18. Leakage path. *P*, Grounded person; *C*, metal instrument case; *PS*, power line connected circuits of instrument; *R*, leakage path from power line to case; *L*, power line connector; *G*, grounding conductor in power cable. An instrument with metal case *C* (which also includes patient contact electrodes) is connected to the 115 V power line conductors 1 and 2 via its power cable and connector *L*. The instrument case is grounded via a grounding conductor *G* in the power cable, which connects to the power system and building ground via the third prong in the power connector. One side of the power wiring circuit (2) is connected according to building code to the building ground at the power distribution point, in the building as shown at *A*. The leakage current path from power line 1 and *PS* to the case *C* through limitations of insulation in the instrument components is represented by *R*. This leakage current can find a return path to line 2 of the power system via ground either through a grounded person, by the dotted path, or through the ground wire *G* in the power cable, by the dashed line path. The grounded wire *G* protects the grounded person *P* because it provides a direct low resistance path for the leakage currents, even if *R* became a low resistance or a short circuit due to a fault; the now dangerous leakage current would flow mainly through *G*, not through *P* because of the much lower resistance of the dashed path through *G*. A routine test for leakage current involves a measurement (under specified conditions) of the normal leakage current that flows in ground wire *G* to ensure that it is below a specified value. Low normal leakage current demonstrates adequate insulation and ensures that innocuous current will flow through *P* if the ground connection *G* should fail.

to capacitance effects and the finite properties of insulation, measurable, small leakage currents can be detected from normally noncurrent carrying parts of power line operated devices when measured to ground. This is due to the presence of power line wiring within the device. For safety purposes then, the metal frame and enclosure of these devices are solidly connected to ground via a third ground wire included in the power cable, which in turn is grounded by the third ground terminal in the power receptacle. This ground connection, mandatory in most power line operated electrical appliances, provides a safe path to ground for these leakage currents and potentially dangerous currents from a fault in the appliance, which would otherwise flow through a grounded subject who touched metal parts of the appliance. A properly grounded power receptacle should always be used, and the power cable and plug should be promptly repaired or replaced if damaged or shows signs of wear.

Some safety standards refer to a so-called "first fault" test whereby the leakage current flowing in the safety ground connection is measured under specified conditions. This leakage current would flow through a person if the ground connection failed (first fault condition) and must be below a minimum value (50–500 μA). This low leakage current indicates that the insulation separating the power line circuits from accessible parts of the equipment is intact (Fig. 15.18).

A "double insulated" class of appliances is constructed with sufficient insulation and spacing between power line connected parts and the remainder of the unit as to make contact extremely unlikely and, therefore, require no ground connection.

Leakage current measurement and electrical safety acceptance should be made by persons trained and equipped to make the requisite tests. Care should be exercised when connecting accessory electrical devices to the EMG or the patient to ensure that these devices, which may not meet modern leakage standards for medical devices, do not by their interconnection dangerously increase the leakage currents in the system or in the grounded patients.

REFERENCES

1. BROWN, P. B., MAXFIELD B. W., AND MORAFF, H.: *Electronics for Neurobiologists* ch. 1, 2, Cambridge, Mass.: MIT Press, 1973.
2. CLIFFORD, M.: *Basic Electricity and Beginning Electronics No. 628*, Summit, Penn.: Tab Books, 1973.
3. LEACH, P.: *Basic Electric Circuits,* New York: John Wiley & Sons, 1969.
4. NIGHTINGALE, A.: *Physics and Electronics in Physical Medicine,* ch. 1, 4–10, Appendices 1–5, 8, New York: Macmillan, 1959.
5. SUCKLING, E. E.: *Bioelectricity,* ch. 1, 2, New York: McGraw-Hill, 1961.
6. WHITFIELD, I. C.: *An Introduction to Electronics for Physiological Workers,* New York: Macmillan, 1953.
7. Technical factors in recording electrical activity of muscle and nerve in man. Report of Committee on EMG Instrumentation, IFSECN, 1969. *Electroencephalogr. Clin. Neurophysiol., 28:* 399, 1970.
8. GEDDES, L. A.: *Electrodes and the Measurement of Bioelectric Events,* ch. 1–3, New York: John Wiley & Sons, 1972.
9. GEDDES, L. A.: *Electrodes in the Measurement of Bioelectric Events,* p. 78, New York: John Wiley & Sons, 1972.
10. JASPER, H., AND BALLEM, G.: Unipolar electromyograms of normal and denervated human muscle. *J. Neurophysiol., 12:* 231, 1949.

11. ADRIAN, E. D., AND BRONK, D. W.: The discharge of impulses in motor nerve fibers. Part II. *J. Physiol.,* 67: 119, 1929.
12. POLLAK, V.: The waveshape of action potentials recorded with different types of EMG needles. *Med. Biol. Eng.,* 9: 657, 1971.
13. BUCHTHAL, F., GULD, C., AND ROSENFALCK, P.: Volume conduction of the spike of the motor unit potential investigated with a new type of multielectrode. *Acta Physiol. Scand.,* 38: 331, 1957.
14. BASMAJIAN, J. V., AND STECKO, G.: A new bipolar electrode for electromyography. *J. Appl. Physiol.,* 17: 849, 1962.
15. FLECK, H.: Action potentials from single motor units in human muscle. *Arch. Phys. Med. Rehabil.,* 43: 99, 1962.
16. STÅLBERG, E. AND EKSTEDT, J.: Single fibre EMG for the study of the microphysiology of human muscle. In *New Developments in Electromyography and Clinical Neurophysiology,* vol. 1, pp. 89–112, ed. by J. E. Desmedt, Basel, Switzerland: Karger, 1973.
17. GAJDUSEK, D. C., ET AL.: Precautions in medical care of, and in handling materials from, patients with transmissable virus dementia (Creutzfeldt-Jacob disease). *N. Engl. J. Med.,* 297: 1253, 1977. Letters, *N. Engl. J. Med.,* 298: 976, 1978.
18. GEDDES, L. A.: *Electrodes and the Measurement of Bioelectric Events,* p. 124, figs. 3–11, New York: John Wiley & Sons, 1972.
19. Technical factors in recording electrical activity of muscle and nerve in man. Report of Committee on EMG Instrumentation. IFSECN, 1969 (Fig. 7). *Electroencephalogr. Clin. Neurophysiol.,* 28: 399, 1970.
20. GARUTS, V., AND SAMUELS, C.: Measuring conventional oscilloscope noise. *Tekscope, 1:* 2, 1969, Tektronix, Inc., Beaverton, Ore.
21. NISSEN-PETERSON, H., GULD, C., AND BUCHTHAL, F.: A delay line to record random action potentials. *Electroencephalogr. Clin. Neurophysiol., 26:* 100, 1969.
22. DAWSON, G. D., AND SCOTT, J. W.: The recording of nerve action potentials through the skin in man. *J. Neurol. Neurosurg. Psychiat., 12:* 259, 1949.
23. DAWSON, G. D.: A summation technique for the detection of small evoked potentials. *Electroencephalogr. and Clin. Neurophysiol., 6:* 65, 1954.
24. *Basic Aspects of the Safety Philosophy of Electrical Equipment Used in Medical Practice, IEC #513,* International Electrotechnical Commission, Geneva 20.
25. *Electricity In Patient Care Facilities, 76B7,* National Fire Protection Association, Boston, Mass. 02210.
26. *Electro-Medical Equipment, CSA Standard C22.2 No. 125,* Canadian Standards Association, Rexdale, Ontario #M9W 1R3.
27. *Good Manufacturing Practices,* Food and Drug Administration, Silver Springs, Md. 20910.
28. *Safe Current Limits Standard, SCL 12-78,* AAMI, Association for the Advancement of Medical Instrumentation, Arlington, Va. 22209.
29. *Safety Code for Electro-Medical Apparatus. Hospital Technical Memorandum No. 8,* Department of Health and Social Security, London, Revised 1969.
30. *Safety Of Electrical Equipment Used In Medical Practice, IEC Standard IEC 601-1 1978,* International Electrotechnical Commission, Geneva 20.
31. *Standard For Medical and Dental Equipment, UL 544,* Underwriters Laboratory, Inc. Melville, N.Y. 11746.

16

Action Potential

JOHN L. MELVIN, M.D.

Cells are capable of developing and maintaining potential differences between the intracellular and interstitial compartments. Some cells, namely muscle and nerve fibers, have membranes which can be described as excitable. Such cells are usually quite long as compared to their diameters. A stimulus is able to initiate transiently depolarization and then repolarization of the membrane of such an excitable cell.

These transient changes in membrane voltage produce what is called an action potential. In elongated cells, the action potential can be propagated in either direction from the point where it is initiated. The stimulus which leads to propagation is the initial depolarization along the membrane which local currents produce in advance of the action potential. These local currents are produced by the action potential.

Needle EMG involves observing electrical potentials which occur within muscle. The size of the exploring electrode is large compared to individual muscle fibers. Therefore, the electrical changes described with sophisticated electrophysiologic equipment need to be correlated with the grosser techniques of EMG. For instance, the intracellular electrode records a transmembrane potential of -90 mV while the EMG needle records the amplitude of a fibrillation potential, presumably usually from a single cell, as up to 150 μV.

EMG basically provides observations on two phenomena. The first is the stability of muscle membranes. Generally, electrical activity is generated only during movement of the needle electrode through muscle unless motor unit disease is present. In various disease states, the membrane may either spontaneously generate potentials or have a low threshold for their development. Not only may potentials occur, but they may be repetitive once initiated, indicating significant changes in membrane excitability.

The second phenomena noted during EMG relates to observations of muscle fibers activated through volitional control. In such circumstances, one almost universally sees the summated effect of the action potentials generated by many muscle fibers. Information is gained not about the membrane per se, but about the number of action potentials present and their relationships with each other.

In clinical nerve conduction studies, many nerve fibers are depolarized, producing a compound action potential, i.e., one that is the summated electrical effect of many action potentials from different nerve fibers. Observations can be made regarding the characteristics of this nerve compound action potential. An action potential propagated along a nerve fiber depolarizes the muscle fibers innervated by that nerve fiber. The characteristics of such muscle compound action potentials can also be studied. Many of the same relationships between action potentials noted during volitional EMG are noted during nerve conduction studies. In addition, clinical nerve conduction studies reveal the velocities of action potential propagation in peripheral nerves.

As can be seen from the above discussion, the bases of the observations made during clinical EMG and nerve conduction studies are the action potentials generated in the excitable cells of peripheral muscles and nerves. A more detailed understanding of the physiological basis of the action potential can assist the electromyographer in conceptualizing what is occurring during these electrodiagnostic procedures and hopefully provide a rational basis for new or improved techniques.

The following provides some discussion regarding the characteristic properties of excitable membranes, particularly as they are explained on the basis of changes in sodium permeability.

Resting Potential

CELL MEMBRANE STRUCTURE

Closely packed cells and the surrounding interstitial fluid compose human tissues such as muscle or brain (1). The cell membrane forms the functional boundary between the intracellular and interstitial fluids. It is a thin structure of about 60 Angstroms (6×10^{-9} meters) formed from a highly organized, bimolecular lipoprotein layer. This structure severely restricts the exchange of materials between the intracellular and interstitial fluid compartments.

The intracellular and interstitial fluids both consist mostly of water and of a roughly equal number of dissolved particles per unit volume. However, the concentrations of ions within them differ significantly. There also is a difference in electrical potential between the two fluids of approximately -70 to -90 mV, negative on the inside of the cell.

The protein portions of the lipoprotein molecules face the aqueous intracellular and interstitial fluids, whereas the inner part of the membrane is made up of the closely packed lipid portions. These densely arranged lipid layers are hydrophobic and act as a barrier to movement of dissolved particles and water. Special structures exist within the lipid bilayer portion of the membrane with permit ionized substances to cross. These are pore channels, of which there are many different types depending upon the specific ion which can pass through them.

ION CONCENTRATIONS

All cells maintain a steady potential across their membranes, negative inside. In nerve and muscle fibers, it is often referred to as the resting potential in order to contrast it with the action potential (2). The size of this potential largely is dependent upon the ratio of the ability of the potassium ions to that of sodium ions to pass through the membrane. The greater this ratio the larger is the resting potential. In nerve and muscle, this ratio is greater than 50:1. These tissues exhibit resting potentials of −70 to −90 mV.

The concentration of ions in the intracellular and interstitial fluids differ greatly (1). Mammalian muscle cells reveal approximately the following intracellular fluid ion concentrations in micromoles/cm^3: $[Na^+]$ 12, $[K^+]$ 155, $[Cl^-]$ 4, and $[A^-]$ 155. $[A^-]$ is used to indicate largely unknown organic anions. In contrast, one finds these ion concentrations in micromoles/cm^3 when analyzing interstitial fluid: $[Na^+]$ 145, $[K^+]$ 4, $[Cl^-]$ 120, and $[A^-]$ 0. Thus, the intracellular fluid has high concentrations of potassium and negatively charged organic ions but low concentrations of sodium and chloride ions. The interstitial fluid demonstrates the opposite, high concentrations of sodium and chloride ions and low concentrations of potassium and organic anions. A number of factors share responsibility for the production of these observed differences.

PERMEABILITY

The ease by which a substance penetrates or moves across a structure is the permeability of that structure to that substance. Ions within an aqueous solution are able to move through fluid structures relatively easily. However, the cell membrane permits very slow diffusion of ions as compared to the aqueous solutions on either side. Thus, the permeability of an aqueous medium is high, while that of muscle or nerve membranes is quite low.

The permeability of the membrane determines how many particles per second cross the membrane for a given driving force (1). It is proportional to the number of pores per square centimeter of membrane. Because of the specificity of the pores for individual ions, the membrane can be differentially permeable to such ions, most notably $[Na^+]$ and $[K^+]$ (3).

Factors which determine the rate of ion movement through cell membranes include molecular concentration differences, transmembrane potential differences, membrane resistance (the reciprocal of its permeability), and active transmembrane movement of sodium and potassium ions.

TRANSMEMBRANE ION DIFFUSION

Individual molecules exhibit constant random motion, which leads them to be constantly intermixing if dissolved in a fluid medium. Such molecules tend to move from regions of higher to lower concentration. Over time, any concentration differences tend to disappear unless other influences exist. This tendency for ions to diffuse because of concentration differences is present across the muscle or nerve membrane, although severely limited by it (1).

If the dissolved molecule should be ionized, the transmembrane potential affects its rate of diffusion through the membrane. The existence of a membrane resting potential indicates that electrical charges are separated by the membrane. Thus, work must be done to move charged particles through the membrane. The charged ions on either side of the membrane exert forces on the ions within the membrane and its vicinity. Cations (+) are attracted into the cell by the negative charges on the inside and are repelled by the positive charges on the outside of the membrane. Similarly, anions (−) tend to be driven through the membrane from inside to outside. These electrochemical effects are important in the mechanisms of action potential generation.

TRANSMEMBRANE ION ACTIVE TRANSPORT

Sodium Ions

The large interstitial concentration of sodium ions influences these ions to diffuse intracellularly. Also, the negative intracellular potential attract sodium ions. However, the relative impermeability of the membrane to sodium ions minimizes the expected leakage of these ions into the cell. Some significant leakage does occur, which is countered by a mechanism which causes sodium ions to leave the cell as fast as they enter. Work must be done to expel sodium ions under such circumstances, thereby utilizing energy from cellular metabolism. The process is referred to as active Na^+ transport, or the Na^+ pump. The Na^+ equilibrium potential, as calculated by standard formulas relating conditions of ionic equilibrium to concentration gradients (the Nernst equation), is +66 mV instead of the observed −90 mV (inside negative) (1). The active sodium transport mechanism must remove sufficient Na^+ to maintain the normal resting potential, despite the tendency of this electrochemical force to produce an increase of the intracellular Na^+ concentration.

Potassium Ions

The negative intracellular potential attracts potassium ions. This is counterbalanced by the outward migration produced by the high intracellular potassium concentration. These two factors almost balance one another, but the Nernst equation shows a K^+ equilibrium potential of −97 mV (1). This closely approximates the observed resting potential of −90 mV, indicating that the influence on diffusion by concentration and electrochemical effects roughly equal one another. However, there is evidence of some metabolic work being used to actively transport a small amount of potassium into the cell. Therefore, active transport of ions across excitable membranes is at times referred to as the sodium-potassium pump, denoting the involvement of both ions in this process.

Chloride Ions

The high interstitial fluid concentration of chloride produces a tendency for its ion to penetrate the cell. This is countered by the negative resting potential. Utilizing the Nernst equation, one finds the equilibrium potential of chloride ions equals the observed resting potential. This would indicate that these ions are partitioned passively and do not require an active transport component.

IONIC PORES

Evidence for Ionic Pores

Although Hodgkin and Huxley (4) produced a largely complete analysis of the ionic permeabilities which are responsible for the action potential, they did not describe molecular detail or whether ions cross the membrane by way of pores or carriers. In the last few years, evidence for the existence of ionic channels (pores) has become more persuasive. A pharmacologic agent (nonyltriethyl-ammonium) is a potent blocker of potassium current across the membrane. An analysis of data from experiments with this chemical provides strong evidence that potassium ions pass through the membranes by means of pores. Observations noted during such experiments are easy to explain if pores are postulated to exist but are difficult to justify via a carrier model (3).

Other evidence includes the observation that each unit of area in a conducting living membrane can transport ions more quickly than known carriers. Also, the observed energy barrier for ion transport through nerve membrane is close to that calculated for a pore of reasonable dimensions but significantly different from that of ion carriers (3).

Pore Characteristics

The density of ion channels in membranes is very low. The density of sodium conducting channels appears to be significantly greater in giant axons than in small fiber preparations. Sodium and potassium channels are separate (3). Experiments show that alterations in sodium channel characteristics occur without affecting potassium current or permeability. Ion channels or pores function as though they have gates at their internal openings (3). Each Na channel has two gates, one designated as sodium activation and the other as sodium inactivation. The function of the Na inactivation gate can be destroyed without affecting activation. A potassium channel has only one gate designated as K activation.

The gates of the sodium and potassium pores open and close in response to changes of the membrane voltage (3). This would indicate that gating structures are charged and able to move in the membrane field. When the activation gates of the sodium pores close after repolarization, there is an inward current probably caused by the movement of the gating structure.

This is referred to as the gating current. The study of various ions such as Ca^{++} in relationship to the gating of sodium and potassium pores may expand knowledge of the mechanisms related to the initiation of action potentials. Studies to date would suggest that Ca^{++} alters the electrical field within the external surface of the membrane but does not alter gating directly.

INITIATION OF THE ACTION POTENTIAL

Variations in Membrane Potential

DuBois-Reymond (5) in 1843 first described changes in the excitability of nerve-muscle preparations following the application of subthreshold stimulating currents. He first used the term "electrotonus" to refer to such phenomena. This term frequently has been used in the physiologic literature to denote the cable properties of nerve (2). Such properties are a function of the geometry of nerve and muscle fibers. They are roughly cylindrical and have lengths which are great compared to their diameters. The major characteristics of note are a high resistance of cell plasm to current flow, a high membrane resistance of approximately 1,000 ohms/cm^2 which decreases to 25 ohms/cm^2 during activity (6), and a relatively high membrane capacitance of 1 μF/cm^2 which remains stable during activity (7). These electrical properties act to reduce the effect of current flow on membrane potentials after the passage of time or at distances from its application.

As long as current flow does not raise a membrane's potential to the threshold level, no significant change occurs in the membrane's resistance to the flow of ions. The only movement of ions through the membrane despite variations in its potential is the amount normally seen. However, the voltage at a given place on the membrane can change and current can flow through the membrane without actual ion penetration. A negative ion inside the cell membrane can be neutralized by a positive one which has migrated from elsewhere in the cell plasm. As a result, a positive ion just on the outside of the membrane is no longer held by the influence of the negative charge opposite it and can move into the interstitial fluid. Thus, the local potential observed at an excitable membrane may vary through such lateral ion movement rather than necessarily by ion penetration of the membrane, as long as the membrane potential is subthreshold. Such current flow is called capacitative current.

When a short duration (less than 0.1 msec) current raises the membrane voltage to less than threshold levels, the resultant increased membrane potential decays back to its prior resting level exponentially. The membrane during this time of decay has a potential which is part of that needed to reach threshold. Therefore, less additional current would be needed to raise it to threshold, making the membrane more easy to excite. The membrane in the above example is said to be more excitable or to have increased excitability. Excitability is defined as the reciprocal of threshold (2).

THRESHOLD

Threshold is that potential of an excitable membrane where the all or none firing of the membrane occurs. Once such firing begins, additional stimulus strength does not change the form of the initiated action potential. A series of changes occurs at threshold which produce an action potential and, subsequently, the status where additional action potentials can be generated. The action potential is more than simple depolarization of the membrane of zero but includes a change at its peak to about 25 mV positive inside (7).

Immediately after threshold is reached, there is a period of time where the membrane is inexcitable to any stimulus, the absolutely refractory period. Later, above normal stimuli may be necessary to produce additional action potentials of usually reduced amplitudes. The return to normal resting excitability from this stage is exponential. The time between the absolute refractory period and the normal resting excitability is described as the relative refractory period.

As discussed, prior to threshold potential there is relatively little change in the permeability of the membrane to sodium and potassium ions even with variations in membrane voltage. Once initiated, an action potential is propagated in both directions from the point of origin. During this propagation, circulating currents which exceed threshold currents precede the action potential and are the normal means of transmission (8, 9). These are commonly referred to as local currents. These local currents depolarize the membrane through largely capacitative current to the threshold level of approximately −50 to −55 mV. It is at this point that further depolarization and repolarization of the membrane occurs through selective changes in sodium and potassium ion conductance.

The Action Potential

The action potential is composed of the sequential changes in membrane potential which occur following the development of a generating potential, which raises its voltage to threshold potential. It begins at the membrane resting potential and rises to a value exceeding zero membrane potential. Prior to 1 msec, it reverses and returns to below the original membrane resting potential, from which it rises slowly to that of the resting potential. These changes in membrane potential relate in time with changes in the conductance of sodium and potassium ions

DEPOLARIZATION

As discussed previously, the rise in membrane potential to threshold voltage is accomplished without changes in the sodium and potassium conductances. Unless generated by an externally applied influence, this portion of the action potential develops from the local currents of adjacent action potentials. These currents depend upon the lateral movement of sodium and potassium ions in the intracellular and interstitial spaces, and no significant net flow of these ions through the membrane occurs. Changes in potential at local areas of the membrane resulting from such mechanisms occur primarily in response to capacitative current, i.e., local currents.

At threshold, a large increase in the conductance of sodium ions occurs. It does so because the membrane becomes specifically more permeable to sodium ions during the upstroke of the action potential (10). The process is one which is self-regenerative, i.e., as more sodium penetrates the membrane from the combined driving forces of molecular diffusion and voltage gradients it becomes more depolarized and thus further permeable to sodium ions (11). This continues until two factors cause an end to the depolarization phase of the action potential. One is the spontaneous onset of a reversal in the increased permeability of the membrane to sodium ions called sodium inactivation. A second is the increase which occurs in the permeability of the membrane to potassium ions, allowing them to leave the cell and to initiate the process of repolarization. The sodium conductance reaches its peak prior to the maximum increase in the membrane voltage and drops from its peak much more rapidly than the return of the membrane voltage to its resting level. This indicates that sodium inactivation is a significant contributor to membrane recovery independent of the process of repolarization alone.

REPOLARIZATION

During the return phase of the action potential, the membrane voltage decreased both because there is a reduced diffusion of sodium ions into the cell and an increased diffusion of potassium ions out of the cell. As the membrane potential return towards normal, it reduces the sodium conductance farther and later leads to a reduction in potassium conductance. Because the latter is delayed, at the time when the membrane potential reaches its resting value there is still an increase in potassium conductance over its normal level. This produces an influence for membrane hyperpolarization which does not disappear until the potassium conductance slowly returns to its resting value. The delayed rise in potassium conductance as compared to sodium conductance is responsible for the rapidity of repolarization. Even if potassium conductance did not increase during activity, the membrane potential would return to its resting value because of sodium inactivation. However, the rate of return would be significantly delayed (2).

Summary

Basic to EMG and nerve conduction studies are observations made regarding the electrophysiologic changes in the excitable membranes of muscle and nerve. These changes occur because a series of events produces an action potential, i.e., a change in the transmembrane potential from -90 to $+20$ mV and back to the resting level after a phase of hyperpolarization. These changes are dependent upon variations in the sodium and potassium conductances of the excitable membrane. The resting potential itself is a function of many factors, including the membrane's selective permeability to potassium ions over sodium ions, the concentration and electrochemical diffusion gradients, and the active metabolic pumping of sodium ions out of the cell and potassium ions into it.

The excitability of a given muscle or nerve cell can vary depending upon the relationship of its membrane potential to its threshold potential. It seems reasonable to assume that, as more is known regarding the changes in excitability produced from motor unit disease, more will be understood about the repetitive discharges (positive waves and fibrillation potentials) which follow insertional activity. Thus, it seems prudent for electromyographers to monitor advances in electrophysiology in order to understand better their observations and to develop improved procedures.

REFERENCES

1. WOODBURY, J. W.: The cell membrane: Ionic and potential gradients and active transport. In *Physiology and Biophysics*, pp. 1–25, ed. by T. C. Ruch and H. D. Patton, Philadelphia: W. B. Saunders, 1965.
2. WOODBURY, J. W.: Action potential: Properties of excitable membranes. In *Physiology and Biophysics*, pp. 26–72, ed. by T. C. Ruch and H. D. Patton, Philadelphia: W. B. Saunders, 1965.
3. ARMSTRONG, C. M.: Ionic pores, gates and gating currents. *Q. Rev. Biophys., 7:* 179, 1975.
4. HODGKIN, A. L., AND HUXLEY, A. F.: A quantitative description of membrane current and its application to conduction and excitation in nerve. *J. Physiol. (Lond), 117:* 500, 1952.
5. DAVIES, P. W.: Classical electrophysiology. In *Medical Physiology*, 11th ed., pp. 916–933, ed. by P. Bard, St. Louis: C. V. Mosby, 1961.
6. DAVIES, P. W.: The action potential. In *Medical Physiology*, 11th ed., pp. 946–969, ed. by P. Bard, St. Louis: C. V. Mosby, 1961.
7. HODGKIN, A. L., HUXLEY, A. F., AND KATZ, B.: Measurement of current-voltage relations in the membrane of the giant axon of loligo. *J. Physiol., 116:* 424, 1952.
8. HODGKIN, A. L.: Evidence for electrical transmission in nerve. Part I. *J. Physiol., 90:* 183, 1937.
9. HODGKIN, A. L.: Evidence for electrical transmission in nerve. Part II. *J. Physiol., 90:* 211, 1937.
10. HODGKIN, A. L., AND KATZ, B.: The effect of sodium ions on the electrical activity of the giant axon of the squid. *J. Physiol., 108:* 37, 1949.
11. HODGKIN, A. L.: Ionic basis of electrical activity in nerve and muscle. *Biol. Rev., 26:* 339, 1951.

17

History

SIDNEY LICHT, M.D.

Until recently the history of electrodiagnosis was closely associated with wars. During the First World War large numbers of casualties survived and carried residuals of nerve injuries. The use of clinical electrodiagnosis increased markedly, and the surge continued for several years after the war. There followed a relative lull until the Second World War began. There were even larger numbers of peripheral nerve casualties. Although interest in electrodiagnosis was slow in starting, there grew a postwar interest which received an even greater stimulus from newer electronic technology. We believe that fragments of history from previous centuries are of sufficient interest to warrant retelling.

The ancients saw and felt the contraction of muscles which followed contact with those aquatic animals we now recognize as capable of electrical discharge.[1] Electricity as a force or even a name was not described until

---

[1] Several ancient physicians wrote on the subject. Scribonius Largus (*Compositiones medicamentorum.* Argentorati, 1786) wrote, "Cap. I. The live black torpedo when applied to the painful area relieves and permanently cures some chronic and intolerable protracted headaches, providing that the pain is localized and lacks feeling. However, there are many varieties of torpedo and it may be necessary to try two or three varieties before numbness is felt; numbness is the sign of the cure" .... "Cap. XLI. The live black torpedo, when available and placed under the feet carries off the pain of arthritis. The patient must stand in the water just off the shore, and the torpedo must numb the whole foot and leg up to the knee. When that happens the pain is relieved and the cure is permanent. Thus was cured Anthero, hereditary freedman of Tiberius." Dioscorides (*Les Six Livres de Dioscoride.* Lyon, 1559) said that "The marine torpedo eases prolonged headache when applied to the top of the head and it also relieves all other chronic pains of the body." According to Dujardin-Beaumetz (*Dictionnaire de Thérapeutique.* Paris, 1885), Galen stated, "I therefore applied a living torpedo to the head of a person suffering from headache because I thought the remedy would have a calming effect as do all things which numb sensation, and I have seen that it was so." In his *Natural History,* Book XXII, Cap. I, Piny wrote, "From a considerable distance even, and if only touched with the end of a spear or staff, this fish has the property of benumbing even the most vigorous arm, and of riveting the feet of the runner, however swift he may be in the race." (Coulter, J. S. *Physical Therapy.* New York, 1932.) The subject was also mentioned by Paulus Aeginata in his seventh book (Turrell, W. J. History of electrotherapy. *Arch. Radiol. Electrother., 24:* 277, 1919).

1600 when William Gilbert[2] of Colchester published *De Magnete* and used the Latin adjective *electrica* to label the force excited in *electrum* (the Latin form of the Greek word for amber) (1). In 1666, Francesco Redi suspected that the shock of some fishes was muscular in origin and wrote, "It appeared to me as if the painful action of the electric ray was located in these two sickle-shaped bodies, or muscles, more than in any other part" (2). Until the time of invention of the Leyden jar (1745), frictional electricity was seldom available in quantities shocking to man, but soon after its discovery the sensation of powerful static electricity became well known to many scientists, including the French botanist Michael Adanson, who, in 1751 while travelling through Africa, became acquainted with the *Malapterus* and likened its discharge to that of the Leyden jar. In 1772, Walsh proved that the *Torpedo* discharge was electrical and showed that the back and belly of the fish gave different electrical reactions (2).

In 1658, Jan Swammerdam amused his patron of science, the Duke of Tuscany, with the twitches of an isolated frog muscle, by pinching and cutting its nerve. He described this performance as a "most delightful and indeed equally useful experiment."[3] In the light of later developments, some authors had considered those muscle contractions as the response to electrical stimuli because metal instruments had been employed, but an examination of Swammerdam's illustrations fails to reveal the possibility of a closed circuit. In 1700, Duverney, a French anatomist, tried for the first time what is now perhaps the most universally performed experiment of the physiology classroom: the electrical stimulation of frog muscle (3).

Toward the middle of the 18th century, the results of several investigators were published on their studies of tissue stimulation.[4] Interest in the subject of experimental muscle physiology was universally aroused by the publication of Haller's numerous observations, which established the fundamental principles of peripheral nerve function.[5]

---

[2] Gilbert's (or Gilberd's) work was remarkable not only for its frequent examples of inductive philosophy, which preceded the publication of Bacon's *Novum Organum,* but also for its experimental approach to science. The first mention of the electric is in Chapter II of Book II (De Magnete). "The feeble power of attraction ... we may observe in mid-winter ... when the electrical effeuvia of the earth offer less impediment, and electric bodies are harder." Gilbert also wrote, "Men of acute intelligence, without actual knowledge of facts, and in the absence of experiment, easily slip and err."

[3] Swammerdam, Jan. *Biblia Naturae.* Leyden, 1938, v. 2, p. 839; Table XLIX, Fig. V.

[4] Francis Glisson (1667) contracted the muscles of recently killed animals by simulating them with corrosive fluids and cold. He was the first to mention irritability as a property of tissue (*Tractatus de Ventriculo et Intestinis,* Lugduni Batavorum, 1691, p. 168). Whereas Glisson included even blood among irritable tissues, Haller limited it to the "capability of muscle to contract when stimulated as the result of vital force." John Brown called the capability of tissue response to stimuli, "excitability" (*The Elements of Medicine.* London, 1803). From, Verworn, M. *Irritability.* New Haven, 1913.

[5] Albrecht von Haller in his *Mémoires sur la Nature Sensible et Irritable* (Lausanne, 1756) described experiment 179: "I cut the nerves of the thigh posteriorly. The thighs lost their sensation entirely, as well as their voluntary movement, but the muscles they supplied remained irritable."

The first report on purposeful muscle contraction with static electricity was made in 1745 by Kratzenstein[6] while he was still at Halle (4). In the years which followed, there were many reports of muscular contraction induced by electricity for the purpose of curing paralysis and other diseases. Jallabert (5), in 1749, stated that muscles "could be made to move at my will in a very pronounced manner." A few years later, Whytt wrote that "the power of (electric) stimuli in exciting the muscles of living animals into contractioɴ is greater than any effort of will" and "what will prove a strong stimulus to the nerves of one part will more weakly effect those of another and vice versa" (6). In 1758, Beccaria noted that the contractions arising from electrical stimulation were stronger than those observed from mechanical stimuli (7). Seven years later, the Abbot Felice Fontana (8), curator of the largest anatomical museum in Italy, in trying to explain the conduction of stimulus to the muscle, guessed that "if it be not electricity, it may be something however very analagous to it." In 1784, Cotugno recorded the story of a student who insisted that he had received a strong electrical shock when the scalpel with which he was disssecting a mouse touched one of its nerves (9). Two years later Galvani (10) began his series of observations on muscle contraction in the frog, which he published in 1791.

Galvani noted a relationship between electricity and muscle contraction. He believed that electricity was generated by the body and called the production "animal electricity." The animal electricity of which he spoke was not derived from the muscles but from the nervous tissue, especially the brain. He correctly assumed that the nerves were good conductors and that their oily envelopes prevented the dispersion of electricity, but he considered muscles, which he likened to Leyden jars, as the receptacles for the animal electricity. Thus, the "frog current," as it came to be called popularly, was a nerve current and not a current of muscular origin.

Galvani's *Commentary* fired the scientific minds of Europe, and many rushed to repeat his experiments. The immediate reaction among most was confirmatory admiration. Vali (11) questioned Galvani's identification of nervous fluid with electricity but Volta (12) was sufficiently impressed when he first read the *Commentary* to write in 1792 that "it contains one of the

[6] Christian Gottlieb Kratzenstein was born in Wernigerode on February 2, 1723. He studied at the University of Halle where the Professor of Medicine, J. C. Krueger, suggested in a lecture to the students that electricity might be used in the treatment of paralysis. In the following year (1744), the 21-year-old physics graduate applied static electricity to the contracted finger of a woman which straightened out in 15 minutes. In March of that year he wrote the first chapter of *Schreiben von dem Nutzen der Electricität in der Arzneiwissenschaft* which was published at Halle in 1746, and is thus the first report on electrotherapy. He arrived in Copenhagen in 1752 and was made Royal Professor of Physics there in the following year. The King of Denmark ordered him to take patients for electrotherapy even though his primary interest was the basic sciences. He wrote extensively on many subjects, including geology, chemistry and milk. He also wrote what is possibly the first book on the navigation of aircraft (*L'Art de Naviguer dans l'Air*. Copenhagen, 1784), in which there is a full description of how to build and fly a balloon. He died on July 7, 1795. (*Dansk Biogrefisk Leksikon*. Copenhagen, 1938).

most beautiful and surprising discoveries and the germ of many others." But by the following year he objected with, "It is thus that I have discovered a new law, which is not so much a law of animal electricity (most of the phenomena would appear from the work of Galvani to belong to forms of spontaneous animal electricity) but they are in reality the effects of a very weak artificial electricity which is excited in a manner of which there is no doubt, by the simple application of two plates of different metals" (13).

Monro (*Secundus*), the famous Edinburgh anatomist, agreed with Volta that metals had to be connected to one another and to the muscle in a complete "circle," and Fowler (14) confirmed that "convulsions are not excited unless the metals are in contact with the animal substance or the water making part of the circle." In 1794, Galvani stimulated muscle contraction by placing the free end of a nerve across a muscle without the intervention of metals, which proved that electricity could be generated by animal tissue.

In 1795, Humboldt blistered his own shoulder and applied electricity to the denuded area to prove on his own muscles that their contraction resulted from direct stimulation. He also indicated that the nerve must be intact to achieve such a response (15).

In 1799, Volta[7] constructed a dependable source of continuous electric current. With his "pile"[8] he noted that "a contraction takes place only at the first flow of electricity, and sometimes also at the breaking of the circuit" (16). In his search for a stimulation threshold, he concluded that the muscle response was a more delicate instrument for measuring minute quantities of electricity than the electrometer, which was deflected only 0.0001 degrees by an equivalent charge (15). The genius and novelty of Volta's new invention all but extinguished any arguments in favor of electricity of muscular origin, since with the battery all those things could be produced which Galvani attributed to animal electricity. Virtually nothing further was heard about the subject of animal electricity (which Galvani proved in 1794) until 1838.

Ritter applied electricity to a muscle, using a tapped series battery of one hundred cells, in 1801 (17). He increased the current very gradually by inserting one cell after another until full strength was reached, then reduced it slowly through a water resistance, and concluded that, if the exciting stimulus were not applied with briskness, the muscle would not contract.

The initial impetus given to electrophysiology by the work of Galvani decayed because of the slow improvement in the methods of producing and detecting electricity. It was not until the end of the third decade of the 19th century that Nobili improved the galvanometer and not until 1836 that

[7] Volta, A. On electricity excited by the mere contact of conducting substances. *Philos. Trans., 90: 403,* 1800.

[8] Volta, A. *Collezione dell 'Opere del Cavaliere Conte Alessandro Volta.* Florence, 1816, v. 2, p. 158.

Daniell improved the wet cell. Electrical studies on muscle were kept alive in the country of their origin. Stefano Marianini, Volta's favorite pupil, went to Venice, where he became Professor of Physics. There in 1829 he found that the ascending (negative) current caused a greater contraction than the descending, which was also more painful (16). He spoke of two kinds of muscle contractions: the idiopathic or direct muscle stimulation response and the sympathetic, resulting from stimulation of its nerve. He was the first to state that, "When the electric fluid penetrates the nerve in a direction contrary to its ramifications, a sensation is produced."

Plaff (18) had pointed out certain regular differences in the action of the ascending and descending currents. Ritter developed this concept by distinguishing six stages of excitability based on the degree of contraction following make and break with these currents. Nobili of Reggio (19) recognized only four stages of excitation easily identified with those later rediscovered by Heidenhain (20) and subsequently used clinically by Erb.

Carlo Matteucci of Pisa, the last of the great Italian electrophysiologists, demonstrated that proximal stimulation of the ligated or sectioned nerve did not elicit a contraction. In 1838, he proved that electrical currents did originate in muscles. In September of 1848 he wrote, "The interior of a muscle placed in connection with any part whatever of the same animal . . . produces a current which goes in the animal from the muscular part to that which is not so" (21). It was the work of Matteucci which stimulated the interest of DuBois-Reymond, who in 1842 identified the muscular origin of the current (3). DuBois-Reymond registered action currents from the arm of a man who contracted his muscle by using jars of liquid as electrodes in 1851 (22).

Galen (23) divided nerves into sensory and motor. In 1810, Bell differentiated between the anterior intensible nerve roots and the sensible posterior roots. But it was Magendie in 1822 who made the final distinction between motor and sensory nerves (24). Magendie's protégé, Sarlandière (25), proposed the heroic therapy of electropuncture in 1825. He plunged large needles into muscles along the lines of the ancient Japanese practice of acupuncture. "I know I am in the muscle by the fact that all of the muscle contracts when I apply the smallest sparks. . . . I believe that I have often stimulated nerves directly. The magnitude of the contraction following the application of very weak sparks convinced me of that." Magendie tried to introduce the needle directly into nerves (26), but the method was too painful to remain popular. Before its use was abandoned, critical observers like Hamilton (27) announced that the procedure was useless in many patients with facial palsy. Hamilton employed batteries of 50 cells and noted that the magnitude of contraction depended upon the number of cells used.[9]

---

[9] Most observers of the 19th century agreed that an increase in electrical stimulation to a muscle excited increased contraction because the impulses transmitted by the nerves were increased.

In 1833, Duchenne de Boulogne[10] became so interested in the procedure of electropuncture that he devoted much of the remainder of his long life to electrical stimulation. He soon found that he could stimulate muscles electrically without piercing the skin and devised cloth-covered electrodes for percutaneous stimulation, the basic design of which is still used. Duchenne called his method of application "localized electrization" (26) and was one of the first to use the alternating current for treatment. He suggested the word "Faradic" to describe that current.[11]

Although Duchenne knew that "there are certain spots along the surface of the body and limbs that give peculiar responses to the electrode in producing ample muscle contraction," he offered no written explanation of what he was accomplishing. In the early days of his work, while he was attempting to establish a routine of treatment, he produced contractions with large electrodes using current of such high intensity that, in one instance at least, he admits having produced a fracture of the cervical vertebrae.

Remak (28) explained those "spots or border points" where the muscles were most easily stimulated. The priority controversy between these two men was one of the bitter academic battles of the century, heightened by the spirit of nationalism, which in their own generation was to result in war. In October of 1852, Duchenne invited Remak and other famous German clinicians to Paris to witness a seance of localized electrization. Although he was able to throw two different muscle groups into contraction at will, he did not explain the technique or rationale to his visitors. When Remak returned to Berlin, he said to its medical society, "One could almost complain of his (Duchenne's) intention to preserve his secret." To this Duchenne replied, "When I experiment in the presence of students, I

[10] Guillaume B. A. Duchenne was born in the Channel port of Boulogne in 1806. He was so proud of his City that when he went to practice in Paris in 1842 he virtually changed his name to Duchenne de Boulogne. Although his major interest in medical electricity was therapeutic, by his development of electrodes and apparatus, he furnished the tools and stimulated the interest which made the birth of electrodiagnosis possible. He was a difficult person and as a result was given a difficult time by the University physicians, but his perseverance, intelligence and industry have made his name better and longer remembered than the names of most of his detractors. For a complete story of his life see the article about him by Mote in *Archives d'électricité médicale, 4:* 133, 1896.

[11] In 1819 Oersted discovered "that a metallic wire which communicates with the two extremities of a voltaic cell, acquires the remarkable property of acting at a distance on a magnetic needle." Ampère, who was present when Oersted's work was presented in Paris, repeated the experiments of Oersted and soon after announced the concept of current flow. In 1831, Henry described the augmenting action of a long coil of wire on the direct current, and in that same year Faraday induced current flow in a coil of wire wound on the same iron ring as another coil of periodically charged wire. In the following year Pixii made Faraday's discovery practicable by constructing a rotary magneto-electric generator. Both Golding Bird and Neef claim credit for adding the primary coil circuit breaker, but it was the laboratory assistant Ruhmkorff who designed the inductorium (1851) which was so widely used in experimental physiology during the century which followed.

habitually remember to explain anatomical reasons that induce me to place the electrode on this or that point of election, but before the select audience of which Remak formed part, I should have thought it out of place to deliver a lesson in anatomy. Remak saw me produce contractions of a large number of muscles. This great critic obtained no glimpse of the particular methods that allowed me to obtain them. With whom then is the blame? Did I trust too much to his anatomical knowledge? Remak who has thus represented me as a prestidigitator, says again, 'He owes his knowledge of the points perhaps to chance or rather to trials, by which he arrived at this method.' Then Remak for the honor of science sets himself to work, and discovers these famous points of election are the points of entry of the muscular nerves" (26).

While this argument was raging, von Ziemssen (29) in 1857 carefully mapped out the whole surface of the body, marking the motor points on the skin of agonal patients with silver nitrate, and proved by dissection imme- diately after death that his clinical markings corresponded with the entrance of nerves into muscles.[12] Duchenne's unworthy recognition of this master- piece was, "We must not praise this work too much, for the writer has fallen under the influence of Remak."

It is unfortunate that Duchenne, a lonely, proud and bitter man, thus repeatedly lowered world opinion of himself. His contributions to neurology, kinesiology, and electrical stimulation were great indeed. He is regarded by many as the founder of electrodiagnosis. It would be more accurate to say that he stimulated the founders.

Chauveau,[13] the great veterinarian, confirmed the thoughts of his many predecessors (Bellingeri, Lehot, Phillippe, Michaelis, to mention a few) that the negative is more exciting than the positive pole (30). He introduced the monopolar method of stimulation into physiology shortly before the time that Brenner (31) introduced it into clinical practice.

In 1801, a French physician named Hallé found that the static spark did not make muscles contract in a patient with facial palsy, but when he applied the galvanic current, the muscles did contract (32). However, it was not until 1840 that the introduction of electricity into muscles was recom- mended as a diagnostic aid. Marshall Hall (33) used the galvanic current, and with it found that, in paralysis of cerebral origin, the paralytic limbs were always moved by a smaller amount of electricity than that needed for normal limbs. He asserted that in paralysis of spinal (peripheral) origin the excitability of the muscles was diminished or absent.

---

[12] Von Ziemssen, H. *Die Electricität in der Medizin*. Berlin, 1866. The entrance of nerves into muscles was first studied histologically by Doyère in 1840. Kühne showed that all striated muscles possess distinct and similar nerve endings which he called "end-plates." In 1868, Krause was the first to suggest that the impulse of stimulation had to pass through the end- plates to produce contraction.

[13] In 1859, Chauveau showed that irritation takes place only at the poles (Estorc, A. *Contribution a l'Étude de l'Électrodiagnostic*. Montpellier, 1883).

Heidenhain had noted that, occasionally in the presence of disease, a muscle might respond better to continuous current even though it did not respond to faradic. Baierlacher (34) reported that the paralyzed muscles of a woman of 28 responded to galvanic but not to faradic current and is thus credited by Erb with the discovery of electrodiagnosis. Schulz (35) and Moritz Meyer, as well as others, confirmed the value of Baierlacher's observations, but it was the obscure E. Neumann (36) of Königsberg, in 1864, who explained the phenomenon. He conceived the idea of rapidly interrupting the continuous current by means of a mechanical device and noted that, if the interruptions exceeded a certain speed, no effect was produced on the paralyzed muscle. From this he made the first truly important conclusion in electrodiagnosis—that the duration of the current was the deciding factor in eliciting contraction.

Wilhelm Erb agreed with Neumann and called the abnormal pairing of nerve reactions to both currents in nerve interruption the reaction of degeneration (*Entartungsreaktion*). In 1882, he suggested a further qualification, the partial reaction of degeneration (37), which Wernicke later correctly attributed not to partial degeneration of the nerve but to degeneration of part of the nerve fibers. Erb also studied muscle response quantitatively in relation to current strength. He demonstrated that approximately the same amount of electrical energy was needed to contract symmetrical muscles. During the progress of these studies, he found instances of increased and decreased muscle irritability as evidenced by the quantity of electrical energy required to elicit contraction.[14] He found increased irritability in early spinal and peripheral nerve lesions, "but of great interest and importance is the marked increase of electrical excitability in proven forms of spasm; I was the first to demonstrate this in tetany" (38). Mann (39) later showed the critical value to be 5mA with the anodal opening stimulus. In 1860, Pflüger had shown in animals that the shock of the closing current is stronger than that of the opening, with the anodal opening stimulus. In his book on Thomsen's disease, Erb listed ("extraordinary sluggishness and long persistence of the galvanic contraction") its electrical characteristics, although a beginning in this direction had been made by Sëeligmüller in 1878.[15] Erb is best remembered for the enunciation of his polar contraction formula which Biedermann later explained by pointing out that in disease, a virtual cathode forms in the region of the anode and, in that event, electrical action starts from that point. Erb's formula, and its inversion, remained prominent in electrodiagnosis for more than 50 years,

[14] This was announced before the present electrical units were accepted at the Congress of Paris in 1881. Erb's notations of electromotive force were recorded in terms of the number of battery elements; resistance as the number of feet of 1 mm copper wire; amperage in degrees of deflection of the galvanometer needle.

[15] Sëeligmuller in 1878 noted tonic contraction in muscles of patients with Thomsen's disease. (Bobonneix., Le syndrome électrique de la réaction myotonique. *Arch. Elect. Med., 24:* 116, 1914).

even though careful investigators such as Burke (40) recognized its inconsistency and urged that it be dropped as a criterion in 1916.

Nobili had tetanized muscle by rapidly interrupting direct current application (41). Jolly (42) found that if the tetanizing current was applied interruptedly to the orbicularis oculi muscle of a patient with myasthenia gravis, "the tetanus becomes less complete after each successive stimulus" until it finally can no longer be elicited.

Geigel (43) discovered that compression of the circulation to a nerve resulted in a negation of the Erb formula (Rich reaction).[16] Ghilarducci (44) noted that the motor point moved toward the tendinous insertion of muscle after degeneration, sometimes as much as 20–30 cm. Soon after this pronouncement in 1896, Doumer (45) pointed out that he had a prior claim to this discovery in 1891, at which time he had called it the *longitudinal reaction*, and that the finding had not only been confirmed but named "displacement of the motor point" by Wertheim-Salomonson (46) in 1895. Lewis Jones later announced that there was no shift of the motor point, but that, whereas in health the motor point is the electrically most sensitive point on the muscle, during degeneration all points on the muscle become equally sensitive.

Several other "specific" electrical reactions have been described but have not proven of clinical importance. In 1874, Hartwig (47) noted that during the paralytic attack in periodic familial paralysis the electrical response of muscle to stimulation was virtually absent. In 1922, Soderbergh (48), while examining a proven case of Wilson's disease, found an unusual response to electrical stimulation which he later called the myodystonic reaction: "The muscle responded to faradic current normally, but the relaxation was abnormally slow and disconnected."

According to Richardson and Wynn Parry (49), Bordet was the first, in 1907, to use accommodation measurements to identify denervation. Intact nerves adapt themselves to stimuli which reach their maximum only after some time, a property not possessed by muscles deprived of their nerve supply. The difference between the accommodation of innervated and denervated muscle resulted in the development of two electrodiagnostic tests: galvanic-tetanus ratio and the progressive current ratio.

The Time Factor

The French speak of that period in electrodiagnosis which first became concerned with the time factor as "modern." Neumann was the first to suggest the importance of time; Lapicque was its chief historian and a major contributor (50). He begins its story by condemning DuBois-Reymond and

---

[16] Schiff, working on compressed nerves, noted that the nerve responded to stimuli above the site of compression thus dissociating the individuality of two nerve properties—excitability and conductivity. Battez showed that stimulation of a traumatized, but continuous, nerve above the lesion would elicit contraction in the muscle supplied (Reaction of Conductibility).

his followers for perpetrating the scientific crime of prohibiting others for many years (through the influence of their authority) the correction of the statement made in 1848 that "It is not the absolute value of current density in the nerve, at any given moment, that determines the response of a muscle, but the variations of this value from moment to moment." The satellites of DuBois-Reymond continued the study of neurophysiology, and it probably occurred to some of them that the master was wrong, but no retraction was published. When one of his pupils, Bezold, dedicated his book (17) to his "teacher and dear friend DuBois-Reymond," he included the length of the latent period of muscle stimulation but failed to mention "the law" of DuBois-Reymond.

Fick used an apparatus in which a metal contact point on a stretched rubber band flew across a supporting plate (under the elastic recoil of release) and thus closed the circuit, which enabled him to administer stimuli lasting less than one ten-thousandth of a second (17). He learned that the briskness of stimuli could vary within certain limits and that "The current, to produce excitation must flow a certain length of time." He concluded that, "for the striated muscle of the frog, the law of DuBois-Reymond is not the last expression of truth." In 1867, Brücke showed that nerve and muscle could be excited separately. In 1870, Engelmann worked with the ureter muscle of a rabbit, which contracts slowly enough to be observed easily. He found a regular relationship between intensity and duration of current flow (strenth-duration curve) and called the time factor of stimulation the "physiological time" (17). König obtained brief stimuli with a pendulum constructed for him by Helmholtz. In spite of the admission that "the electric current must continue to act during a certain time to produce molecular changes in the nervous substance" he found no disagreement with "the law." Lapicque investigated the medical and university politics of the time and indicted Helmholtz for his influence of König and friendship with DuBois-Reymond with the lamentation, "Helmholtz sacrificed scientific truth for friendship not ambition."

In 1871, Tiegel (51) suggested the use of condenser discharges as a method of obtaining short-lasting stimuli; but the condenser discharge for clinical electrodiagnosis was not to be used for another 40 years.[17]

The inadequacy of "the law" was not seriously challenged[18] until 1892, when a Dutch physics teacher, Hoorweg (52), boldly asserted, "I must consider it an effort in vain to save the old classical law . . . nerve excitation

---

[17] Cluzet, J. J. Radiol. Electrol., 1: 121, 1914. "The procedure which I described for the first time in 1911." (*Lyon. Med.*, Nov. 26, 1911).

[18] Cybulski and Zanietowski had been paralleling the work of Hoorweg and were quite bitter to learn that their publication had been ignored. Their results had been published in a Polish journal which did not enjoy an international audience. Perhaps this was fortunate, for their conclusions were based on an experimental error resulting from defective wire insulation (55).

is not evoked by changes in current ... " but " ... is a function of the time and intensity."

Augustus Waller[19] at first considered stimulation as a quantity of energy but later (53), realizing the importance of the time element, spoke of the duration-intensity relationship as the "optimal minimal stimulus." Lucas (54) carried this work forward by "choosing arbitrarily an increasing series of potentials to which condensers were to be charged and seeking for each potential the minimum capacity which yielded a contraction of muscle." He proposed to adopt as a label for each excitable substance in tissue the excitation time.

In 1901, Weiss (55) studied the minimal energy needed to excite. But with the condenser method "one does not know at what moment one can consider the effective discharge as ended." Weiss not only recognized the difficulty of trying to determine what part of the diminishing discharge was effective (*temps utile*) but set about to produce a rectangular wave of electrical energy with his ballistic rheotome, which was an ingenious departure from the devices previously introduced.[20] With this instrument, he developed a simple formula of excitation[21] which, like others before and since his time, has failed to prove mathematically accurate.

Madame and Louis Lapicque carried on the tradition of experimental neurophysiology at the Sorbonne withWeiss's apparatus, but soon found that a more flexible instrument was needed. Lapicque (50) developed a precision gravity-operated pulley circuit breaker, which allowed greater accuracy. In 1909, he named the threshold of excitation "the rheobase," so-called because it is the base above which the variation of intensity as a function of time during which the current passes is developed. From the Greek *chronos* for time and *axia* for value, he derived the word *chronaxie* (in this book we shall use the Anglicized version of the Greek, chronaxia, and the French, chronaxie: chronaxy) to denote the minimal value of current duration at double the rheobase intensity needed to excite (56). The concept was not new, but it was the first expression embodying time and intensity which caught on.

Hoorweg and others had used condenser discharges in man to arrive at an excitation formula. Cluzet was the first to use a battery of condensers for clinical electrodiagnosis in 1911. At about the same time, Doumer (45) was

---

[19] Waller was the first to describe nerve degeneration and with it the one general law of biology—the portion of a cell which is separated from its nucleus dies.

[20] The instrument was simple but tedious. For each determination a projectile was fired from a coiled spring through two successive wires. As the bullet cut the first wire it closed the circuit and when it cut through the second it opened it. The distance between the wires could be varied to alter impulse duration.

[21] Davis, H. and Forbes, A. Chronaxie. *Physiol. Rev.*, *16*: 407, 1936. These authors collected about forty excitation formulae from the literature and concluded that no simple theory or equation could cope with the complexity of electrical excitation.

studying the "time constant" in man, and in the following year Bourguignon began the study of chronaxy in man, even though Lapicque had doubted its clinical value.[22]

H. Lewis Jones (57) was the first to introduce condenser discharges as a differential diagnostic procedure to the English-speaking world. He used a battery of condensers with which he was able to achieve "the ready recognition of twelve different degrees of muscle excitability." His apparatus was soon improved by Hernaman-Johnson (58), who varied the voltage as well as the capacity and thus brought the apparatus to the approximate state which Bourguignon suggested in the same year when he wrote for the first time on chronaxy in man (56).

Strength-duration curves had been determined on laboratory animals by Engelmann in 1870, but it was not until 1916 that Adrian reported on strength-duration curves in healthy and diseased human muscle (59). He plotted minimal current excitation strength against minimum excitation duration and developed curves which in health were roughly parabolic. He noted a shift of the curve in degeneration and certain fairly constant changes in regeneration. "The curve for recovering muscle is complex and is always made up of two distinct curves of which the slower corresponds more or less with that for denervated muscles and the more rapid with that for intact muscle. In the earlier stages of recovery the more rapid curve does not appear until the current strength is several times the minimal value. As recovery progresses the rapid curve becomes evident with weaker and weaker current strengths until eventually it would seem to oust the slower curve altogether."

Chronaxy determination is a relatively tedious procedure when performed on many different muscles and especially when the examiner considers it critically important to determine time differences to the fifth decimal place. Strength-duration curves are even more time consuming. There was little time and less interest during and after World War I for the busy clinician to perform routine chronaxy and S-D measurements with the equipment then available. If it had not been for Bourguignon and his many pupils, clinical

---

[22] Bourguignon, G. *La Chronaxie Chez l'Homme*. Paris, 1923. The question of priority in clinical use of chronaxy is complicated by the following satement of Lapicque written in 1915: "I have for a long time thought that the notion of measuring chronaxy in the hospital would be very useful in making electrodiagnosis more accurate. Such is also the opinion of electrotherapists such as Doumer and Cluzet, who without using the word chronaxy, have tried to determine the excitation time constant with condenser discharges. Dr. Bourguignon and my excellent pupil and friend Dr. Laugier have, by comparing the opening and closing thresholds with the induction coil according to the method of Lapicque and Weil, sought an index of speed, permitting an appreciation of the variations in chronaxy .... But I do not believe that these studies have furnished a practical procedure. The techniques are laborious, require much calculation and permit only generalizations. Now that so many nerve lesions are present among our wounded I find that interest has become urgent." He constructed a rotating rheotome which he called a chronaximeter. Lapicque, L. Présentation d'un chronaximètre clinique. Compt. Rend. Soc. Biol., *78:* 695, 1915.

chronaxy might have been completely abandoned, as it was in many countries. Electrodiagnosis was resurrected during the Second World War, as it has been in previous wars with their concomitant peripheral nerve injuries. The conventional method of generating brief electrical impulses was based on the condenser discharge. In the fourth decade of the 20th century there was a gradual introduction of electronics into electromedical equipment.

In 1941, Bauwens (60) designed a constant, current impulse generator based on earlier electronic discoveries,[23] and since that time others (61) have continued in the development of a more versatile impulse generator for the determination of chronaxy values and strength-duration curves.

Elihu Thompson showed that if the number of waves in an alternating current exceeded a frequency of 10,000/sec, neither sensory nor motor response would be elicited by it (62). In 1888, Roth used an alternating current of audio frequency and observed that the threshold potential of muscle excitation rises as the frequency is increased.[24] This was verified by d'Arsonval and later by Renqvist and Koch (64), who used frequencies up to 40,000 cycles/sec and found a minimum threshold for intensity and frequency. During the fourth decade of the 20th century interest was developed in the diagnostic possibilities of high frequency currents. Coppée named the threshold frequency "isopotential," (63), and Frappier (65) advanced its clinical application, but the method did not assume clinical importance.

Skin Resistance

The best accounts of the history of electrical skin resistance are those of Prideaux (66) and Landis and DeWick (67). Up to the time of Landis' report, the electrical phenomena of the skin were used almost exclusively by psychologists, many of whom saw a reflection of emotional status in ohmic variations. Vigoroux (68) found a diminution of skin resistance in patients with exophthalmic goitre[25] and an increase in hysterical patients on the side of anæsthesia. He attributed the findings to changes in the superficial circulation and not to the state of the epidermis. Feré (69) placee electrodes of the same diameter on the anterior surface of the forearm and the posterior surface of the thigh and passed a current through them and a galvanometer. He noted a brisk deviation in the indicating needle after visual, auditory,

[23] Eccles, W. H. in *Radio Review, 1:* 143, 1919, described a circuit which would give a rapid rise and fall of plate current. Abraham, H. and Block, E., in *Annals of Physics, 12:* 237, 1919, described a multivibrator which produced similar current impulses.

[24] Roth, *J. Pflüger's Arch., 42:* 91, 1888, in Coppée (63). Kronecker in 1868 found that if the frequency of a tetanizing current was sufficiently increased the muscle would respond with a brief jerk instead of tetanus. Wedensky (1883) showed that stimuli sufficient to produce contraction of a muscle indirectly when given through its nerve, may fail when they are repeated at certain relatively rapid rates.

[25] In 1887, Eulenberg said that the lowered skin resistance in thyroid disease was due to the perspiration. Castex, E. *Résistance Électrique des Tissues et du Corps Humain.* Montpellier, 1892.

painful, and other stimuli. He thought that this verified the hypothesis of decreased skin resistance secondary to increased circulation. Tarchanoff explained the reaction as an active state of the sweat glands which produces a secretory current (66). Veraguth (70) named the phenomenon "psycho-galvanic-reflex." Waller (53) dropped the prefix "psycho," because there is nothing central about it. Lauer (71) lists 54 variations of the name given to the phenomenon and concludes that it is "largely non-psychic in nature, only at times is it galvanic, and there is considerable doubt as to whether it is reflex."

At about that time, Richter was one of the psychologists investigating the galvanic skin reaction. He decided that more study was required on the basic conductivity of the skin. He found that section of the nerves in monkeys caused an increase in the resistance of the skin area they supplied. He also found that sympathectomy did the same thing (72). Some years later he was able to demonstrate the same results in man (73). Jasper improved the apparatus Richter designed for ESR (Electrical Skin Resistance) in 1945 (74), and a further improvement with mechanization was suggested in 1951 by Thomas and Korr (75).

Gildemeister[26] stressed the interference in skin electrical measurement of the counter electromotive force produced in human skin by the polarization which follows the passage of direct current. Brazier (76) suggested the use of alternating current to avoid the polarizing effect. She disregarded the accepted electrical structure of the human body and considered it as a dielectric. Dielectrics are measured by a specific physical property called the dielectric loss angle, which is independent of the size and the shape of the object measured. The dielectric loss angle, or angle of impedance (I.A.), is a measure of a physical property of the human tissues and not of the skin alone. By measuring the impedance angle in many normal subjects and patients, Brazier showed its specific diagnostic value in thyrotoxicosis.

Action Potentials

The subject of muscle-generated electricity first opened by Redi and, in 1794, championed by Galvani was sent into rapid oblivion when Volta discovered the electric pile. The words *animal electricity* were not even mentioned in historical articles for the next 30 years until, in 1827, Nobili spoke of the "frog current" which he thought was a thermoelectric effect (21). In 1838, Matteucci began using Nobili's improved galvanometer[27] on

---

[26] Gildemeister, M. Über elektrischen Widerstand, Kapazität und Polarisation der Haut. *Pflügers Arch., 176:* 84, 1919. Bordier had recognized the influence of polarization under the testing electrodes and considered the body as a condenser with a capacity estimated at 0.0025 microfarads.

[27] The first practical galvanometer based on Oersted's discovery, was made by Schweigger in 1820. In 1825, Nobili improved upon it by compensating for the torque of the earth's magnetism (*Ann. Chem. Phys., 3:* 225, 1828). In 1858, Lord Kelvin perfected the device with a highly sensitive reflecting galvanometer. The moving coil galvanometer was based on the

frog preparations and proved conclusively what Becquerel called "one of the most important properties of muscle in the empire of life," the generation of electricity by contracting muscle (21). It was the work of Matteucci which interested DuBois-Reymond in electrophysiology. In 1842, DuBois-Reymond wrote a letter to Poggendorff in which he confirmed the work of Matteucci: "These currents are produced by muscles" (77). In 1851, DuBois-Reymond registered action currents from the contracting arm of a man. He used jars of liquid as electrodes (22) and thus performed what was virtually the first human EMG at a time when electrical measuring devices were primitive. According to Piper (78), human action potentials were detected by Bernstein in 1867 and by Hermann 11 years later.

More precise knowledge of muscle action currents had to await the perfection of apparatus which could record the small and rapidly fluctuating potentials developed by muscles. In 1872, Lippmann (79) offered the capillary electrometer, which continued to be used for more than 30 years for recording tissue potentials. The reflecting coil galvanometer of d'Arsonval constructed in 1882 was another helpful tool, which Einthoven (80) modified in 1901 by substituting a single straight fiber of silvered quartz for the loop. This enabled the recording of millivolt potentials with speed, accuracy, and permanence. The string galvanometer, however, is sensitive only to fluctuations up to 2000/sec, and, although it can be used for EMG, it became necessary to seek a device in which the "writing" was done by a virtually weightless device.[28]

Action potentials have been recorded from nervous tissue and from all muscles of the body. In 1910, Theilhaber (81) studied the electric potential of the human uterus by placing one electrode on the cervix and the other in the rectum. In 1954, Steer (82) described electrohysterography with skin electrodes on women during labor and was able to show that variations in the potential tracings occurred in abnormal labor. Action potentials have also been studied in the other smooth muscles.

---

discovery by Ampère in 1820 that a conductor carrying current tended to move transversely across a magnetic field. On this principle Sturgeon built a galvanometer in 1836 which was finally perfected by d'Arsonval in 1882 as the reflecting coil galvanometer. Joubert devised the ondograph or ink-writing pen and this was made more sensitive by Blondel in 1891 and Duddell in 1893 (*Encylopaedia Britannica*).

[28] In 1897, Braun (*Ann. Phys. Chem., 60:* 552) invented the cathode ray tube which was improved 8 years later by Wehnelt. Dufour and A. B. Wood introduced photography to record its luminescent tracing. But the tube could not be used for the high voltages demanded by amplification requirements until Langmuir invented a method of *hardening* it in 1912. A patent was not granted on the process until 1925 which restricted its use markedly. In 1920, Forbes and Thacher (*Amer. J. Physiol., 52:* 409) were the first to use the electron tube to amplify action currents. With it and a string galvanometer they were able to produce excellent electromyograms. In 1922, Gasser and Erlanger used the cathode ray oscilloscope in place of the galvanometer and thus set the pattern for future electromyographic apparatus (*Amer. J. Physiol., 73:* 613, 1922).

Electromyography

Piper (78) recorded voluntary contractions in the forearm flexors of man in 1907 with the string galvanometer. He found distinctive rhythms for each muscle, which he thought indicated the rate of stimuli received from the central nervous system. Buchanan (83) tried to confirm his findings on the same muscles with the capillary electrometer but found that there was no regular muscle potential rhythm. Instead she found an irregular response of potentials at a rate of up to 120/sec. As might be expected, the string galvanometer was used in the country of its invention for EMG. Chief among the investigators of human EMG in Holland was Wertheim-Salomonson (84) who thought that with it he could differentiate between tetanic and tonic muscle spasm. Until the third decade of the 20th century, most human EMGs were made by physiologists attempting to correlate laboratory findings with "normal" human muscle potentials. Wertheim-Salomonson examined patients with tetany, chorea, and hemiplegia, but the first attempt to obtain tracings in peripheral nerve paralysis was that of Proebster (85), in 1928, and to him most authors give the credit for beginning clinical EMG. He described spontaneous irregular action potentials in the denervated muscles of a boy with a traumatic plexus birth lesion and in another patient with long-standing poliomyelitis. Proebster used a recording galvanometer and tested muscles in voluntary as well as in electrically induced contractions.

Until 1929 human EMGs showed the potentials developed in relatively large portions of muscle. In that year, Adrian made two more great contributions to the field of electrodiagnosis. With the introduction of the coaxial needle electrode (86) he made it possible to pick up the potential developed by a single muscle fiber. With the introduction of the loud-speaker he added the sound record, which some workers find a necessary adjunct to EMG, "for the ear can pick out each new series of slight differences in intensity and quality which are hard to detect in the complex electrometer record." Adrian and Bronk found that in completely relaxed normal muscle, even at amplifications up to 2×10^6, there was no spontaneous electrical activity. They noted the rate and range of action potentials in voluntary contraction.

One of the major difficulties in recording minute muscle action potentials was the intrusion of extraneous electrical activity. To minimize its confusing effect, screening of the test area was necessary until Matthews (87) suggested differential amplification.[29]

In 1935, Lindsley (62) made the first tracings of a patient with myasthenia gravis and noted the marked fluctuations in amplitude of motor unit responses to contraction. In 1938, Denny-Brown and Pennybacker (88),

---

[29] Instead of grounding one lead and attaching the other to the grid, Matthews connected each of the bipolar leads to parallel grids which offered immunity from feedback in later stages and comparative freedom from electrical interference as well as reduction in stimulus escape when electrical stimulation was employed (*J. Physiol., 81:* 28P, 1934).

using bipolar needle electrodes with tracings on bromide paper, differentiated between fasciculation and fibrillation.[30] In 1941, Denny-Brown and Nevin (89) recorded the characteristic potentials of myotonia. In that year, Buchthal and Clemmesen (90) validated with clinical EMG the findings in muscle atrophy, and Hoefer (91) obtained rhythmic potentials in rigid muscles at rest in patients with Parkinsonism.[31]

Until 1944, EMG had been used by few clinicians. The equipment was expensive and custom built, the procedure and identification of diagnostic patterns were not well organized and its possibilities not widely appreciated. In that year, Weddell, Feinstein and Pattle (92) published a complete report on clinical EMG, which became the working reference for many workers. It discusses and analyzes muscle potentials in normals and all the neuromuscular entities ordinarily encountered. In the same year, Jasper and Notman (93) introduced the monopolar needle electrode. In 1950, Bayer, according to Lenman (94), showed that the muscle potential increases with the force of contraction. With the increasingly useful information offered by EMG, its use spread with considerable speed. Although Bauwens (95) used EMG in his clinic in 1941, the procedure was regarded primarily as a research method until 1950. In that year, only a handful of physical medicine specialists had personally conducted examinations with an EMG by 1960, most physical medicine specialists considered it required equipment for a good department.

Up to the middle of the present century, most electrodiagnostic exploration was conducted at the muscle. In 1948, Hodes, Larrabee and German (96), influenced by the work of Harvey and Kuffler (38), stimulated nerves at two different levels and noted the temporal difference in muscle response. By correlating the difference with the distances measured or estimated, they were able to determine conduction time or velocity. In the second half of the sixth decade of this century, conduction velocity became increasingly popular as a research project until Christie and Coomes called velocity measurements "suspect." They concluded that, "For routine electrodiagnostic investigation of nerve conduction the measurement of latency is probably

---

[30] When the motor nerve to a muscle is completely divided there is immediate loss of voluntary contraction. Individual muscle fibrils retain their terminal nervous supply for a matter of days to weeks. When nerve degeneration is complete, the denervated fibrils begin to contract spontaneously (fibrillation). Schiff was the first to associate fibrillation with paralysis (*Arch. Physiol. Heilkunde, 10*: 579, 1851). He cut the nerves to the tongues of animals and noted spontaneous twitches in them from about the 3rd day until their complete atrophy about 6 months later. Langley and his co-workers revived interest in this phenomenon, once more by inspection, in a series of publications between 1915 and 1918 (*J. Physiol., 49*: 410, 1915). The history of fibrillation is covered in detail in *Clinical Electromyography* by A. A. Marinacci, Los Angeles, 1955.

[31] Stanley Cobb had begun electromyographic examinations in 1917 with skin electrodes and a galvanometer. He found a "remarkable regularity of this tremor; average 5.8 per second." (Electromyographic studies of paralysis agitans. *Arch. Neur. Psych., 8*: 247, 1922.)

all that is required."[32] Liberson found that conduction occurs in both directions and that the portion of the impulse which is antidromic returns through the reflex arc to permit still another recording from the muscle supplied by the stimulated nerve.[33]

EMG has enjoyed uses other than clinical diagnosis. It has been used to monitor ventilation by identification of diaphragmatic action potentials.[34] It has also been received as legal evidence in the courts of a growing number of American states.

The history of electrodiagnosis and EMG has been one of increasing quantification on diminishing areas; from the millisecond impulse of the faradic coil to the hundredth millisecond impulse of the electronic generator; from the large percutaneous electrode to the barely visible tip of a needle; from the muscle to the muscle fiber. It would seem that we have reached the limits of minuteness in time and tip. But the one great lesson of the history of science is that the boundaries of knowledge are not fixed.

REFERENCES

1. GILBERT, W.: *De Magnete, Magnetisque Corporibus et de Magno Tellure*, London, 1600. Translation, P. F. Mottelay, New York, 1893.
2. BIEDERMANN, W.: *Electrophysiology*, London, 1898.
3. MORGAN, C. E.: *Electrophysiology*, New York, 1868.
4. KRATZENSTEIN, C. G.: *Schreiben von dem Nutzen der Electricität in der Arzneiwissenschaft*, Halle, 1746.
5. JALLABERT, M.: *Experiences sur l'Electricité avec Quelques Conjectures sur la Cause de ses Effets*, Paris, 1749.
6. HOFF, H.: Galvani and pre-Galvanian electrophysiologists. *Ann. Sci., 1:* 157, 1936.
7. COLWELL, H.: *An essay on the History of Electrotherapy*, London, 1922.
8. FONTANA, F.: Treatise on the Venom of the Viper. London, 1795. (A translation from the Italian, *Richerche Fisiche Sopra il Veleno della Vipera*, Lucca, 1767.)
9. WILKINSON, C. H.: *Elements of Galvanism*, London, 1804.
10. GALVANI, L.: *De Viribus Electricitatis*. Translation by R. Green, Cambridge, 1953.
11. VALLI, E.: *Experiments in Animal Electricity*, London, 1793.
12. VOLTA, A.: *Collezione dell' Opere del Cavaliere Conte Alessandro Volta*, Florence, 1816.
13. VOLTA, A.: *An account of some discoveries made by M. Galvani. Philos. Trans., 83:* 10, 1793.
14. FOWLER, R.: Experiments and Observations Relative to the Influence Lately Discovered by M. Galvani, Edinburgh, 1793.
15. CASSIUS, L., DAUBINCOURT, AND DE SAINTOT: *Precis Succinct des Principaux Phénomènes du Galvanisme*, Paris, 1803.
16. MARIANINI, S.: Mémoires sur la secousse qu'éprouwent les animaux. *Ann. Chem. Phys., 40:* 225, 1829.
17. LAPICQUE, L.: La chronaxie et ses applications physiologiques. In *Physiologie Generale du Système Nerveux*, vol. 5, p. 23, Paris, 1938.

[32] Christie, B. G. B. and Coomes, E. N. Normal variation of nerve conduction in three peripheral nerves. *Ann. Phys. Med., 5:* 303, 1960.

[33] Liberson, W. T. Paper delivered at the Third International Congress of Physical Medicine in Washington, D. C. August 1960.

[34] Fink, B. R., Hanks, E. C., Holaday, D. A. and Ngai, S. H. Monitoring of ventilation by integrated diaphragmatic electromyogram. *J.A.M.A., 172:* 1367, 1960.

HISTORY / 421

18. PFAFF, G.: Ueber thierische Elektricität, Leipzig, 1795. In Morgan (3).
19. HUMPHREYS, A.: Development of the conception and measurement of electric current. *Ann. Sci., 2:* 164, 1937.
20. HEIDENHAIN: In Biedermann (2).
21. MATTEUCCI, C.: *Traités des Phenomènes Electro-Physiologiques,* Paris, 1844.
22. LUCAS, K.: *Vade Mecum d'Electrodiagnostic,* Paris, 1916.
23. GALEN, C.: *Epitome Galeni Pergameni Operum,* p. 184, Basle, 1571.
24. CORRESPONDENCE. *Lancet, i:* 697, 1911.
25. SARLANDIERE. *Mémoires sur l'Electropuncture,* Paris, 1825.
26. DUCHENNE, G. B.: *Treatise on Localised Electrisation,* London, 1871.
27. HAMILTON, J.: Trial of acupuncture with galvanism. *Dublin J. Med. Sci., 6:* 78, 1835.
28. REMAK, R.: *Galvanotherapie,* Berlin, 1858.
29. VON ZIEMSSEN, H.: *Die Elektricität in der Medizin,* Berlin, 1866.
30. CHAUVEAU, M. A.: Théorie des effets produits par l'électricite. *J. Physiol.* (Paris), *2:* 490, 1859; *3:* 274, 1860.
31. BRENNER, H.: Versuch zur Begrund einer, etc. *Petersburg Med. Zeitschr., 3:* 257, 1882.
32. ESTORC, A.: *Contribution à l'Electrodiagnostic,* Montpellier, 1883.
33. HALL, M.: On the condition of muscular irritability in paralytic muscles. In *Electricity in Relation to Medical Practice,* M. Meyer, New York, 1872.
34. BAIERLACHER, E. BAYREUTH: Aerzt. Intelligenzblatt, 1859. In Neumann E. (36).
35. SCHULZ, B.: Ueber das Verhalten der Muskeln bei Paralysis Nervi facialis gegen den inducirten und konstanten elektrischen Strom. *Wien. Med. Wchnschr., 27:* 417, 1860.
36. NEUMANN, E.: Ueber das verschiedene Verhalten gelähmter Muskeln gegen der konstanten und inducirten Strom und die Erklärung desselben. *Deutche Klinik, 16:* 65, 1864.
37. ERB, W.: *Handbook of Electrotherapy,* New York, 1883.
38. HARVEY, A. M., AND KUFFLER, S. W.: Motor nerve function with lesions of peripheral nerves. *Arch. Neurol. Psych., 52:* 317, 1940.
39. MANN, L.: Untersuchungen über die elektrische Erregbarkeit im frühen Kindes alter mit besonderer Beziehung auf die Tetanie. *Monschr. Psychiatr. Neurol., 7:* 14, 1900.
40. BURKE, N. H.: The reaction of degeneration in medical literature. *Arch. Radiol. Electrol., 21:* 54, 1916. Also, Roberts, R.: Degeneration of muscle following nerve injury. *Brain, 39:* 297, 1916.
41. GARRATT, A.: *Electrophysiology and Electrotherapeutics,* Boston, 1861.
42. JOLLY, F.: Myasthenia gravis pseudoparalytica. *Berl. Klin. Wchnschr., 32:* 33, 1895.
43. GEIGEL, R., AND VOIT, F.: *Lehrbuch der klinischen Untersuchungs-Methoden,* Stuttgart, 1895.
44. GHILARDUCCI, F.: Sur une nouvelle forme de la réation de dégénérescence. *Arch Elect. Méd., 4:* 17, 1896.
45. DOUMER, E.: Note sur un nouveau signe électrique musculaire. *Compt. Rend. Soc. Biol., 9:* 656, 1891.
46. WERTHEIM-SALOMONSON, J. K.: Bijdrage tot de diagnostick der Kleinhersen aandoenigen. *Neder. Tidj. Geneesk., 31:* 978, 1895.
47. HARTWIGS: In Oddo and Darcourt: *Les réactions électriques dans la paralysie familiale périodique. Arch. Elect. Méd., 10:* 1, 1902.
48. SODERBERGH, G.: The myodystonic reaction. *Acta Med. Scand., 56:* 585, 1922.
49. RICHARDSON, A. T., AND PARRY, C. B. WYNN: The theory and practice of electrodiagnosis. *Ann Phys. Med., 4:* 3, 1957.
50. LAPICQUE, L.: Première approximation d'une loi nouvelle de l'excitation électricque. *Compt. Rend. Soc. Biol., 1:* 615, 1907.
51. TIEGEL, F.: Ueber den Gebrauch eines Condensators zum Reizen mit Induction-sapparaten. *Pfluger's Arch., 14:* 330, 1877.
52. HOORWEG, J.: Ueber die elektrische Nervennerregung. *Arch. Ges. Physiol., 52:* 87, 1892.
53. WALLER, A.: *Proc. Roy. Soc., 45:* 214, 1899.
54. LUCAS, K.: The excitable substance in amphibian muscle. *J. Physiol., 36:* 113, 1907.
55. WEISS, G.: *Technique d'Electrophysiologie,* Paris, 1895.

56. BOURGUIGNON, G.: *La Chronaxie Chez l'Homme*, Paris, 1923.

57. JONES, H. L.: Use of condenser discharges in electrical testing. *Proc. Roy. Soc. Med., 61:* 49, 1913.

58. HERNAMAN-JOHNSON, F.: The use of condensers in diagnosis and prognosis of nerve lesions. *Lancet, 1:* 351, 1916.

59. ADRIAN, E. D.: The electrical reactions of muscles before and after injury. *Brain, 39:* 1, 1916.

60. BAUWENS, P.: The thermionic control of electric currents in electro-medical work. *Proc. Roy. Soc. Med., 34:* 715, 1941.

61. RITCHIE, A. E.: Electrical diagnosis of the peripheral nerve injuries. *Brain, 67:* 314, 1944.

62. LINDSLEY, D. B.: Myographic and electromyographic studies in myasthenia gravis. *Brain, 58:* 470, 1935.

63. COPPÉE, G.: Une nouvelle caracteristique chronologique de l'excitabilite. *Arch. Intern. Physiol., 38:* 251, 1934.

64. RENQVIST, Y., AND KOCH, H.: *Skand. Arch. Physiol., 59:* 279, 1930. In Coppée (63).

65. FRAPPIER, H.: *Essai d'Electrodiagnostic par l'Emploi des Courants Alternatifs à Hautes Fréquences Variables*, Paris, 1934.

66. PRIDEAUX, E.: The psycho-Galvanic reflex, *Brain, 42:* 51, 1920.

67. LANDIS, C., AND DEWICK, H. N.: The electrical phenomena of the skin. *Psychol. Bull., 26:* 64, 1929.

68. VIGOROUX, R.: Sur le rôle de la résistance électrique des tissus dans l'electrodiagnostic. *Compt. Rend. Soc. Biol., 31:* 336, 1879.

69. FERE, C.: Note sur des modifications de la résistance électrique sous l'influence des excitations sensorielles et des émotions. *Compt. Rend. Soc. Biol., 5:* 217, 1888.

70. VERAGUTH, O.: *Das psychogalvanische Reflexphânomen*, Berlin, 1909.

71. LAUER, A. R.: A new type of electrode for the galvanic skin reflex. *J. Exp. Psychol., 11:* 248, 1928.

72. RICHTER, C.: Physiological factors involved in the electrical resistance of the skin. *Am. J. Physiol., 88:* 596, 1929.

73. RICHTER, C., AND KATZ, D.: Determination of the peripheral nerve injuries by the electrical skin resistance method. *J.A.M.A., 122:* 648, 1943.

74. JASPER, H.: An improved clinical dermohmmeter. *J. Neurosurg., 2:* 257, 1945.

75. THOMAS, R. E., AND KORR, I. M.: The automatic recording of electrical skin resistance patterns of the human trunk. *Electroencephalography, 3:* 361, 1951.

76. BRAZIER, M.: Impedance angle test for thyrotoxicosis. *West J. Surg., 43:* 429, 1935.

77. MOTTELAY, P. F.: *Biographical History of Electricity*, London, 1922.

78. PIPER, H.: *Elektrophysiologie menschlicher Muskeln*, Berlin, 1912.

79. LIPPMANN, G.: *Unités Electriques Absolues*, Paris, 1899.

80. EINTHOVEN, W.: Ein neues Galvanometer. *Drude's Ann. Physik.*, 1901.

81. THEILHABER, A.: Insufficientia uteri, atonia uteri. *Monatsch. Geburtheil. Gynäk., 31:* 727, 1910.

82. STEER, C. M.: The electrical activity of the human uterus in normal and abnormal labor. *Am. J. Obstet. Gynecol., 68:* 867, 1954.

83. BUCHANAN, F.: The electrical response of muscle to voluntary, reflex and artificial stimulation. *Q. J. Exp. Physiol., 1:* 211, 1908.

84. WERTHEIM-SALOMONSON, J. K.: Tonus and the reflexes. *Brain, 43:* 369, 1920.

85. PROEBSTER, R.: Über Muskelaktionsströme am gesunden und kranken Menschen. *Zeitschr. Orthop. Chir., 50:* 1, 1928.

86. ADRIAN, E. D., AND BRONK, D. W.: The discharge of impulses in motor nerve fibers. *J. Physiol., 67:* 119, 1929.

87. MATTHEWS, B. H. C.: A special purpose amplifier. *J. Physiol., 81:* 28, 1934.

88. DENNY-BROWN, D., AND PENNYBACKER, J. B.: Fibrillation and fasciculation in voluntary muscle. *Brain, 61:* 311, 1938.

89. DENNY-BROWN, D., AND NEVIN, S.: The phenomenon of myotonia. *Brain, 64:* 1, 1941.

90. BUCHTHAL, F., AND CLEMMESEN, S.: On differentiation of muscular atrophy by electromyography. *Acta Psychiatr., 16:* 143, 1941.

91. HOEFER, P. F. A.: Physiology of motor innervation in the dyskinesias. In *Physiological Foundations of Neurology and Psychiatry*, Gellhorn, E., Minneapolis, 1953.

92. WEDDELL, G., FEINSTEIN, B., AND PATTLE, R. E.: The electrical activity of voluntary muscle in man under normal and pathological conditions. *Brain, 67:* 178, 1944.

93. JASPER, H., AND NOTMAN, R.: In *Clinical Electromyography*, A. A. Marinacci, Los Angeles, 1955.

94. LENMAN, J. A. R.: Quantitative electromyographic changes associated with muscular weakness. *J. Neurol. Neurosurg. Psychiatr., 22:* 306, 1959.

95. BAUWENS, P.: Electrodiagnosis and electrotherapy in peripheral nerve lesions. *Proc. Roy. Soc. Med., 34:* 459, 1941.

96. HODES, R., LARRABEE, M. C., AND GERMAN, W.: The human electromyogram in response to nerve stimulation and the conduction velocity of motor axons. *Arch. Neurol. Psychiatr., 60:* 340, 1948.

97. ERB, W.: Historisches von der Entartungsreaktion. *Berl. Klin. Wochnschr., 22:* 765, 1885.

98. ERB. W.: *Die Thomsen'sche Krankheit*, Leipzig, 1886. Also, Thomsen, J. Tonische Krampfe in willkurlich beweglichen Muskeln. *Arch. Psych. Nervenkr., 6:* 706, 1875.

99. RUSHTON, W.: The time factor in electrical excitability. *Biol. Rev., 10:* 1, 1935.

100. GOLSETH, J. G., AND FIZZELL, J. A.: A constant current impulse generator. *Arch. Phys. Med., 27:* 154, 1945.

101. THOMSON, E.: In Weiss. (55).

Glossary of Some Technical Terms Relating to Apparatus for EMG

STUART REINER, M.E.E.

Active Elements. Components of a circuit which provide amplification or which control direction of current flow, for example, diodes, transistors and vacuum tubes.

Address. In digital data storage systems, the description of a location (stated in system notation) where information is stored. Also, as a verb, to select or designate the location of information in a storage system.

Alternating Current (AC). A flow of current in which the direction of current flow reverses periodically. When the reversal occurs cyclically, two current reversals are termed one cycle. The number of complete cycles per second is the frequency and it is stated in Hertz.

Amplifier. A device which multiplies its input voltage, current, or power by a fixed or controllable factor, usually without altering its wave form.

Amplifier, AC. Will respond to alternating current (AC) signals only and will not respond to an input potential that does not vary. This type of amplifier is used in EMG apparatus. Sometimes termed RC or AC coupled amplifier.

Amplifier, DC (or Direct Coupled). Responds to direct current (DC) signals, pulsating DC and alternating current signals. This type of amplifier is not used in clinical EMG. It is used in force and tension measurements as well as in the recording of intracellular resting potentials where fixed, slowly and rapidly changing phenomena are measured.

Amplifier, Differential. Used in EMG preamplifiers. It has two recording electrode input terminals (instead of the single input terminal of a conventional amplifier) and a ground or zero-potential terminal. It rejects unwanted potentials originating at a distance and presenting at both input terminals (common-mode or in-phase potentials).

Amplitude Modulation (AM). Systems of signal transmission, recording or processing, that utilize an alternating current carrier potential of peak amplitude which varies proportionally with the instantaneous amplitude of the signal.

Analog. Applied to signals and devices capable of or accommodating continuous change and assuming an infinite number of values with finite limits. An analog signal may be a current or a voltage that varies in time continuously, simulating a natural phenomenon it represents.

Analog-to-Digital Converter (A-D Converter). A device which converts an analog signal, usually a varying voltage or current, to digital output (See Digital System.)

Anode. A positive terminal. The terminal through which "electron current" enters a device. "Conventional current" flow, however, is said to be away from the anode and toward the cathode (opposite or negative) terminal.

Artifact. All unwanted potentials which originate outside the tissues examined. They are also called "noise" when they appear in measurement. An artifact may arise from biological activity, the electrode or apparatus used in the examination, the power line, or extrinsic electricity (surrounding the apparatus or patient). (See Noise.)

Attenuator. In electrical circuits, an arrangement which introduces a definite reduction in the magnitude of a voltage current or power. Attenuators may be fixed or adjustable continuously or in steps.

Averager Signal. A signal processing method that aids in the recording of small stimulus evoked potentials which are obscured by noise or artifact. The stimulus is repeated a number of times and the responses are subjected to a special summation technique that causes the random noise portion of the response to become smaller in proportion to the evoked potentials which are coherent in time with each stimulus.

Beam Switching. A technique for producing a multitrace display on a single beam cathode ray tube by rapidly commutating the beam to a number of signal sources. This system is also called Chopped Display and Electron Switched Display.

Bias. A fixed electrical or mechanical input to a device or a system that is distinct from the input signal. The bias brings the system to a desired operating range.

Binary Coded Decimal (BCD). A binary numbering system coding decimal numbers in groups of four bits for each decimal digit.

Binary Logic. A digital logic system which operates with two distinct states variously called "one and zero," "high and low," and "on and off."

Bit. A binary numeral, the "one and zero" or "high and low," and so on, of binary logic. A group of bits comprise a binary word.

Blocking. An effect that results when a large transient input potential is applied to an amplifier, temporarily causing the disappearance or severe distortion of the output signal.

Calibrator. A device which identifies units of measurement by reference to a known standard.

Calibrator, Amplitude. An accurate source of voltage of known amplitude, usually within the range of EMG motor activity, for example, between 10 and 1,000 μv, which can be applied or switched to the input terminals of the apparatus.

Calibrator, Time. An alternating or pulsatile wave form of accurately known frequency that can be applied to the cathode ray display of an EMG so as to permit accurate adjustment of "time per division" on the horizontal graticule scale of the EMG screen.

Capacitance. A measure of electric charge that can be stored within the insulation separating two conductors when a given voltage is applied to the conductors. A capacitor or a condenser uses conductors of large surface area separated by air or by various insulators (dielectrics) which enhance capacitive effects. The unit capacitance is the farad. Direct current is not conducted by capacitors; alternating current or pulsating direct current signals are conducted to an extent proportional to frequency.

Carrier. A potential, usually alternating current, of sine or pulse wave form used in signal transmission or recording or processing systems that in itself carries no information but is modified most commonly in amplitude (amplitude modulation), frequency (frequency modulation), or timing by the signal. The carrier is at least a number of times higher in frequency than the highest frequency component in the signal.

Cathode. A negative terminal; the terminal through which "electron current" leaves a device. Conventional current flow is said to be toward the cathode, or away from the anode (positive) terminal.

Cathode Ray Tube (CRT). A vacuum tube used to visualize electrical wave forms. It generates X-Y traces on its screen by means of a moving fluorescent spot on its screen.

Clipping (Limiting). Occurs when signals of excessive amplitude are applied to an amplifier with a resultant wave form at the amplifier output that faithfully reproduces the shape of the input wave form only up to a level at which the signal becomes excessive (clipping level). All portions of the wave form that exceed the clipping level will appear at the output at a fixed level unvarying with time and, therefore, seriously distorted.

Common Mode Rejection. An important property of differential amplifiers that expresses their ability to discriminate against artifact potentials that appear equally at both amplifier input terminals (common mode signals) and to amplify the desired potentials (differential or series-mode signals) that appear as different signals at the two input terminals.

Commutation. A system that cyclically switches a number of signals sequentially to a single device amplifier, transmission, or recording channel. Also termed Multiplexing.

Conduction Time Indicator. A movable time index on the trace of the cathode ray tube arranged to be positioned on the screen by a dial accurately calibrated in time, measured either from the start of the sweep or from a shock artifact to the index position.

Crosstalk. The incursion of information from one channel into any other channel of a multichannel information-handling system. The presence of crosstalk in a multichannel EMG study can be seriously misleading.

Cycle. A complete sequence of values of an alternating quantity repeated as a unit. CPS—cycles per second, called Hertz.

Decibel (dB). A dimensionless unit for comparing the ratio of signal levels on a logarithmic scale. Positive decibel values represent a signal increase with respect to a reference. Negative decibel values represent signal decrement with respect to a reference signal.

Delay Line. A short term electrical dynamic storage device that delays potentials applied to its input so that they appear at its output as if they had occurred (1–20 msec) later in time. This permits events preceding action potentials to be seen on the cathode ray tube screen when the sweeps are triggered by the potentials.

Differentiator. A device or circuit whose output wave form is proportional to the rate of change (speed, velocity, etc.) of the input wave form.

Digital System. A system or circuit for handling or processing information in terms of numbers and utilizing circuits which operate in the manner of switches, having two (on-off) or more discrete positions. The simplest and most common digital system is the binary system.

Digital-to-Analog Converter (D-A Converter). A circuit that accepts the discrete coded signal voltages of a digital system and generates, at its output, voltages of amplitudes analogous to the numbers represented by the digital codes at its input. The analog output may then be directly interpreted by viewing a cathode ray tube, on a meter, or by graphic recording.

Diode. A two-terminal device which permits the flow of electric current in one direction only.

Direct Current (DC). A unidirectional current. An intermittent or time-varying current which has a net flow in one direction is called pulsating direct current or direct current with an alternating current component.

Dynamic Range. The ratio of the maximum input signal capability of a system without overloading to the minimum usable signal (noise level).

Electrode. A conductor of electricity. In clinical electrodiagnosis, it is generally a metal device which introduces or picks up electricity from tissue.

Electrodes, Recording. Electrodes used to measure electrical activity from tissue.

Bipolar, Bifilar Needle Electrodes. Variations in voltage are measured between the bared tips of two insulated wires cemented side by side in a steel cannula. The bare tips of the electrodes are flush with the bevel of the cannula. The latter may be grounded.

Concentric Needle Electrode. Variations in voltage are measured between the bare tip of an insulated wire, usually stainless steel, silver, or platinum, and the bare shaft of a steel cannula through which it is inserted. The bare tip of the central wire (exploring electrode) is flush with the bevel at the end of the cannula (reference electrode).

Monopolar Needle Electrode. A solid wire, usually stainless steel, coated except at its tip with an insulating varnish or plastic. Variations in voltage between the tip of the needle (exploring electrode) in the muscle and a metal plate on the skin surface or bare needle in subcutaneous tissue (reference electrode) are measured.

Multilead Electrode. Three or more insulated wires inserted through a common steel cannula have their bared tips arranged linearly at an aperture in the wall of the cannula which is parallel with its axis, the bare tips being flush with the outer circumference of the cannula.

Surface Electrodes. Metal plate or pad electrodes placed on the skin surface should be described (material, size, and separation).

(From the report of sub-committee of the Pavia Committee on Terminology on Electromyography presented at the International Meeting on Electromyography, Glascow, June 29–July 1, 1967. Reprinted in *Electroencephalogr. Clin. Neurophysiol.*, 26: 224, 1969.)

EMG Analyzer. A term applied to a wide range of EMG computer processing techniques that attempt to display one or a number of attributes of the EMG wave form in a more explicit manner than the conventional voltage-time graph of the usual EMG trace.

Feedback. An effect which occurs when a portion of the output of a system or a circuit is connected back to the input. When the fed-back signal reinforces the original input, the feedback is positive; when the fed-back signal tends to reduce the input signal, the feedback is negative.

Negative feedback acts to stabilize the performance of electronic instrument systems and to make the operation and calibration of such systems stable and independent of changes in many of the system components.

Positive feedback appears in oscillating circuits. Unintentional positive feedback occurs, for example, when a microphone, which is the input to an amplification systems, is brought too close to the loudspeaker output. When this occurs, positive feedback often produces an oscillatory howl. Similar undesirable positive feedback may occur when the input electrodes of an EMG system are brought too close to the loudspeaker output or the cathode ray tube output of an EMG system.

Filter. In an EMG system, circuits usually comprised of capacitors and resistors that modify or adjust the high and low frequency limits of the amplifier frequency response curve.

Frequency. The rate in cycles per second that an alternating current signal alternates. The unit of frequency is the Hertz.

Frequency Analyzer. Analyzes the EMG to produce a spectrum of sine wave frequencies (harmonics) that will uniquely describe the original EMG wave form.

Frequency Modulation (FM). Systems of signal transmission, recording, or processing that utilize a constant amplitude carrier potential with instantaneous frequency proportional to the instantaneous amplitude of the signal.

Frequency Response. Describes the speed range (slowest to fastest) of potential wave form changes that will be displayed by the EMG apparatus. Stated as a range (band) of frequencies of sine wave test signals for which the amplification will be uniform. Amplification will decrease progressively for sine wave test signals at frequencies above and below the frequency response band. The frequency between the lower and upper frequency is called bandwidth. The amplifier frequency response bandwidth is often defined by two frequencies, one at the low end, the other at the high end, where the amplification falls to 70% of its midband value.

Gain. The increase at the output of an amplifier in voltage, current, or power of the signal applied to its input is called the amplifier voltage, current or power gain, or amplification.

Gate. A circuit used in digital systems as decision elements and having two or more inputs and one output. The output depends upon the combination of digital states of the signals at the input. A gate circuit in an analog system acts like a switch that permits or stops the flow of signals. The gate opens or closes in response to a control voltage (or gating signal).

Graticule. The ruled scale on the face of the cathode ray tube. Time and voltage display calibrations are usually adjusted with reference to the X and Y rulings on the graticule.

Ground. The lowest potential reference terminal in a system. In power distribution systems, a terminal that is usually physically connected to a conductor in intimate contact with the earth. Sometimes referred to as the earth terminal. Frame and chassis portions of electrical systems are almost always connected to ground to avoid the possibility of their assuming other random potentials which might be either dangerous or cause electrical interference within the system.

Ground Loop. The condition that sometimes exists when the ground connections of two interconnected electronic instruments or circuits are not at the same potential. This may result in power line interference.

Hertz (Hz). Cycles per second.

Impedance. Hindrance to electrical current flow in an alternating current circuit, hence comparable in simplified terms to resistance in direct current circuits. It includes the effects of resistance, capacitance, inductance, and frequency.

Integrated EMG. The integrated EMG is a time-varying potential with instantaneous amplitude equal to the total area (voltage × time) accumulated from a designated start point under an EMG wave form. It provides a measure of total electrical activity.

Interface. An expression or device which embodies all technical considerations in interconnecting two portions of a system, such as proper mating connectors, shielding of connecting leads, establishment of compatible voltage and impedance levels, and such problems as ground loops.

Interference. Generally applied to unwanted signals outside the system. Power line frequency most common. (See Artifact.)

Linear Circuit. A circuit whose output is congruent with its input, with the exception of possible amplification or attenuation.

Microphonics. An effect noted in sensitive electronic systems and their connecting cables, where incidental mechanical vibration applied to portions of the system gives rise to spurious electrical outputs.

Noise. Any potential other than that being measured. Commonly applied to spurious potentials originating within the apparatus or electrodes. (See Artifact, Interference, Root Mean Square Voltage.)

Off Line. Any signal or data processing function that is deferred with respect to the original recording or generation of signal or data.

On Line. Any signal or data processing function that occurs simultaneously with the original recording or generation of the signal or data.

Overload. A general condition in which the input to an amplifier circuit is so large as to exceed the capability of the circuit to perform its intended function.

Parallel. Circuit elements connected in parallel (as different from series) are all subjected to the same voltage. The current flow to elements connected in parallel will be inversely proportional to the impedance (resistance) of the elements. The word "shunt" is sometimes used to refer to parallel connections. In digital systems, the word parallel refers to a technique of transmission, storage, or logical operation on all bits of binary data words simultaneously using separate facilities. (See also Serial.)

Parameter. Any specific characteristic of a device. When considered together, all the parameters of a device describe its operation or its physical characteristics.

Peak-to-Peak Voltage (or Current). A statement of the magnitude of an alternating voltage (or current). It is the total excursion from the most negative peak of the wave to the most positive peak of the wave.

Polarity Sense, Display. Many neurophysiological records are published with an upward deflection denoting a negative potential on the active electrode. Engineering convention dictates an upward deflection for a positive potential.

Polarization. Electrolytic effects that occur at the metal-tissue interface of electrodes which increase the resistance of the junction and give rise to direct current potentials (which may fluctuate) that can be many times larger than EMG potentials.

Potential, Action. The voltage which results from activity of muscle or nerve. It can be spontaneous, volitional, or evoked by stimulation. Action potentials may be named for their appearance (high frequency, positive sharp, biphasic, monophasic, polyphasic, tetraphasic, triphasic) or their origin (endplate, fasciculation, fibrillation, motor unit, muscle, nerve). The term potential is also used to refer to action potential.

Preamplifier. The first stage or stages of an EMG amplifier system. It must have a high input impedance, common mode rejection, and low noise, as well as a large dynamic range.

Pulse. A signal of very short duration. It can be described according to its characteristic rise, duration, and decay.

Raster. A predetermined pattern of lines generated on a cathode ray tube (CRT) display which provides uniform coverage of an area. Also display on the CRT screen of an EMG where each successive sweep is displayed below or above the previous sweep, thus permitting the observer to see more information on the screen than is possible when successive sweeps are superimposed (same base line). Also a similar mode of graphic recording.

Rectifier Circuit. A circuit utilizing unidirectional current flow properties of diodes which converts an alternating current into a pulsating direct current.

Resistance. A property of matter to hinder the flow of electric current. Resistance is expressed in ohms and is derived by dividing the voltage impressed by the current which flows. Resistance (R) = Voltage (E), divided by the Current (I).

Ringing. A short duration, transient, usually low amplitude, damped oscillation that occurs in the output of certain electronic circuits, especially some filters, wideband amplifiers, and certain delay lines, immediately after the input wave suddenly changes in amplitude.

Rise Time. Used in describing rectangular pulses and square wave forms or amplifiers or circuits transmitting them. Rise time is the elapsed interval between the time at which the amplitude of the rapidly changing transition part of the wave reaches specified percentages of its lower and upper limits. The rise time of an amplifier is a function of its high frequency response.

Root Mean Square (RMS) Voltage or Current. The root mean square value is a means of stating numerically the magnitude of an alternating voltage or current. It equals a direct current that has the same heating effect in a resistor as an alternating current of the same RMS magnitude.

Semiconductor. A material which exhibits relatively high resistance in a pure state but much lower resistance when minute amounts of impurities are added.

Serial. A term applied to digital circuits where each bit is acted upon sequentially. (See Parallel.)

Series. Electrical components are in series when they are so connected that a common current flows through each of them. (See Parallel.)

Shield. Shielding. An electrostatic shield is an electrically-conductive sheath or an enclosure not in contact with the circuit or device shielded. It is comprised of electrically-conductive material connected directly to ground or by a low impedance to ground. It is used to prevent undesirable capacitative coupling of external voltages to the elements within the shield (or to contain potentials within the shield).

Magnetic shielding requires an enclosure of iron or other magnetically permeable alloys and provides protection against interference from magnetic fields that surround nearby current-carrying conductors or permanent magnets.

Signal. Any potential, wave form, or intelligence which is communicated, detected, transmitted, or processed with a system. It is usually in the form of a voltage or current within the system.

Silence, Electrical. The absence of signals from the tissues being studied.

Solid State. Electronic devices utilizing semiconductors. Electric currents, as well as light, heat, and magnetic fields, may interact in solid state devices. The transistor and integrated circuit are solid state devices.

Stabilized Current or Voltage Generator. A source of direct current or alternating current or voltage in which the output current or voltage remains at a predetermined, usually adjustable, value independent of wide variations of load resistance or impedance or of variations of power supply voltages. The stabilized current source will exhibit wide fluctuations in output voltage in response to changing load conditions, whereas the stabilized voltage source will exhibit wide variations in output current in response to load changes.

Stimulator, Ground Free (Isolated). Used in nerve conduction studies to minimize stimulus artifact. Ground free stimulus output circuit has no connection to the common system ground, thereby removing a possible path for injection of undesirable artifact via the patient to the EMG amplifier input terminals.

Storage, Display. A means for retaining, usually on the screen of a cathode ray tube, a transient wave form for study or analysis, together with a means for erasing such information to permit the storage of new data. Such storage can be accomplished by means of special cathode ray tubes (CRTs) that embody, in addition to other design features, special screens with electrostatic storage surfaces which store the desired wave form as a pattern of electric charges on their surfaces. The pattern is then visualized by flooding the storage screen with an unfocussed beam of electrons which pass through the storage screen and strike the phosphor screen on the face of the CRT only at those points where charge was stored. Transient wave forms may also be displayed on conventional CRTs by electrically storing the transient wave in some signal storage means, such as digital storage circuits or magnetic recording systems. The signal is then displayed by rapid, repetitive read-out of the storage device and superimposed display on a conventional CRT.

Strain Gauge. An electrical transducer which generates or modifies an electrical signal proportional to a mechanical deformation due to application of a mechanical load.

Strain Relief. Mechanical restraint, usually applied to the jacket of insulated cables where they join fixed mechanical assemblies or where they join connectors or other terminations, especially where the cable might be subjected to repeated flexing or mechanical stress. The purpose of the strain relief is to minimize possibility of failure of the electrical conductors within the cable or connector.

Sweep. The horizontal (X axis) linear time axis of a cathode ray tube display generated by the left-to-right movement of the trace spot at constant preselected speeds across the face of the cathode ray tube. Sweep velocities are usually specified in reciprocals of speed: time per division on the graticule.

Telemetry. The transmission of data, typically from preamplifiers located on a subject (free to move about the laboratory) via a radio link to a receiver and then to the remainder of the recording system.

Time Constant. A factor that is an index to a speed with which voltage and currents respond to changes in the input to resistor-capacitor circuits. This term is used to describe the dynamic performance of EMG amplifiers (which contain resistor-capacitor coupling networks).

Time Scale, Electronic. A discontinuous wave form, usually short pulses, spaced in time at 1 msec, 0.1 msec, or some other convenient time interval, applied to a trace of a cathode ray tube along with the EMG information to provide an independent timing reference.

Trace. The line of light on the face of a cathode ray tube generated by the moving spot of light generated by the electron beam striking the phosphor-coated screen.

Transducer. A device that changes the energy form applied to its input to another form of energy at its output, such that a proportionality exists between input and output. Transducers include loudspeakers, microphones, strain gauges, and photocells.

Transistor. An active semiconductor device used as an amplifier or switching device.

Trigger. A short pulse used to initiate some action within an electronic system. Also used as a verb. (See Sweep.)

Wave. A generic term loosely applied to a time-varying voltage, current, or other quantity, the amplitude of which varies with time.

Z Axis Modulation (Intensity Modulation). Applies to cathode ray displays where information is applied to the beam-generating electrodes so as to instantaneously vary the brightness of the trace during the course of the sweep.

appendix

II

Test

ERNEST W. JOHNSON, M.D.

Only *1* answer is correct! The figures correspond to the questions directly above them.

1. Dawson and Scott are two famous names in EMG. Which of the below conditions is best diagnosed by using their contribution?
   a) amyotrophic lateral sclerosis
   b) carpal tunnel syndrome
   c) Charcot-Marie-Tooth disease
   d) Duchenne muscular dystrophy
   e) familial spastic paraparesis
2. In a newborn infant (birth weight, 4 kg) the following conduction studies were obtained at 2 days of age: median nerve 20 m/sec; peroneal nerve 25 m/sec. What is the diagnosis?
   a) baby is premature
   b) baby is dysmature (low weight—normal term)
   c) baby has peripheral neuropathy secondary to drug ingestion during pregnancy
   d) normal term baby
   e) none of the above
3. Assume a patient who complains of a pain in the neck, posterior shoulder and forearm: paresthesias of index and middle finger. In which muscles would you expect to find EMG abnormalities on the needle examination?
   a) brachialis and triceps
   b) serratus anterior and abductor pollicis brevis
   c) pronator teres and supinator
   d) flexor carpi ulnaris and biceps brachii
   e) latissimus dorsi and pronator quadratus
4. Trains of positive waves varying in frequency and amplitude are generally considered diagnostic of which of the below diseases?
   a) Roussy-Levy disease
   b) Aran-Duchenne disease
   c) Thompson disease
   d) Eaton-Lambert syndromes
   e) Frederich Ataxia

5. In orthodromic technique for determining the distal sensory latency of ulnar nerve, if the cathode is placed distally on little finger and the anode proximally, what are the consequences?
   a) latency will be falsely shortened
   b) there will be an interfering motor artifact
   c) conduction velocity could *not* be calculated
   d) anodal block may occur
   e) this is *correct* technique

6. The most frequently found EMG pattern in arthrogryposis multiplex congenita is:
   a) myopathic
   b) chronic (remote) neuropathic
   c) acute neuropathic
   d) nonspecific but abnormal
   e) normal

7. Which of the below EMG abnormalities would be *least* likely in a 12-year-old Duchenne muscular dystrophy patient?
   a) fasciculation potentials
   b) positive waves
   c) fibrillation potentials
   d) bizarre high frequency discharges
   e) polyphasic motor unit potentials

8. In "Myasthenic Syndrome" (Eaton-Lambert), often associated with small cell carcinoma of the lung, the evoked muscle action potential after a *single* supramaximal shock will differ from that in myasthenic gravis how?
   a) higher amplitude
   b) lower amplitude
   c) both will be normal amplitude
   d) both will be lower than normal
   e) none of the above

9. The *earliest* EMG abnormality in *mild* L5 radiculopathy would be:
   a) prolonged H reflex latency
   b) reduced number of motor unit potential in extensor digitorum longus
   c) positive waves in appropriate level of paraspinals
   d) fibrillation potentials in limb muscles
   e) reduced number of motor unit potentials in paraspinal muscles at L5

10. A 25-year-old lady has a sudden onset of left facial palsy. Ten days later you examine her. There are *no* voluntary motor unit potentials with needle EMG and no positive waves or fibrillation potentials. With surface electrodes over frontalis, facial nerve stimulation evokes a muscle action potential of 2 mv after 5.2 msec. Your conclusion?
    a) hysterical paralysis
    b) bad prognosis
    c) good prognosis

d) unable to determine

e) none of the above

11. Three children of a known Charcot-Marie-Tooth (mother) patient had the following peroneal nerve conductions: Jane, age 1 year: 37 m/sec; Joe, age 1 month: 22 m/sec; Alice, age 9 years: 19 m/sec. Who has the disease?

a) all have it

b) all are free of it

c) only Alice has it

d) only Joe has it

e) Alice and Joe have it

12. In a known diabetic patient who develops severe pain and atrophy of unilateral thigh muscles, the EMG will likely show:

a) marked reduction in conduction velocity of femoral nerve.

b) EMG abnormalities (fibrillation potentials and positive waves) in two or more lumbar roots distribution

c) widespread fibrillation potentials in upper and lower extremities

d) marked reduction of conduction velocity in all nerves

e) no EDX abnormality

13. Which of the conditions below are most similar (and thus confusing) on the EMG exam?

a) myotonic dystrophy and active polymyositis

b) McArdle's syndrome and normal muscle

c) amyotrophic lateral sclerosis and idiopathic polyneuritis

d) Pompe's disease and fiber type disproportion

e) Duchenne muscular dystrophy and benign congenital hypotonia

14. Assume a 45-year-old man with insidious onset of a foot drop. Which of the below EDX procedures would *not* be of help in differential diagnosis?

a) needle EMG in limb muscles

b) needle EMG in paraspinal muscles

c) motor nerve conduction studies

d) H reflex in anterior compartment muscles

e) none of the above

15. Identify the difference between the fibrillation potential and the positive sharp wave (besides it's shape).

a) fibrillation signifies denervation while positive wave is nonspecific

b) positive wave is often present in myopathies while fibrillation potentials are not

c) positive wave is associated with endplates and fibrillation potential indicates no endplates or separation from endplates

d) conceptually the positive wave is an artifact produced by the needle tip

e) fibrillation indicates more severe disease

16. A retired postman complains of burning pain in the right foot, worse at night. Conduction studies of right tibial nerve: proximal conduction

velocity, 51 msec; distal latency to abductor digiti quinti pedis, 7.9 msec distal latency to abductor hallicus, 5.6 msec. Probable diagnosis:

a) classic tarsal tunnel syndrome
b) entrapment of lateral plantar nerve
c) entrapment of medial plantar nerve
d) these are normal findings
e) none of the above

17. Which of the below identifies a motor unit potential as a fasciculation potential?

a) its number of phases
b) its amplitude
c) its rate and rhythm
d) its association with positive sharp waves
e) its presence with patient at rest

18. Introducing a low frequency filter (100 Hz and below) into the amplifying system will distort which of the below the most?

a) fibrillation potential
b) polyphasic motor unit potential
c) fasciculation potential
d) positive sharp wave
e) endplate spike

19. Assume a supramaximal stimulus during the determination of an H reflex in the tibial nerve and recording from the medial gastrocnemius. What will differentiate the F wave from the H reflex?

a) H wave will have a longer latency since it involves a synapse
b) F wave will usually be longer latency since the "echoing" axons are small diameter, high threshold, lower velocity axons
c) F wave will be higher amplitude
d) F wave shape will vary
e) H latency will always be shorter since it involves fast conducting axons

20. Which of the below sweep is appropriate for a distal sensory latency determination?

a) 1 msec/mm
b) 5 msec/cm
c) 2 msec/cm
d) 0.01 sec/inch
e) 50 msec/0.1 mm

21. Normal "jitter" is of the order of:

a) 50 μsec
b) 0.1 msec
c) 10 msec
d) 1–2 msec
e) 200 μsec

22. "Neurogenic jitter" occurs in:
    a) only neuropathic conditions
    b) reinnervation states of the motor unit
    c) far advanced myasthenia gravis
    d) fiber type dystrophies
    e) the "myasthenic syndrome"
23. Most probable explanation of the absence of smaller muscle action potential when stimulating the peroneal at the ankle than when stimulating at the fibular head (record over extensor digitorum brevis) is:
    a) submaximal stimulus
    b) edema at ankle
    c) accessory peroneal nerve
    d) misplacement of electrodes
    e) atrophied extensor digitorum brevis
24. Which is the *least* accessible muscle for needle EMG exploration?
    a) posterior tibial muscle
    b) serratus anterior muscle
    c) teres major
    d) abductor hallicus
    e) extensor digitorum longus
25. Which muscles are usually supplied by the median nerve?
    a) abductor pollicis brevis and medial two lumbricales
    b) flexor pollicis brevis (deep head) and lateral two lumbricales
    c) opponens pollicis and opponens digiti minimum
    d) flexor pollicis brevis (superficial head) and first dorsal interosseous
    e) none of the above

26. Consider the record of peroneal nerve stimulation below. Top two traces are at fibular head; bottom two are at ankle. Recording electrodes are over extensor digitorum brevis. What accounts for shape of M response?

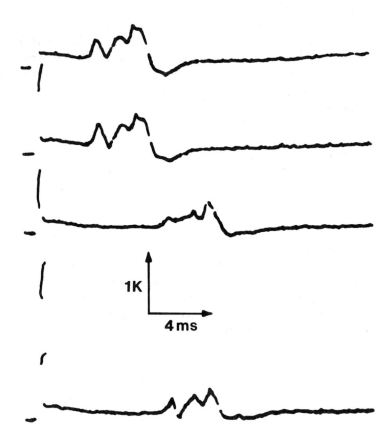

a) submaximal stimulus
b) accessory peroneal nerve (anomaly)
c) idiopathic polyneuropathy
d) muscular dystrophy
e) poor contact with recording electrode

27. Same as 26. The neurophysiologic explanation for shape of the M response is most likely:
a) slowing of conduction along distal axonal twigs
b) loss of motor units and/or muscle fibers
c) disease atrophy with all muscle fibers smaller in caliber
d) blocking at myoneural junction
e) defect of repolarization of muscle cell membrane

28. Motor conduction study of ulnar nerve. Bottom trace is stimulus just above elbow; middle trace is at the ulnar groove; top trace is at the wrist. Recording electrodes are over abductor digit minimum. Diagnosis:

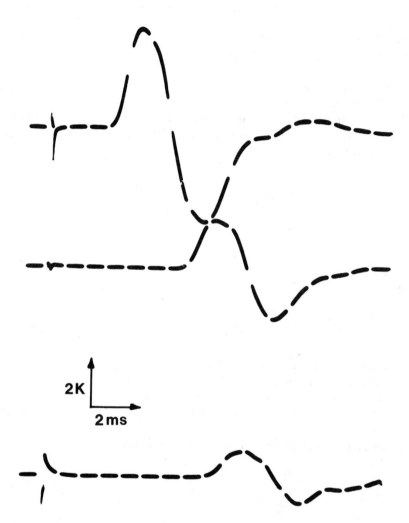

    a) compromise of ulnar nerve at the elbow
    b) peripheral neuropathy (demylinating type)
    c) peripheral neuropathy axonal type
    d) this is normal conduction study
    e) none of the above
29. "Classic" term to describe the neurophysiologic condition in 28.
    a) neurapraxia
    b) axonocachexia

    c) axonostenosis
    d) Wallerian degeneration
    e) axonotmesis
30. Which complaint would be most likely in this patient? Assume 2 weeks duration.
    a) "I bumped my elbow"
    b) "gradual onset of weak hand"
    c) "pain in the neck"
    d) "my arm aches"
    e) "I feel bad all over"
31. This is a single finger median nerve distal sensory latency. Width of time signal is 20 μV; each dot is 0.1 msec. Which of the below statements are supported by the recording?

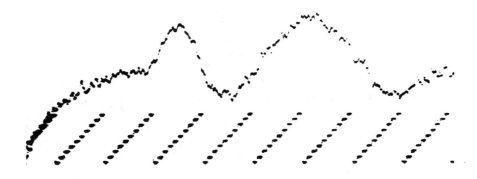

    a) antidromic technique was used
    b) definite diagnosis of carpal tunnel syndrome
    c) no sensory nerve action potential has been recorded
    d) latency and amplitude are mean normal valves for most clinical electromyographers
    e) there is a high probability of a sensory neuritis

32. Consider the muscle action potential recorded over the thenar eminence after a supramaximal stimulus at the elbow. Why is the shape of the M response irregular on the initial negative deflection? Calibration: width, 2K; each dot, = 0.1 msec.

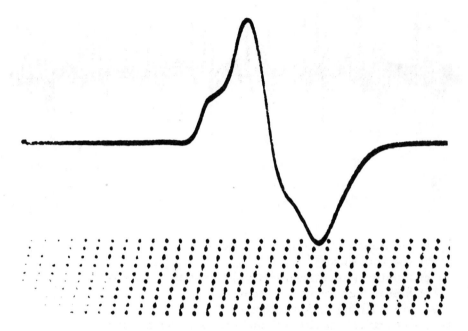

a) recording electrode is proximal or distal to the motor point
b) volume conducted response from ulnar innervated muscle
c) poor contact with recording electrode
d) movement artifact
e) recording electrode over motor points of two adjacent muscles

33. What is the recording?

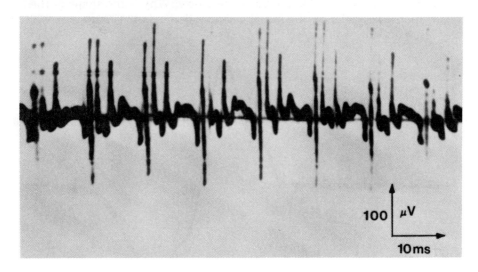

    a) "neuropathic" interference pattern
    b) endplate spikes
    c) iterative (repetitive discharge) potentials in alkalosis
    d) bizarre high frequency discharge
    e) grade III fibrillation potentials
34. This electrical activity is thought to be associated with:
    a) exploring electrode in vicinity of myoneural junction
    b) reinnervation (sprouting) motor unit
    c) intrafusal muscle fibers
    d) spontaneous discharges of denervated muscle fibers
    e) shortening of relative refractory period
35. Calibration: width, 1K; each dot, 1 msec. What is the cause of interference seen on this recording?

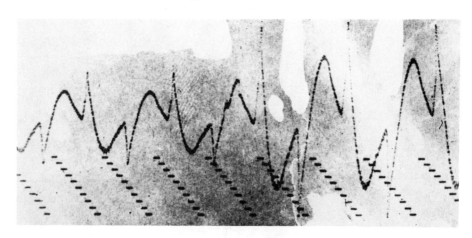

a) 60 c/sec power line
b) poor electrode contact
c) electric motor in vicinity
d) short wave diathermy
e) fluorescent lights

36. Calibration: width of signal, 2K; each dot, 0.1 msec. Median nerve stimulation (motor fibers). Recording over thenar eminence; top trace, stimulus at elbow; bottom, at wrist. Forearm segment measures 20 cm. Distal, 8 cm. Calculate the conduction velocity.

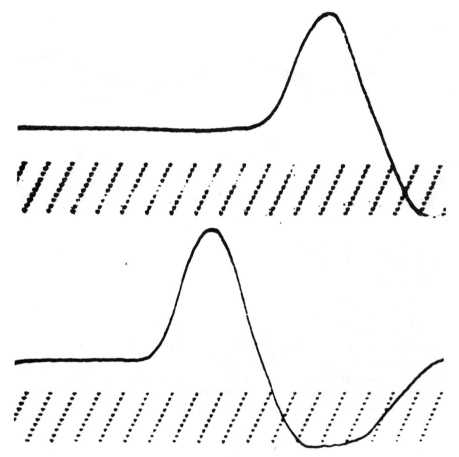

a) 58 m/sec
b) 36 m/sec
c) 48 m/sec
d) 72 m/sec
e) 110 m/sec (Martin-Gruber Anastomosis)

37. With the distal motor latency indicated, if one would have determined the distal sensory latency, what would you expect it to be? (14 cm, orthodromic)

    a) 4.0 msec
    b) 10 msec
    c) 8 msec
    d) 6 msec
    e) it would be absent (without using averaging techniques)

38. Calibration: width of time signal, 50 μV; each dot, 1 msec. Positivity indicated by downward deflection. These potentials were recorded in the paraspinal muscles at the S1 level in a suspected radiculopathy 10 days after abrupt onset of pain in back and leg. They are:

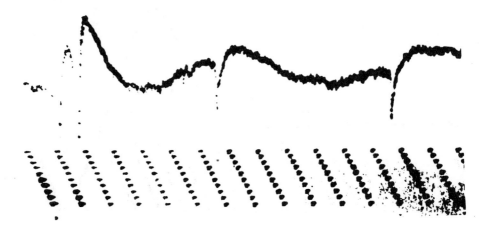

    a) fibrillation potentials
    b) endplate spikes
    c) fasciculation potentials
    d) positive sharp waves
    e) none of the above

39. They would have the following clinical significance:
    a) electrode was in vicinity of intrafusal muscle fibers
    b) supports diagnosis of radiculopathy
    c) would disappear if patient stopped drinking coffee and coca cola
    d) would be associated with a feeling of pain at the tip of electrode
    e) would be present simultaneously with a cramp

40. Consider tracing below. Calibration: time signal width, 1K; each dash, 1 msec. Surface recording over medial gastrocnemius and low intensity stimulus over tibial nerve popliteal area. (45-year-old man)

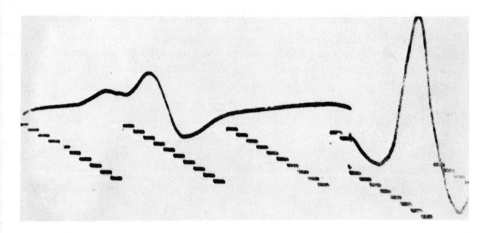

a) this represents an F wave
b) this is a definitely prolonged H wave latency
c) this is an iterative discharge of the gastrocnemius
d) normal H wave and latency
e) demyelination neuropathy

Index